NURSING SERIES

Death, Dying, and Bereavement:

Providing Compassion During a Time of Need

2nd Edition

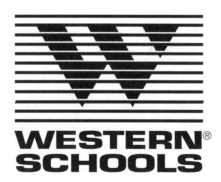

WESTERN® SCHOOLS

By
Barbara Rubel, BS, MA, BCETS, CPBC

30 contact hours will be awarded upon successful completion of this course.

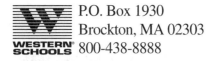 P.O. Box 1930
Brockton, MA 02303
800-438-8888

ABOUT THE AUTHOR

Barbara Rubel, BS, MA, BCETS, CPBC, is a dynamic keynote speaker, trainer, consultant, and widely acclaimed, nationally recognized author. Barbara received a BS in Psychology and a MA in Community Health, with a concentration in thanatology, from Brooklyn College. She is a Board Certified Expert in Traumatic Stress; Diplomate, American Academy of Experts in Traumatic Stress; Certified Bereavement Specialist and Certified Pastoral Bereavement Counselor. As a bereavement specialist, Barbara has supported terminally ill individuals, provided support to those who were impacted by 9/11, facilitated anticipatory and sudden loss bereavement support groups and taught graduate and master's level courses at Brooklyn College. Barbara currently presents trainings on traumatic death and compassion fatigue and, through ShareGrief, supports the bereaved internationally. Barbara is the author of the best-selling book, *But I Didn't Say Goodbye: Helping Children and Families After a Suicide* (2nd Ed), co-author of the Department of Justice, Office for Victims of Crime Training Curriculum Compassion Fatigue, and is currently writing her next book on the topic of bereavement support groups. Barbara's website is www.griefworkcenter.com.

Barbara Rubel has disclosed that she has no significant financial or other conflicts of interest pertaining to this course book.

ABOUT THE CONTENT EDITOR

Barbara Head, PhD, RN, CHPN, ACSW, is currently an assistant professor at the University of Louisville School of Medicine. She has over 25 years of experience in hospice and palliative care. Currently, she serves on the social work faculty for the University's Palliative Care Fellowship, teaching on death and grief to graduate students and to end-of-life care nurses. Dr. Head does research in oncology, palliative care, and symptom management during life-threatening illness.

Barbara Head has disclosed that she has no significant financial or other conflicts of interest pertaining to this course book.

Nurse Planner: Amy Bernard, MS, BSN, RN-BC

The planner has disclosed that she has no significant financial or other conflicts of interest pertaining to this course book.

Copy Editors: Kathleen Zander and Dorothy Terry

Indexer: Sylvia Coates

Western Schools' courses are designed to provide nursing professionals with the educational information they need to enhance their career development. The information provided within these course materials is the result of research and consultation with prominent nursing and medical authorities and is, to the best of our knowledge, current and accurate. However, the courses and course materials are provided with the understanding that Western Schools is not engaged in offering legal, nursing, medical, or other professional advice.

Western Schools' courses and course materials are not meant to act as a substitute for seeking out professional advice or conducting individual research. When the information provided in the courses and course materials is applied to individual circumstances, all recommendations must be considered in light of the uniqueness pertaining to each situation.

Western Schools' course materials are intended solely for *your* use and *not* for the benefit of providing advice or recommendations to third parties. Western Schools devoids itself of any responsibility for adverse consequences resulting from the failure to seek nursing, medical, or other professional advice. Western Schools further devoids itself of any responsibility for updating or revising any programs or publications presented, published, distributed, or sponsored by Western Schools unless otherwise agreed to as part of an individual purchase contract.

Products (including brand names) mentioned or pictured in Western Schools' courses are not endorsed by Western Schools, the American Nurses Credentialing Center (ANCC) or any state board.

ISBN: 978-1-57801-421-7

COURSE INSTRUCTIONS
IMPORTANT: Read these instructions *BEFORE* proceeding!

COMPLETING THE FINAL EXAMINATION

Enclosed with your course book you will find a FasTrax® answer sheet. Use this answer sheet to respond to all the final exam questions that appear in this course. If the course has less than 100 questions, leave any remaining answer circles on the FasTrax answer sheet blank.

Be sure to fill in circles completely using **blue or black ink.** The FasTrax grading system will not read pencil. If you make an error, you may use correction fluid (such as Wite-Out®) to correct it.

FasTrax answer sheets are preprinted with your name and address and the course title. If you are completing more than one course, be sure to record your answers on the correct corresponding answer sheet.

A PASSING SCORE

The final exam is a multiple choice exam. You must score 70% or better in order to pass this course and receive a certificate of completion. Should you fail to achieve the required score, an additional FasTrax answer sheet will be sent to you so that you may make a second attempt to pass the course. You will be allowed three chances to pass the same course without incurring additional charges. After three failed attempts, your file will be closed.

RECORDING YOUR HOURS

Use the Study Time Log provided in this course book to monitor and record the time it takes to complete this course. Upon completion, tally your total time spent and use this information to respond to the final question of the course evaluation.

COURSE EVALUATIONS

The Course Evaluation provided in this course book is a critical component of the course and must be completed and submitted with your final exam. Responses to evaluation statements should be recorded in the right hand column of the FasTrax answer sheet, in the section marked "Evaluation." Evaluations provide Western Schools with vital feedback regarding courses. Your feedback is important to us; please take a few minutes to complete the evaluation.

To provide additional feedback regarding this course, Western Schools services, or to suggest new course topics, use the space provided on the Important Information form found on the back of the FasTrax instruction sheet included with your course. Return the completed form to Western Schools with your final exam.

SUBMITTING THE COMPLETED FINAL EXAM

For your convenience, Western Schools provides a number of exam grading options. Full instructions and complete grading details are listed on the FasTrax instruction sheet provided with this course. If you are mailing your answer sheet(s) to Western Schools, we recommend you make a copy as a back-up.

COURSE COMPLETION TIME FRAMES AND EXTENSIONS

You have two (2) years from the date of purchase to complete this course. If you are not able to complete the course within 2 years, a six (6) month extension may be purchased. If you have not completed the course within 30 months from the original enrollment date, your file will be closed and no certificate will be issued.

CHANGE OF ADDRESS?

In the event that your address changes prior to completing this course, please call our customer service department at 1-800-618-1670, so that we may update your file.

WESTERN SCHOOLS GUARANTEES YOUR SATISFACTION

If any continuing education course fails to meet your expectations, or if you are not satisfied for any reason, you may return the course materials for an exchange or a refund (less shipping and handling) within 30 days. Software, video, and audio courses must be returned unopened. Textbooks must not be written in or marked up in any other way.

Thank you for using Western Schools to fulfill your continuing education needs!

WESTERN SCHOOLS
P.O. Box 1930
Brockton, MA 02303
800-438-8888
www.westernschools.com

WESTERN SCHOOLS
STUDY TIME LOG

DEATH, DYING, AND BEREAVEMENT: PROVIDING COMPASSION DURING A TIME OF NEED

INSTRUCTIONS: Use this log sheet to document the amount of time you spend completing this course. Include the time it takes you to read the instructions, read the course book, take the final examination, and complete the evaluation.

Date	Time Spent	
	Hours	**Minutes**
_____	_____	_____
_____	_____	_____
_____	_____	_____
_____	_____	_____
_____	_____	_____
_____	_____	_____
_____	_____	_____
_____	_____	_____
_____	_____	_____
_____	_____	_____
_____	_____	_____
_____	_____	_____
_____	_____	_____
_____	_____	_____
_____	_____	_____

TOTAL*

Hours   Minutes

* Please use this total study time to answer the final question of the course evaluation.

WESTERN SCHOOLS
COURSE EVALUATION

DEATH, DYING, AND BEREAVEMENT: PROVIDING COMPASSION DURING A TIME OF NEED

INSTRUCTIONS: Using the scale below, please respond to the following evaluation statements. All responses should be recorded in the right-hand column of the FasTrax answer sheet, in the section marked "Evaluation." Be sure to fill in each corresponding answer circle completely using blue or black ink. Leave any remaining answer circles blank.

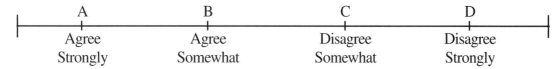

A	B	C	D
Agree Strongly	Agree Somewhat	Disagree Somewhat	Disagree Strongly

OBJECTIVES: After completing this course, I am able to

1. Discuss the historical evolution of attitudes toward death and methods the nurse can use to develop positive attitudes and helping skills when confronting death.
2. Identify the components and functions of the death system.
3. Describe the ways that individuals and family members cope with dying.
4. Discuss hospice and palliative care as treatment approaches for end-of-life care.
5. Describe the significance of advance care planning and various methods for conveying one's wishes for end-of-life care.
6. Describe how individuals grieve after experiencing a loss.
7. Recognize the impact of public tragedies and methods for assisting survivors during and after such tragedies.
8. Discuss the magnitude and significance of suicide as a public health concern and related implications for healthcare professionals.
9. Explain how bereaved individuals cope with mourning.
10. Describe how bereaved children and adolescents express their grief and cope with the death of significant people in their lives.
11. Discuss the impact of stress on the nurse who cares for the dying, and coping strategies to prevent compassion fatigue and burnout.

COURSE CONTENT

12. The course materials were presented in a well organized and clearly written manner.
13. The course content was presented in a fair, unbiased and balanced manner.
14. The course expanded my knowledge and enhanced my skills related to the subject matter.
15. I intend to apply the knowledge and skills I've learned to my nursing practice. (Select the appropriate response below.)

   A. Yes   B. Unsure   C. No   D. Not Applicable

ATTESTATION

16. By submitting this answer sheet, I certify that I have read the course materials and personally completed the final examination based on the material presented. Mark "A" for Agree and "B" for Disagree.

v

continued on next page

COURSE HOURS

17. Choose the response that best represents the total number of clock hours it took to complete this **30 hour** course.

    A. More than 32 hours   B. 28–32 hours   C. Less than 28 hours

Note: To provide additional feedback regarding this course, Western Schools services, or to suggest new course topics, use the space provided on the Important Information form found on the back of the FasTrax instruction sheet included with your course.

CONTENTS

FIGURES AND TABLES

PRETEST

1. Begin this course by taking the pretest. Circle the answers to the questions on this page, or write the answers on a separate sheet of paper. Do not log answers to the pretest questions on the FasTrax test sheet included with the course.

2. Compare your answers to the PRETEST KEY located at the end of the Pretest. The pretest key indicates the chapter where the content of that question is discussed. Make note of the questions you missed, so that you can focus on those areas as you complete the course.

3. Complete the course by reading the chapters and completing the exam questions at the end of each chapter. Answers to these exam questions should be logged on the FasTrax test sheet included with the course.

Note: Choose the one option that BEST answers each question.

1. The three most common causes of death for those 65 years old and over in the United States are

   a. chronic lower respiratory disease, influenza, and pneumonia.

   b. diabetes, Alzheimer's disease, and nephritis.

   c. diseases of the heart, cancer, and stroke.

   d. diseases of the heart, accidents, and septicemia.

2. A specific service provided to grieving family members immediately after a death in a hospital is

   a. offering bereavement therapy.

   b. discarding all belongings of the deceased.

   c. calling a chaplain, minister, rabbi, or priest, whether or not the family wants spiritual support.

   d. making a secluded, quiet, nicely furnished room for family privacy immediately available at the time of loss.

3. Burial, cremation, and body donation are associated with

   a. final disposition.

   b. final arrangements.

   c. embalming.

   d. entombment.

4. The type of funeral where a celebrant facilitates the funeral by meeting with family and friends of the deceased, listens to their stories, and creates a shared picture including the beliefs, cultures, and religious values of the decedent and family members, is

   a. cremation.

   b. fun.

   c. traditional.

   d. secular, life-cycle.

5. An occurrence wherein a patient's pulse rate and breathing have stopped, and the patient is either very close to death or clinically dead, is known as a(n)

   a. dying awareness context.

   b. near-death experience.

   c. stage-based approach to coping with dying.

   d. anticipatory grief experience.

continued on next page

6. An open-ended question used to identify the patient's perspective on his or her illness is

    a. "Do you think that you will get better?"

    b. "Do you think your family is keeping anything from you?"

    c. "Have you talked with any other dying patients?"

    d. "How are you coping with all this?"

7. The type of grief that is experienced in anticipation of a future loss, and before an actual death occurs, is

    a. disenfranchised grief.

    b. traumatic grief.

    c. anticipatory grief.

    d. complicated grief.

8. The identification of the physical, psychosocial, emotional, and spiritual needs related to the terminal illness that will be addressed in promoting the patient's well-being and comfort happens during the

    a. initial assessment.

    b. comprehensive assessment.

    c. short term respite.

    d. bereavement assessment.

9. A physician's order not to conduct cardiopulmonary resuscitation in the event of cardiac arrest is known as

    a. informed consent.

    b. a living will.

    c. a do not resuscitate order.

    d. medical power of attorney.

10. According to which faith are there eight stages in the dying process?

    a. Buddhist

    b. Jewish

    c. Muslim

    d. Hindu

11. The sorrow one feels over the loss of a loved one can last

    a. 6 months.

    b. 1 year.

    c. 10 years.

    d. a lifetime.

12. The disaster phase when survivors take inventory and focus on basic needs is the

    a. heroic phase.

    b. honeymoon phase.

    c. disillusionment phase.

    d. reconstruction phase.

13. According to the American Association of Suicidology, compared to other age groups in the United States, the rate of suicide among elderly adults is close to

    a. the same.

    b. 30% lower.

    c. 25% higher.

    d. 50% higher.

14. The most common method of suicide in the United States is

    a. drowning.

    b. carbon monoxide poisoning.

    c. hanging.

    d. firearms.

15. To improve the quality of time spent with a dying patient or with a family member who is experiencing either anticipatory mourning or bereavement, you should

    a. be willing just to be there, without doing anything.

    b. ignore awareness of your energy levels to avoid exhaustion and burnout.

    c. impose your philosophy of dying on the person you are seeking to help.

    d. be dishonest with yourself about what you are willing to give to the dying or bereaved.

16. Grieving people can be helped in support groups by

    a. discussing the changes in their lives since the death.

    b. controlling their feelings in the presence of others.

    c. encouraging unforgiveness.

    d. keeping personal stories private and focusing on others.

17. The understanding that death is final and that, once dead, a person cannot become alive again, is called

    a. non-functionality.

    b. irreversibility.

    c. universality.

    d. causality.

18. The understanding that death is inevitable to living things, and that all living things die, reflects the concept of

    a. personal mortality.

    b. irreversibility.

    c. universality.

    d. causality.

19. Upon the loss of a sibling, adolescents respond to grief by

    a. blaming someone for the death.

    b. engaging in typical grief tasks.

    c. continuing the bond with the deceased.

    d. forming a mature death concept.

20. The draining of emotional energy resulting from an empathetic response to suffering and continuing need for nurses to act and relieve suffering is

    a. compassion stress.

    b. compassion fatigue.

    c. burnout.

    d. vicarious trauma.

PRETEST KEY

1.	C	Chapter 1
2.	D	Chapter 1
3.	A	Chapter 2
4.	D	Chapter 2
5.	B	Chapter 3
6.	D	Chapter 3
7.	C	Chapter 3
8.	B	Chapter 4
9.	C	Chapter 5
10.	A	Chapter 6
11.	D	Chapter 6
12.	A	Chapter 7
13.	D	Chapter 8
14.	D	Chapter 8
15.	A	Chapter 9
16.	A	Chapter 9
17.	B	Chapter 10
18.	C	Chapter 10
19.	C	Chapter 10
20.	A	Chapter 11

CHAPTER 1

CONFRONTING DEATH

CHAPTER OBJECTIVE

After completing this chapter, the reader will be able to discuss the historical evolution of attitudes toward death and methods the nurse can use to develop positive attitudes and helping skills when confronting death.

LEARNING OBJECTIVES

After studying this chapter, the reader will be able to

1. describe the historical evolution of attitudes toward death.

2. describe three categories or types of bodily death.

3. explain the causes and impact of fear of death and death anxiety.

4. describe three positive outcomes of death education.

5. list the most frequent causes of accidental death.

6. describe four steps in the process of death notification.

7. name three actions a nurse can take to support parents during a miscarriage or stillbirth.

INTRODUCTION

Historically, nurses have not received education on how to care for dying patients and their families (Allchin, 2006), yet nurses frequently confront issues of death and bereavement. Nurses, due to the very nature of their work, may come in contact with those who are dying or grieving. They may also be called upon to offer assistance to their own family members who are experiencing loss.

Although Allchin found that nursing students associated caring for the dying with discomfort, anxiety, and sadness, the students believed that taking a death and dying course was beneficial and necessary to becoming a nurse. No matter the amount of education, though, nurses gain much of their death awareness and related attitudes on the job. This chapter will focus on historical perspectives on death, causes of death, attitudes and fears toward death, the value of death education, and methods for confronting and addressing death when it occurs in the nurse's workplace.

DEATH PERSPECTIVES

Historical Perspectives on Death

Human observances of death can be traced back to prehistoric times when survivors would observe special ceremonies when burying their dead. Historically, people thought of the dead as impure and feared proximity to dead bodies. Bodies were buried in cemeteries outside of living areas.

As Christianity became the dominant religion in the West, attitudes began to change. Individuals wanted to be buried near the bodies of the martyrs because they believed the martyrs' relics would

1

protect them at the Second Coming. Basilicas began to be built in these places. As death became an accepted feature of human experience, the dead ceased to inspire fear. People began to move around near the dead with no anxiety. Eventually, most cemeteries were located near churches (Corr, Nabe, & Corr, 2000).

Prior to the discovery of vaccines and antibiotics, people were at the mercy of contagious diseases such as the plague. In the 1330s, an outbreak of bubonic plague took place in China, a busy trading nation. In October 1347, Italian merchant ships returned from a trip to the Black Sea, which was a key link for trade with China. As the ships docked in Sicily, many passengers were already dying of the plague. Within days, the disease spread throughout Sicily. By August 1348, the plague had spread to England, where it was called "the Black Death" because of the black spots it caused on the skin (Byrne, 2004). Rats often carried the disease, which was transferred from person to person by fleas. The plague went dormant until the spring of 1348, when it struck again. After 5 years, 25 million people had died. Recurrences of the plague through the centuries left people living in constant fear of its return. The black plague largely disappeared from Europe in the 1600s.

In the 1800s, the leading causes of death were pneumonia, tuberculosis (TB), and diarrhea. American families would bury their dead in cemeteries that resembled parks. Picnics would be shared near the stones that marked their loved one's final resting place. Photos would be taken of the deceased and sent to family members who could not attend the funeral. Individuals died in their homes surrounded by their families. In the nineteenth century, carpenters and owners of carts and horses became funeral directors, otherwise known as undertakers. Caring for the dead became a profession, rather than a family responsibility. During the Civil War, the role of undertakers across the United States was very significant, as bodies of dead soldiers came home needing to be buried.

In 1900, the leading causes of death were pneumonia, TB, and diarrhea as well as enteritis, which together with diphtheria caused one third of all deaths. Between 1930 and 1950, there was a shift in where people died. Individuals no longer died in their homes surrounded by family but were taken to hospitals where they usually died alone.

Current Perspectives on Death

In 2007, life expectancy at birth hit a record high of 77.9 years, an increase from 77.7 years in 2006. Record high life expectancy was recorded for both white males and black males (75.9 years and 70.0 years, respectively) as well as for white females and black females (80.8 years and 76.8 years, respectively). Currently, the leading causes of death are heart disease, cancer, and stroke (Xu, Kochanek, Murphy, & Tejada-Vera, 2010), with most individuals dying at home, in hospitals, or in long-term care facilities. Table 1-1 details the 10 leading causes of death by age group.

The total number of deaths in the United States in 2007 was 2,423,712, a 2.1% decrease from the 2006 total. Declines in the number of deaths are unusual, and the 2007 decline is largely the result of less influenza mortality in 2007 compared with 2006 (9.0%). Other declines in the number of deaths from 2006 to 2007 were observed for stroke (3.2%), hypertension (1.3%), diabetes (3.4%), heart disease (4.6%), chronic liver disease and cirrhosis (3.4%), cancer (1.3%), homicide (1.6%), and Alzheimer's disease (0.4%) (Xu et al., 2010).

Deaths from AIDS

Another modern cause of death is infection by the HIV virus and AIDS. There were more than a million people – an estimated 1,106,400 adults and adolescents – living with HIV infection in the United States at the end of 2006. Gay and bisexual men of all races, African Americans, and Hispanics/Latinos were most heavily affected

TABLE 1-1: 10 LEADING CAUSES OF DEATH, UNITED STATES 2007, ALL RACES, BOTH SEXES

Rank	<1	1-4	5-9	10-14	15-24	25-34	35-44	45-54	55-64	65+	All Ages
1	Congenital Anomalies 5,785	Unintentional Injury 1,588	Unintentional Injury 965	Unintentional Injury 1,229	Unintentional Injury 15,897	Unintentional Injury 14,977	Unintentional Injury 16,931	Malignant Neoplasms 50,167	Malignant Neoplasms 103,171	Heart Disease 496,095	Heart Disease 616,067
2	Short Gestation 4,857	Congenital Anomalies 546	Malignant Neoplasms 480	Malignant Neoplasms 479	Homicide 5,551	Suicide 5,278	Malignant Neoplasms 13,288	Heart Disease 37,434	Heart Disease 65,527	Malignant Neoplasms 389,730	Malignant Neoplasms 562,875
3	SIDS 2,453	Homicide 398	Congenital Anomalies 196	Homicide 213	Suicide 4,140	Homicide 4,758	Heart Disease 11,839	Unintentional Injury 20,315	Chronic Low Respiratory Disease 12,777	Cerebrovascular 115,961	Cerebrovascular 135,952
4	Maternal Pregnancy Comp. 1,769	Malignant Neoplasms 364	Homicide 133	Suicide 180	Malignant Neoplasms 1,653	Malignant Neoplasms 3,463	Suicide 6,722	Liver Disease 8,212	Unintentional Injury 12,193	Chronic Low Respiratory Disease 109,562	Chronic Low Respiratory Disease 127,924
5	Unintentional Injury 1,285	Heart Disease 173	Heart Disease 110	Congenital Anomalies 178	Heart Disease 1,084	Heart Disease 3,223	HIV 3,572	Suicide 7,778	Diabetes Mellitus 11,304	Alzheimer's Disease 73,797	Unintentional Injury 123,706
6	Placenta Cord Membranes 1,135	Influenza & Pneumonia 109	Chronic Low Respiratory Disease 54	Heart Disease 131	Congenital Anomalies 402	HIV 1,091	Homicide 3,052	Cerebrovascular 6,385	Cerebrovascular 10,500	Diabetes Mellitus 51,528	Alzheimer's Disease 74,632
7	Bacterial Sepsis 820	Septicemia 78	Influenza & Pneumonia 48	Chronic Low Respiratory Disease 64	Cerebrovascular 195	Diabetes Mellitus 610	Liver Disease 2,570	Diabetes Mellitus 5,753	Liver Disease 8,004	Influenza & Pneumonia 45,941	Diabetes Mellitus 71,382
8	Respiratory Distress 789	Perinatal Period 70	Benign Neoplasms 41	Influenza & Pneumonia 55	Diabetes Mellitus 168	Cerebrovascular 505	Cerebrovascular 2,133	HIV 4,156	Suicide 5,069	Nephritis 38,484	Influenza & Pneumonia 52,717
9	Circulatory System Disease 624	Benign Neoplasms 59	Cerebrovascular 38	Cerebrovascular 45	Influenza & Pneumonia 163	Congenital Anomalies 417	Diabetes Mellitus 1,984	Chronic Low Respiratory Disease 4,153	Nephritis 4,440	Unintentional Injury 38,292	Nephritis 46,448
10	Neonatal Hemorrhage 597	Chronic Low Respiratory Disease 57	Septicemia 36	Benign Neoplasms 43	Three Tied 160	Liver Disease 384	Septicemia 910	Viral Hepatitis 2,815	Septicemia 4,231	Septicemia 26,362	Septicemia 34,828

WISQARS™ Produced By: Office of Statistics and Programming, National Center for Injury Prevention and Control, Centers for Disease Control and Prevention. Data Source: National Center for Health Statistics (NCHS), National Vital Statistics System.

Note. From "10 Leading Causes of Death, United States 2007, All Races, Both Sexes," by Centers for Disease Control and Prevention, National Center for Injury Prevention and Control. (n.d.). Retrieved August 23, 2010, from http://webappa.cdc.gov/cgi-bin/broker.exe

(Centers for Disease Control and Prevention [CDC], 2008b). A total of 11,295 people died of HIV/AIDS in 2007, and age-adjusted death rates from the disease declined 7.5% from 2006 (Xu et al., 2010). Between 1981 and 2006, 545,805 known AIDS deaths have been reported in the United States (CDC, 2008b).

DEFINING DEATH

What is death? The first edition of the *"Encyclopaedia Britannica* informed its readership that 'death is generally considered as the separation of the soul and body; in which sense it stands opposed to life, which consists in the union thereof' (1768, v. 2, p. 309)" (Encyclopedia of Death and Dying, n.d.a.). There are various death categories, with the general definition of death being the cessation of life. However, there is no such thing as the moment of death. Death is a process that takes place over time as the body dies cell by cell. Death categories include:

- *Cell Death:* death of individual body cells. During this process, respiration, heartbeat, and brain activity stop.

- *Local Death:* death of a part of the body.

- *Brain Death:* the end of all brain activity, complete unresponsiveness, and no spontaneous breathing. The lack of brain activity is indicated by a flat electroencephalogram (EEG) and there is no muscular movement.

- *Cardiac Death:* the moment the heart stops beating.

- *Spiritual Death:* when the soul, as defined by various religions, departs the body.

- *Functional Death:* end of all vital functions.

Personal Insight

What does death mean to you?

Do you see death as extinction or a new beginning?

ATTITUDES TOWARD DEATH

Death-related attitudes develop in contemplation of one's own death or that of another person. Attitude is defined as a mental position, feeling, or emotion toward a fact or state (Merriam-Webster Dictionary, 2010). Attitudes about what will happen as one dies and attitudes about an afterlife stem from personal experiences and spiritual beliefs as well as discussions with patients, clients, and other healthcare professionals. Two significant death-related attitudes are fear of death and death anxiety.

Fear of Death

Although Hui and Fung (2009) postulated that fear of dying and death may be universal, an individual's emotional reactions to it may be different. Adversely, Freud believed that people did not fear death (1953). He coined the term *thanatophobia* as a disguise for a deeper source of concern. Freud believed that it was not death that people feared because:

> Our own death is indeed quite unimaginable, and whenever we make the attempt to imagine it we…really survive as spectators…At bottom nobody believes in his own death, or to put the same thing in a different way, in the unconscious every one of us is convinced of his own immortality (1953, 304-305).

Twenty years later, Feifel and Branscomb (1973) proposed that everybody, in one way or another, is afraid of death. Fear of death may be due to the experience of letting go, of being in pain, of going to Hell, or of losing control. When individuals are facing the end of their lives, their fears are associated with letting go of earthly affairs and leaving those they love. Moreover, fear of being in pain or dying alone is overshadowed by fear or uncertainty about the future. For some, there is the fear that they may go to Hell and spend eternity with sinners. Physically, individuals become nonexistent and lose control, bringing great fear to those who are not willing to accept those losses. Death is the ultimate loss.

Attitudes toward death have a direct bearing on our approach to helping. If nurses fear death, their opinions, beliefs, and feelings will be reflected in their attitudes about helping those who are dying and those who are grieving. Attitudes about death stem from experiences with loss, formal and informal death education training, and teachable moments experienced throughout life.

Throughout history, societies have been death defying and death denying. In 1933, Franklin Delano Roosevelt said, "The only thing we have to fear is fear itself." We can avoid thinking about death in order not to face our fear. However, it is an illusion to think we can completely shield ourselves from it. Early Egypt defied the idea that death would be the finality of life. As a death-defying society, pyramids were constructed to house bodies as well as possessions to be brought into the next life. This created an illusion of control and continuity, which lessened fear.

Unlike Egypt, America is a death-denying society. Alhough many nurses are comfortable discussing death, for the most part, Americans would rather not talk about death or be around a dying person. Although millions die each year and millions more are affected by these deaths, death in America continues to be a subject that is often avoided and difficult to discuss.

Death Anxiety

Death anxiety is a stressful condition that occurs when individuals are unable to cope with the reality of death. Anxiety is a feeling of apprehension and fear that is often marked by physiological signs, such as sweating, tension, and increased pulse.

Racial differences in death anxiety have been reported. DePaola, Griffin, Young, and Neimeyer (2003) found that elderly African Americans were more anxious in regard to fear of the unknown, fear of consciousness when dead, and fear for the body after they died, than were older Caucasians. As individuals age and accept that death is a natural part of life, they are faced with issues such as where they will spend the last days of their lives. Elderly Caucasians may experience greater death anxiety than African Americans because more Caucasians than African Americans die in hospitals and nursing homes where they are isolated from family. Many of these elderly Caucasians die in pain. Fear of a prolonged and painful death is particularly evident among institutionalized older adults; palliative care interventions at the end of life can alleviate the pain and related fears (DePaola et al., 2003).

Research on personal loss, death education, and occupational exposure suggests that experience with death can have a positive impact on death attitudes and decrease death anxiety. For death experience to be related to lower levels of anxiety, the experiences need to occur in a supportive context with personal involvement and exposure to the dying process and without feelings of personal risk (Bluck, Dirk, Mackay, & Hux, 2008).

High religiosity and having a purpose in life have been associated with lower death anxiety (Ardelt, 2003; Cicirelli, 2001). Conversely, anxiety can develop as a result of fear of the unknown or the ways individuals choose to represent death. Representation is found in death personification, such as viewing death as the grim reaper or a gentle loving angel. Bassett, McCann, and Cate (2008) reported that anxiety can be caused by individual differences in the way death is personified. Kastenbaum and Herman (1997) found gender differences in personification of death; women reported death as a gentle image, whereas men reported death as a cold image. Similarly, Cotter (2003) reported that women were more likely than men to personify death as a gentle comforter and feminine.

Acceptance of Death

Dying is a life long process that begins at conception; it is simply the process of growing older. As individuals grow older they are reminded of their mortality with each loss. Over the course of life, they may encounter all types of losses, helping them to accept their deaths as a part of life.

"The elderly, with their many years of experience, are arguably the least subject to death anxiety" (Richman, 2006-2007, p. 44). Studies often find older individuals to be less afraid of death than younger individuals (Tomer, Eliason, & Smith, 2000). Coming to terms with death may represent a final task of psychological development. As adults age, they have less death anxiety because:

- Death does not threaten as many values.

- There is a continued developmental process through which we come to terms with mortality (Kastenbaum, 2000a, p. 22).

Nurses working in healthcare must face their fears and anxiety about death and dying. Death education is one way for nurses to address their fears.

DEATH EDUCATION

The term thanatology is derived from Greek mythology and refers to a discipline concerned with death and dying. A famous scientist, Metchnikoff, called for the establishment of a scientific discipline devoted to the study of death in 1903. Over one hundred years later, individuals are still interested in learning about death and dying and seek out death education through schools, media, and personal experience.

Nurses are better able to provide support to the dying and bereaved when they have received relevant education and training. Death education includes learning about one's own death attitudes, death meanings, and death anxiety. Such self-knowledge and attitude awareness can enable the nurse to better address the needs and feelings of others.

Corr et al. (2000) note that death education occurs via formal education, informal education, and teachable moments as described below:

- *Formal education:* usually associated with programs of organized instruction, such as elementary and secondary education, college and university curricula, professional and postgrad-

uate education, training and in-service programs for care providers, workshops, presentations, and support groups, both private and public.

- *Informal education:* typically begins at an earlier point in time. May start in the arms of a parent and proceed through interactions within social groups (e.g., travel, media).

- *Teachable moments:* stem from unanticipated events in life that offer possibilities for developing useful educational insights and lessons for personal growth. (p. 9)

> ### *Personal Insight*
> *Are you taking this course because of a previous or ongoing personal experience?*
>
> *Are you taking this course because of your involvement with dying patients?*
>
> *What do you wish to understand better concerning death, dying, and bereavement?*

Formal Education on Death and Dying

"There are numerous effective and valuable ways to approach the teaching of death and dying. Many thanatology courses are discipline based, residing in programs in psychology, health education, nursing, sociology, and philosophy/religion" (Fowler, 2008, p. 54). Students in the health professions are typically offered death-related content in a few lectures; less than one fifth of students in health-related professions are exposed to adequate death education (Wass, 2004). In recent years, colleges have begun to offer specialty programs such as a master's degree program at Brooklyn College in community health with a concentration in thanatology.

During the 1960s and 1970s, end-of-life issues and death education received very little attention in nursing schools in the United States (Dickinson, 2007). Debra Sullivan, RN, notes, "When I completed nursing assistant training 25 years ago, the only topic covered regarding death and dying was postmortem care. I was 22 years old and had no experience whatsoever with a dying person" (Gross, 2004). By the mid 1980s, 80% of baccalaureate nursing programs offered death and dying courses (Dickinson, 2006). Although the number of death and dying courses in nursing schools has been increasing, the amount of the total curriculum content that deals with the wide range of end-of-life issues remains at a minimal level (Walsh & Hogan, 2003). Topics given highest priorities in the nursing curriculum are advance directives, grief and bereavement, attitudes toward death and dying, communications with dying patients and family members, and religious and cultural aspects of dying (Dickinson, 2007).

The Impact of Death Education on Nursing Practice

The primary reason for standards of education for nurses is to ensure that patients receive quality care. Ferrell, Varani, Grant, Coyne, and Uman (2000) examined basic nursing education in a group of 2,033 nurses and found that the vast majority of nurses reported their basic nursing education to be inadequate in all areas of end-of-life care. Neglected topics included pain, end-of-life content, family caregiver needs, symptom management, grief, ethical issues, and care at time of death.

Whether in a classroom setting or online, nurses who continue their education in end-of-life care will become more adept in providing compassion during a time of need. Silverdale and Katz (2003) found that students' personal and interpersonal skills and abilities when responding to a dying person were enhanced due to taking a long-distance death and dying course, and Mooney (2005) found that a death education program was effective in reducing death anxiety in undergraduate nursing students.

Personal Insight
How confident do you feel in providing care to those who are dying?

The more confident nurses are about their skills in providing end-of-life care, the more considerate they will be of the needs of their patients. Silverdale and Katz (2003) found that if healthcare providers are more knowledgeable regarding the experience of a dying person, they will be more confident in communicating with the dying person and will perceive themselves as having the skill to offer individualized care and patient autonomy. The study demonstrated that caregivers exhibited positive attitudes after becoming aware of what the dying person was going through, learning effective ways to provide emotional care, and developing appropriate communication skills. Due to these changes in their attitudes, nurses were able to develop meaningful relationships with their dying patients. Although professionals are taught about loss through formal training, attitudes about death are also influenced by media, personal experiences, and society.

Media

Media is a powerful form of informal education about death. Whether nurses have actually seen someone die or have seen a dead person, they may have seen it in the movies or on television. In our society, television, movies, video games, print media, and the Internet have become significant means of exposing children and adults to death, and such exposure has been blamed for "provoking heightened fear reactions in children" (Cantor, 2001, p. 218). Media exposed thousands of children to the events of September 11, 2001, as the tragedy was repeatedly broadcast. Although viewing the tragedy had a significant negative effect on children's mental functioning (Lengua, Long, Smith, & Meltzoff, 2005; Pfefferbaum et al., 2005), it is possible that watching the events on television helped children and adults who were fearful of death better understand death in our society.

As with children, exposure to death in the media can help adults understand and make sense of loss in society as well as in their personal worlds. The public perception of Princess Diana's tragic death was influenced by media representatives who became the eyes and ears for those around the world seeking information about the public tragedy. Mourners of Diana's death consumed all available media coverage (Bull, Clark, & Duszynski, 2002-2003). One's perceptions and responses to a personal loss such as the death of a loved one are influenced by his or her exposure to media handling of deaths.

People are also influenced by the way media portrays images of death. Individuals who have not experienced a death may derive their images of death from those in television shows or movies. Media plays a significant role in presenting death, dying, and bereavement stories. By presenting these stories in an authentic and compassionate manner, positive attitudes and reduced death anxiety can result for the viewers.

> *Personal Insight*
> *What role do you think media has played in your attitudes about death?*

Personal Experience

According to Cicirelli (2001), personal meanings of death are created primarily as cognitive interpretations of objects and events related to death that result from one's life experience.

> *Personal Insight*
> *When you think of your first death experience, what kind of image comes to your mind?*
>
> *In creating that picture, is the image disturbing or does it cause anxiety?*

Most nurses have experienced the death of a loved one and that image remains with them. Their current attitudes about death stem from past experience. Informal education typically begins at a young age with a parent or guardian. How effective a health professional will be in providing support may stem from past experiences, including those from childhood. Nurses can reflect on their own childhood experiences of death to better understand

their present attitudes. In a study by Knight, Elfenbein, and Capozzi (2000), it was reported that the average age related to the first recalled childhood human death experience was 9.55 years. Adult death anxiety may be based upon the way parents talked with their children about death, what the parents said, and the parents' affect as they discussed it.

Throughout life, there are teachable moments when we learn about death. Earliest moments may include pointing out a dead bird on the side of a road while riding in a car with one's parents and discussing what happened to the bird. Knowledge of death may come through informal education, such as parental explanation of a death in the family. Nurses learn from these childhood experiences. One's understanding of loss stems from what is seen, who is present, and how others respond to feelings, questions and, most of all, fears.

Nursing students reflect on their own experiences of loss as they confront death in the clinical setting. Allchin (2006) reported that when nursing students reflected on their experiences with dying patients, their personal experiences with grief, loss, and death were combined with their clinical experiences. This made the clinical experience to be of value to these nursing students. Whether a nursing student or a seasoned professional, all nurses must recognize the impact of their personal life experiences when confronting death in the workplace.

> *Personal Insight*
> *Did your parents talk about death in your presence?*
>
> *What do you recall about your first death experience?*

ACCIDENTAL DEATHS

There were 123,706 unintentional injury deaths in the United States in 2007 (Xu et al., 2010). Unintentional injury death is the fifth ranking cause of death. It is the leading cause of death for individuals 1 to 44 years of age, the third ranking cause of death for 45 to 54 years of age, the fourth ranking cause for 55 to 64 years of age and the ninth ranking cause for 65 years of age and older (CDC: NCIPC, 2009).

Accidents are unexpected happenings that occur by chance or arise from unknown causes in which there is a loss, bodily injury, or property damage. The most frequent causes of accidental death include drowning, occupational death, and motor vehicle crashes. Reactions of family members and friends to accidents that cause the deaths of loved ones can include a loss of meaning and purpose, questioning good versus evil and one's basic beliefs, and withdrawal from places of worship (McPherson, 2004).

Emergency department nurses are frequently called upon to treat patients when they are injured. In 2006, there were 119.2 million visits to hospital emergency departments (Pitts, Niska, Xu, & Burt, 2008). The class of an accident is established by the location where it occurs, such as: motor vehicle accident, work-related accident, injury at home, and accident in public. Common types of injury-related deaths from accidents are motor vehicle crashes, suffocation, falls, and solid, liquid, gas, or vapor poisoning. Accidents also include medical accidents, in which an avoidable personal injury is caused by a medical treatment or failure to diagnose. Such unfortunate events can result from carelessness, lack of awareness, ignorance, or a combination of causes.

There were 3,443 fatal unintentional drownings in 2007 in the United States, averaging ten deaths per day. Fatal drowning remains the second-leading cause of unintentional injury-related death for children 1 to 14 years of age. More than one in five fatal drowning victims are children 14 years old and younger. For every child who dies from respiratory impairment from submersion or immersion in liquid, another four receive emergency department care for nonfatal submersion injuries (CDC, 2010). Major risk factors for fatal unintentional drowning include:

*   lack of barriers and supervision
*   age
*   recreation in natural water settings (such as lakes, rivers, or the ocean)
*   lack of appropriate choices in recreational boating
*   alcohol use
*   seizure disorders

(CDC, 2008c).

A fatal injury occurs in the home every 14 minutes (Greene, 2006). In 2007 falls took the lives of 22,631 people and 29,846 individuals died by poisoning (Xu et al., 2010).

Unintentional injury accidents can also occur at work. The preliminary findings of fatal work-related injuries in the United States for 2008 included 5,840 fatalities (all sectors), 5,320 fatalities in private industry, 1,188 highway incidents in private industry, and 789 falls in private industry. Fatal occupational injuries took the lives of 514 blacks, 3,560 whites, 131 Asians, 6 Native Hawaiians or Pacific Islanders, and 30 American Indians or Alaska Natives (U.S. Bureau of Labor Statistics, 2010).

Motor vehicle traffic deaths are a leading cause of injury death accounting for 43,100 deaths in 2007 (National Safety Council [NSC], 2009a). In 2005, motor vehicle deaths were the leading cause of injury death for children 5 to 9 years of age and teenagers 15 to 19 years of age (CDC: National Center for Health Statistics [NCHS], 2008). Motor vehicle crashes are the leading cause of death for U.S. teens, accounting for 36% of all deaths in this age group (CDC: NCHS, n.d.). The age group most affected by vehicle crashes is 15 to 20 (NSC, 2009b). Throughout the period 1999 to 2005, motor vehicle traffic injuries accounted for three fourths of all deaths among young people 20 to 24 years of age. In 2005, motor vehicle traffic deaths were the leading cause of injury deaths in this age group, accounting for 38% of all injury deaths; firearms, the second leading cause of injury death, accounted for 27% of all injury deaths (down from 31% in 1999) (CDC: NCHS, 2008). In 2008, speeding was a contributing factor in 31% of all fatal crashes; 11,674 lives were lost in speeding-related crashes. In 2008, 27% of speeding drivers under the age of 21 involved in fatal crashes had a blood alcohol level - of 0.08 g/dL or higher (National Highway Traffic Safety Administration [NHTSA], 2009).

NOTIFYING SURVIVORS AFTER ACCIDENTAL OR SUDDEN DEATH

Nurses (especially those who work in emergency rooms or trauma centers) are often involved in informing survivors of the sudden death of their loved one. Addressing one's own death attitudes, fears, and anxieties is helpful preparation for confronting death in one's professional life. Stewart, Harris Lord, and Mercer (2000) point out that "persons with far less training than mental health professionals in how to respond to acute trauma and loss reactions (e.g., uncontrollable crying) routinely must tell of a death and attempt to help the survivors in their important initial efforts to cope" (p. 625). The authors reported the significance of being compassionate and supportive to survivors after a death, rather than focusing on the notification as a guilt-ridden process in which they have to "admit defeat" in saving a life.

Being compassionate and supportive begins with skillful notification – knowing what to say and how to say it as well as anticipating the likely responses of family members. Iserson (1999) developed a protocol for notifying survivors after an unexpected death that includes four steps: (1) prepare; (2) inform; (3) support, and (4) follow up.

Prepare:

- Anticipate the needs of the bereaved. Have a room available to speak privately and a room to view the body; know the policies and protocol of your facility before meeting with them.

- Identify the person who died, the survivor's name, and the circumstances of death.

- Notify the survivor, medical examiner, and patient's physician and meet them when they arrive.

- Organize groups of survivors; remove them from the corridor into a room; offer drinks, blankets, and tissues; have information regarding lab tests; organize what you are going to say to survivors before saying anything.

Inform:

- Introduce yourself and identify the survivors to make sure you are speaking with the right family.

- Tell the survivor what happened – use the decedent's name, non-technical language, and always use the word "death" or "died." Do not apologize or argue with survivors; it is okay to show your emotions.

Support:

- Tell survivors that everything was done to save their loved one.

- Relieve them, if possible, of any guilt, avoid clichés, and explain some common reactions.

- Assist them by answering questions, ask them what they need, help them to make necessary contacts, and provide access to a phone.

- Answer questions, even those unasked, by providing written material, phone numbers, and information they may need.

- Explain how the decedent's clothes and belongings will be returned.

- Refer to clergy if survivors request.

- Give survivors your contact information so they can communicate with you.

- If survivors want to see the body, explain any injuries before the viewing and be respectful of cultural beliefs.

- Protect survivors from the media and be prepared for violent outbursts.

- Provide support by arranging for a hotel if survivors are from out of town.

- Conclude by asking if they have any questions, and give them copies of all signed documents and the decedent's belongings.

- Call for someone to take them home if they are alone, and walk them to the exit.

Follow-up:

- Debrief by speaking with staff who cared for the patient.

- Express your own feelings to fellow staff members.

- Follow up the next day with survivors, ask if they have any questions, and send a sympathy card.

There are several potential barriers to effective death notification in the emergency room setting. In most cases, the staff in an emergency department does not have a chance to know the family of the deceased. Not knowing the family makes the task of death notification that much more difficult. Those who deliver bad news experience stress along with the survivors. Survivors wait in a strange environment, while the medical staff experiences a sense of failure and stress. Iserson (1999) maintains that potential barriers to effective emergency department notification include medical staff experiencing anger if the decedent caused other injuries or death, dealing with cultural differences, and having a limited time with next of kin due to needing to treat other patients. Stewart et al. (2000) note, "Among all respondents, death from a violent interpersonal crime was ranked as placing the most emotional demands on the notifiers when they contacted the survivors" (p. 621).

Where Iserson's focus was on the emergency room setting, more recently Miller (2008) outlined a practical system of death notification for families of homicide victims in their home. Miller (2008) maintains that death notification begins with being adequately prepared for the visit or call:

Preparation:

- Know the correct name and address of family.

- Unless there is no choice, death notification should never be over the phone.

- Know basic facts of who the survivors are.

- Do not over-rehearse.

- Anticipate possible reactions and appropriate responses.

Initial Contact:

- Whenever possible, go in person.

- Go in pairs or a small group.

- Decide who will be the lead notifier.

- If no one is home, wait a reasonable amount of time, and leave a card with note and number to call.

- When the call is returned, go back to the home for the death notification.

Presenting the Notification:

- Ask for permission to enter.

- Ask family members to sit down.

- Gently probe about what survivors know so far.

- Use straight language and avoid euphemisms.

- Tolerate silence and sudden explosions of grief.

- Repeat answers to questions as many times as necessary.

Practical Assistance:

- Offer to make phone calls to friends and family.

- Don't leave the family alone unless you think they are safe.

- Give information and instructions in writing.

- Give telephone numbers of a victim advocate, prosecutor, medical examiner, social service agency, and/or hospital.

- Explain what will happen next regarding body identification, police investigation, and criminal justice procedures and, if a high-profile case, brief them on how to handle the media.

Parents of murdered children have reported the need to reconstruct the scene. Therefore, when delivering death notification to parents of murdered children, it is important for professionals to provide complete and accurate details of the murder. By providing consistent information, parents will be better equipped to recreate the death scene later (Dannemiller, 2002). Death notification begins by providing information honestly and clearly. The National Organization of Parents of Murdered Children, Inc. has put together information for doctors and nurses on what is appropriate when informing families or survivors of a loved one's death by violence (Table 1-2). Employing agencies may have bereavement protocols and death notification policies. It is essential that nurses review these documents as soon as possible and comply with their agencies' procedures and policies.

In the case of an infant's death, grieving parents should be helped to create a memory of their child. Gensch and Midland (2000) recommend that parents be given the option of holding their infant no matter the gestational age. Other recommenda-

tions include taking photos of the infant. After the baby is measured and weighed, the information can be written on a card and placed in a memory box. The baby's identification band, crib card, sachets of baby powder, and plaster hand or foot prints can be included in the packet that goes home with the grieving parents.

Death notifiers are in a position to ease the pain of loss by being sensitive to the needs of the bereaved. However, they must also be sensitive to their own needs when helping parents after a perinatal loss. Just as with personal loss, it is important to seek help and support for work-related losses. Those who are more experienced offer support and reach out to novice clinicians.

In 2006, there were 6.7 miscarriages for every 1000 live births (CDC: NCHS, 2008), Nurses are often in key positions for supporting parents experiencing a miscarriage. The parents should be informed that a miscarriage is occurring, procedures should be clearly explained, and grief feelings should be acknowledged and validated. Although it may be painful for parents to see the fetus, nurses should ask them if they want to see it, Ujda and Bendiksen (2000) maintain. In addition to choosing their words carefully and with sensitivity, healthcare providers can contribute to the parents' feelings of being supported if they:

- Say how sorry they are.

- Avoid minimizing even the earliest loss.

TABLE 1-2: APPROPRIATE RESPONSE WHEN INFORMING FAMILIES/SURVIVORS OF A LOVED ONE'S DEATH BY VIOLENCE (1 OF 2)

Information for Doctors and Nurses

What is appropriate when informing families/survivors of a loved one's death by violence?

- Provide a quiet, private area.
- Have a telephone, beverage, and restroom easily accessible.
- If possible, have as many of the family/survivors in the room as possible before informing them of the victim's death.
- Have only one professional speak with the group.
- After introducing yourself, obtain the identity of whom you are addressing to assure the correct family/survivors are in the room.

TABLE 1-2: APPROPRIATE RESPONSE WHEN INFORMING FAMILIES/SURVIVORS OF A LOVED ONE'S DEATH BY VIOLENCE (2 OF 2)

- Sit with whom you are addressing; do not stand above them.

- Speak directly to the individual you are addressing, maintaining eye contact.

- Touch the person, such as placing your hand on the person's knee or holding a hand.

- Speak softly and directly; avoid being "wordy."

- Be precise and timely with the information. Family/survivors are understandably impatient in such situations, so lengthy introductions are not appropriate.

- Use the word "dead." It is universally understood. What is suggested is: "I have bad news for you," and then inform them of the victim's death.

- Never use words such as "passed away," "gone to a better place," "with their maker," etc. Such comments are easily misunderstood.

- If the patient is not dead, but death is expected or a possibility, inform the family/survivors the patient is "critical." Inform them of ongoing resuscitation. What is recommended is: "Hope for the best, but be prepared for the worst."

- Be aware of individual and cultural differences regarding the grieving process. Some cultures may respond in a calm manner. Others express anger, disbelief, or respond in a loud, verbal manner.

- **Be aware the moment you are sharing is a moment the family/survivors will never forget. The face and voice of the professional delivering such a message will forever remain in their memory.**

- Offer the family/survivors the opportunity to spend a few moments with the deceased. Prepare them for what they may view and inform them of why items, such as evidence and medical procedures, may not be removed from the victim's body.

- Provide the opportunity for the family/survivors to contact you if additional information is necessary or unanswered questions remain. Such a moment is very emotional and confusing. Questions and the need for additional information may arise during the following days, weeks, or months.

- After leaving the family/survivors, return a few moments later to assure that all information has been provided and additional arriving family/survivors have been adequately informed of what has occurred.

- Provide religious/spiritual support, if indicated or requested.

- Explain potential law enforcement and medical examiner policies that impact and possibly restrict what will happen to the victim's body.

- Provide assistance regarding funeral arrangements, if requested.

- Do not leave family/survivors alone for extended periods of time. Provide constant visitation from a physician, nurse, social worker, etc., so prompt assistance is available.

- If discussing a patient's status with a family member or friend by telephone, be as honest and clear as possible. Do not provide false optimism. If the patient is dead and you have documented the identity of the caller, tell the caller the truth.

- If the family/survivors inquire regarding pain and suffering experienced by the victim, make every effort to respond to their questions in a compassionate, honest, thorough, and professional manner. **Family/survivors need and want the truth.** Therefore, be as straightforward as possible.

For more information on working with survivors of homicide victims, or to schedule a training session in your area, contact POMC at natlpomc@aol.com or call 1.888.818.POMC.

Note. From "Information for Doctors and Nurses," by National Organization of Parents of Murdered Children, Inc. (n.d.a.). Retrieved August 23, 2010, from http://www.pomc.com/doctors.cfm. Reprinted with permission.

- Treat the baby or fetus with respect.

- Avoid using the word "common" to describe the parents' loss experience.

- Offer all parents with perinatal loss written information about their loss and about availability of bereavement resources and counseling.

- Learn to assess patient's coping resources and recognize symptoms such as prior depression and lack of social support that signal the possibility of chronic grief development (p. 280).

Janzen, Cadell, & Westhues, (2003-2004) studied parents' experiences and their advice to professionals regarding death notification. The parents reported nursing interventions that were helpful included:

- Comforting the dying child

- Preparing parents for seeing the child's body

- Providing information about the status of the child

- Offering food, blankets, a cot, and other amenities

- Helping parents get medical attention for themselves

- Explaining procedures and processes

- Providing empathy and support to parents and family

- Ensuring access to the child's body, time, and privacy

- Offering a naming ceremony (stillbirths)

- Respecting that a real baby was born and lost (stillbirth)

- Normalizing and validating feelings. (p. 158)

Ujda and Bendiksen (2000) noted after a perinatal loss, parents found the following actions to be particularly unhelpful:

- Being given a hospital room on the maternity floor where healthy babies could be seen and heard

- Lack of communication with the parents during the miscarriage process

- Asking the supportive person accompanying the mother to leave

- Being asked to transport the miscarried fetus to the laboratory

- Having a dilation and curettage (i.e., a surgical procedure often done with miscarriage) procedure in the emergency room without an anesthetic, without being told what was happening (p. 276)

Personal Insight
If you have had to deliver bad news, what did you say?

How did the person respond to what you were saying?

How did their response make you feel?

Once notified of the death, the grieving individual begins the process of coping with his or her loss. Survivors should be allowed and encouraged to view and touch the body, especially if the death came suddenly. Seeing the body helps with acceptance that a loved one is dead. Touching is an expression of love. After a terminally ill 6-year-old child died, one nurse washed the child and wrapped her in a thick pink blanket. The hospice nurse then tucked in the child's stuffed bunny. She gave the family an opportunity to hold and touch the child. The child's death had a profound effect on the way that nurse practices nursing. The nurse said, "Now I always give family members an opportunity to touch and hold a loved one who died" (Jones, 2001a, p. 45).

Throughout the process, bereavement support should be offered. This support can be as simple as placing a warm blanket around the shoulders. Specific interventions to offer to the survivors include:

1. Providing a private, quiet, nicely furnished area as a place for family privacy.

2. Arranging a visit from a chaplain, minister, rabbi, or priest (if desired).

3. Arranging for a time and place for a private viewing of the body and saying goodbye.

4. Providing assistance in obtaining belongings the deceased brought to the facility.

5. Offering individual, nondirective counseling.

6. Informing survivors of opportunities for participation in support groups.

7. Initiating follow-up correspondence with a family concerning hospital records and procedures.

8. Sending flowers or sympathy cards from the institution and its staff to the family.

9. Placing phone calls to the family expressing sympathy and asking if further needs or unresolved issues exist.

10. Making referrals to community agencies.

CASE STUDY

Marty Owens, a 71-year-old Caucasian male resident with Alzheimer's disease, died on Monday at 8:00 a.m. at a long-term care facility. Marty had been a resident for only a short time since the recent death of his wife. Although the administrator attempted to call his only child, Matt, he did not answer his phone. She left a message on the answering machine: "Mr. Owens, this is the nursing home. Please come as soon as possible."

Matt hurried to the nursing home unaware that his father had died. As he walked toward his father's room, the receptionist at the front desk pointed him out to the nursing home administrator who had never met him.

The administrator ran up behind Matt, put her hand on his shoulder, and said, "I'm sorry to inform you that your father expired."

The son was clearly confused. He slowly asked "Do you mean my father is dead?"

Repeating the phrase, the administrator said, "He expired."

Marty's son, still confused by what she said, once again asked, "Did Dad die?"

The administrator said, "Yes. He expired."

The son, now irate, said, "My dad is not a carton of milk. I hope the next time you have to inform a son that his father is dead, you are more comfortable saying it like it is."

The administrator did not respond to what Matt said, nor did she offer any apology. She then asked if he wanted her to take him to see his father's body. He told her that he did and together they walked toward the room where his father's body was located; neither spoke a word.

Questions

1. How would you have informed the resident's son that his father was dead?

2. What intervention would you offer this family member after notifying him that his father was dead?

3. What additional information would you provide the resident's son after you notified him of his father's death?

Discussion

Although in most hospitals and long-term care facilities physicians and administrators are responsible for death notification, nurses are commonly called upon to offer support to grieving family members. Nurses are in a crucial position: What they say or do not say and what they do or do not do will have a profound effect on the bereaved. The death of a family member is one of life's most difficult moments. Although family reactions may vary from denial to hysteria, the professional's presence will alleviate fear, doubt, and confusion when done effectively.

The administrator did not effectively notify Marty's son. Being that she did not have a relationship with this family member, she should have taken the time to be more compassionate and caring. She should have introduced herself to him immediately upon meeting him in the hall.

Marty's son was not prepared by the administrator and it is clear that she did not anticipate his needs. Instead of remaining in the hall, she could have brought him into a private room or her office to speak with him. She did not ask the receptionist to find Marty's nurse to describe how his father died, if he was alone when he died, and if he was in any pain.

Rather, the focus was on the ineffective phrasing of the death notifier. Clearly, the phrase, "he expired" is upsetting to hear. It sounds like the administrator was not comfortable talking about death. It appears as though she was not trained in death notification. Phrases such as "gone away" or "passed away" or "lost" can be confusing to family members. Marty's son most definitely was not comforted by the words "he expired." Instead of focusing on his father's death, he was angry at the phrasing that was used. That is why, when supporting family members during death notification, it is critical to avoid clichés. Nurses must be mindful of the words they use, and recognize that it is not only how loved ones die that becomes a part of the survivor's story; how they are told of the death is also important.

Death notification is difficult and stressful. No one wants to inform next of kin that their loved one is dead. If nurses are faced with the challenging task of death notification or supporting survivors after notification, they must know what to do. This is not the time to come up with platitudes or clichés. It is the time to focus on the immediate needs of the survivors. Even if there are other patients waiting for assistance, nurses should not appear rushed in any way. Being compassionate and caring to survivors is sometimes difficult. It is easier to get back to work and treat other patients than attempt to offer support immediately after a death.

In some situations, there are no words. Nurses can then focus on the gift of presence. If acceptable to the survivor, hold their trembling hand, shake your head, and make eye contact. It is okay to cry along with the survivor. Offer a hug, when appropriate. These are simple ways to show survivors the healthcare system cares. Survivors often mention compassionate nurses who helped them through the first terrible moments of death notification.

SUMMARY

This chapter began by describing historical and current perspectives on death. It discussed the importance for nurses to identify where they obtained their beliefs about and fears of death and dying, addressing the role of media, and personal experiences in shaping a nurse's attitudes about death. As nurses become more comfortable facing any death fears and death anxiety, they will be better able to support those in death and dying situations. Death education is paramount. Often, nurses are present when persons die and must assist with notifying and supporting the bereaved survivors. Knowing an effective and supportive process for death notification and interventions will help the nurse in situations in which news of a death must be conveyed. Parents experiencing a miscarriage or the death of an infant need to be supported with honest explanations and the opportunity to touch and see their child as desired.

WEB RESOURCES

To gain insight into your personal attitudes about death, take the quiz, "Self-Assessment of Your Beliefs About Death and Dying" from *On Our Own Terms – Moyers on Dying.* http://www.pbs.org/wnet/onourownterms/articles/quiz.html

Association for Death Education and Counseling http://www.adec.org

Palliative Care from About.com http://www.dying.about.com

EXAM QUESTIONS

CHAPTER 1
Questions 1-9

Note: Choose the one option that BEST answers each question.

1. From a historical perspective, death observances of humans can be traced to

   a. prehistoric times.
   b. England during the Black Death.
   c. the spring of 1348.
   d. the Civil War.

2. The death category or type of death that best describes when the soul – as defined by various religions – departs the body is

   a. cell death.
   b. brain death.
   c. cardiac death.
   d. spiritual death.

3. In a death-denying society, dying is looked upon as

   a. a natural and inevitable part of life.
   b. a topic that should not be discussed.
   c. an automatic referral for life-sustaining treatment.
   d. an abnormal part of human existence and opposed to life.

4. A trait that increases death anxiety is

   a. experience with death.
   b. high religiousity.
   c. having a purpose in life.
   d. fear of the unknown.

5. Positive outcomes of death education include

   a. longer life expectancy.
   b. professional support of assisted suicide.
   c. increased death anxiety.
   d. compassionate care for patients facing the end of life.

6. The most frequent causes of accidental death include

   a. drowning, falls, and motor vehicle crashes.
   b. HIV/AIDS deaths.
   c. plane crashes and homicides.
   d. heart attacks and strokes.

7. The four steps of death notification are

   a. support, inform, assist, protect.
   b. anticipate, inform, debrief, support.
   c. prepare, inform, support, follow-up.
   d. prepare, inform, provide, support.

8. According to Iserson, for survivors, during the inform stage, a death notifier should

   a. communicate with clergy if they request it.
   b. protect them from the media and be prepared for violent outbursts.
   c. use the decedent's name and use non-technical language.
   d. arrange for a hotel if the next of kin is from out of town.

9. When supporting parents after a stillbirth, it is important to

    a. remove the infant's body as soon as possible to avoid upsetting the parents.

    b. assure the parents that they will be able to have other children.

    c. offer a naming ceremony.

    d. ask everyone besides the parents to leave the room to allow the parents to grieve.

CHAPTER 2

THE DEATH SYSTEM

CHAPTER OBJECTIVE

After completing this chapter, the reader will be able to identify the components and functions of the death system.

LEARNING OBJECTIVES

After studying this chapter, the reader will be able to

1. describe the five components of Kastenbaum's death system.

2. list decisions made during funeral planning.

3. name three common symbols of death.

4. recognize two common euphemisms used for death.

5. specify two roles of the warning and prediction function of the death system.

6. describe one way social consolidation can be achieved after a death.

7. define assisted suicide.

8. identify uses for a death certificate.

INTRODUCTION

As long as there is life, there will be death and a system to prevent chaos in times of loss and tragedy. Nurses often work in the trenches of the death system. They frequently come in contact with death and dying. They work in places where people take their last breath. They recognize anniversaries of significant losses in their personal and professional lives. There are times, when through ritualization, they honor those patients who have died. They keep mementos and objects that remind them of patients and rely on their customs and faith to sustain them in death and dying situations. Being that no society can escape death, nurses are an important part of the network that makes up the death system.

FIVE COMPONENTS OF THE DEATH SYSTEM

Kastenbaum (2000b) maintains, "We may think of the death system as the interpersonal, socio-physical, and symbolic network through which an individual's relationship to mortality is mediated by his or her society" (p. 66). Kastenbaum's Contemporary American Death System model includes five components: people, places, times, objects, and symbols.

People

The first component of the death system is the people who come in contact with death or dying. Some of the people who work with dying and the dead or come in contact with those grieving include nurses, nursing assistants, social workers, bereavement counselors, home health aides, physicians, medical examiners, emergency medical technicians, cemetery workers, florists, police officers, clergy, life insurance salesmen, counselors, and members of the military. Educators who teach death and dying courses, writers, and researchers are also some of the people that make up the system model. Funeral directors and their staff are the most recognized group of professionals working in the death system.

A funeral can be preplanned by the individual or family or planned by family members with the funeral director after the death. The staff gathers demographic information and reviews details for decisions, such as:

- location for the service
- religious preference
- participating organizations to be involved (e.g., military, fraternal)
- flag preference, if used: draped or folded
- type of viewing: none, public, or private
- open or closed casket at the service
- type of casket
- type of vault
- whether body will be shown
- cremation versus burial
- if cremation, type of urn or disposition of ashes
- music, floral, and clothing preferences
- personal accessories to stay on the body or be returned to significant other
- pallbearers selection
- eulogy
- newspaper notices and names in the notices
- preference of memorial park or cemetery
- type of memorial marker: upright monument, memorial plaque, other
- preference for a graveside or memorial service
- preference to be buried near a particular person.

During the meeting, paperwork is signed with the current date or date of death. Even if everything

 was preplanned, it is a state law to have a current "General Price List" and a current "Statement of Funeral Goods and Services." This is done in case there is anything mourners wish to append to the funeral that was not originally set in the prearrangements.

Places

The second component of Kastenbaum's death system model is places. A cemetery, funeral home, or battlefield are places in the death system. Acute-care facilities, long-term care facilities, and home and hospice inpatient units are places where people see their loved ones alive for the last time. These places are where people hear the news of their terminal illness, where they make frequent trips for treatment, or where they reside in order to receive necessary care. Such places serve as reminders of one's own mortality, especially for older adults (Corr et al., 2000).

Times

The third component of the death system includes ceremonial or holiday times allowing a society to honor and remember the dead. Memorial Day in the United States and the Day of the Dead in Mexico are two holidays that mark society's mourning. Prayers for the dead are offered throughout the year, especially on anniversaries of tragic events. A year after the tragedy of September 11, 2001, communities came together to mourn those who died, and fall continues to be a time of the year when people recognize the anniversary of the day when thousands of people lost their lives because of a terrorist attack.

Objects

The fourth component of the death system is objects: Caskets, tombstones, and death certificates sorrowfully remind the bereaved of their loved one's death. Other objects such as personal items belonging to the deceased can bring comfort. When individuals are in mourning, they are comforted by reminders of their loved ones and certain objects the bereaved owned become very significant. Ho and Brotherson (2007) reported that object linking was found to bring comfort to grieving Chinese parents. Such linking is a concrete and physical way for bereaved parents to feel closer to their deceased child and maintain a connection with them.

A Chinese mother responded: "However, I still feel that she is around us in the house. Sometimes I take her pictures out and share the memory with my eldest daughter." Another parent expressed her object linking by using her dead son's belongings to feel a connection to him: "Normally, I feel a connection by looking at his pictures and the gifts he gave me. I kept his stuff with me. For example, I'm using his cell phone. I have his photos in my wallet and the wallet was a gift from him on my birthday." (p. 10)

Ho and Brotherson (2007) note that parents in Chinese families did not differ significantly from bereaved parents of other races who also use object linking to feel such connections (Rosenblatt, 2000). Maintaining a sense of connection with the child is "a way to find solace and an acknowledgment of loyalty and the inseverability of connection" (Rosenblatt, 2000, p. 123). Therefore, object linking becomes a connection with the deceased, and this strategy seems to cross cultural boundaries (Ho & Brotherson, 2007).

Caskets are other objects that make us very much aware of death. When we look at caskets, we are immediately reminded of death. Other examples of objects in the death system are obituaries in local newspapers, the electric chair, and tombstones.

Symbols

The last group of components of the death system are symbols identified with death represented through behaviors, actions, and language. Fast (2003) describes traditional, local, and derived symbols used after the Columbine incident. Traditional symbols used were crosses and angels. Local symbols that expressed loyalty to the school included the Columbine flowers and doves. Derived symbols were the mourning wall and commemorative quilt that linked the mourners of Columbine with past losses in the community. The author notes how in time these symbols will become the foundations for traditions needed to express grief after future tragedies. They will become reminders of past losses as well as present ones. Traditional symbols as well as symbolic actions can bring solace to the bereaved or simply be reminders of death. A few common symbolic actions associated with death include:

Customs: wearing black (European) or white (Asian) to symbolize mourning.

Faith: Jewish mourners wear a torn piece of black ribbon on their lapel; the Sacrament of the Sick or last rites for dying Catholics.

Traditional Figures: the grim reaper, who wears a long robe and skull mask and carries a scythe (a curved, sharp blade at the end of a long handle).

Culture: human skull and skeleton.

Animals: crows, vultures and bats.

Architecture: tombs and tombstones.

Government: flags at half-mast.

Common verbal expressions that refer to death are:

- dead ringer
- scared to death
- dead serious
- talk a subject to death
- dead ahead
- dead as a door knob
- dying to meet you.

Other verbal symbols identified with death are called euphemisms. Euphemisms often replace the words "death," "dead," and "dying" and appear to be a more pleasant word or phrase. However, Corr et al. (2000) note that the excessive use of euphemisms when talking about death provides a distancing from this basic life event. Some nurses still use certain terms such as "passed on" or "expired" instead of using the word "dead." Other common euphemisms include:

- resting in peace
- bought the farm
- pushing up daisies
- called home
- gone away
- merely sleeping
- down for the long count
- kicked the bucket.

> **Personal Insight**
> *What parts of the death system have you come across in your personal and professional life?*

FUNCTIONS OF THE DEATH SYSTEM

There are seven functions of the death system: warning and predicting death, preventing death, caring for the dying, disposing of the dead, achieving social consolidation after death, making sense of death, and killing (Kastenbaum, 2000b). Nurses are involved in many functions of the death system. They provide patients with test results and administer medications. During the dying process, nurses provide support to family members. After a patient's death, nurses communicate with family members and help them cope. Nurses may prevent someone from dying, assist the dying, or help family members make sense of the death. Whatever function nurses serve, they must be mindful of the death system and their roles in it.

Warning and Predicting Death

The first function of the death system is warning and predicting. Members of society must be protected from harm and death when possible. Media venues have procedures in place that can warn many individuals about impending dangers at one time. Examples of such warnings include:

- tornado watch
- flash flood warning
- warning labels on cigarette packs
- Code Orange airport security threat level.

This function of the death system can warn millions of people of danger. However, living in a free society we can choose to ignore the warning and the predictions, as was the case in Louisiana. Although many individuals were warned of the impending flood during Hurricane Katrina, many individuals did not leave their homes. Their choice cost some of them their lives. The warning and predicting function of the death system also includes laboratory staff who interpret and report patients' test results.

Preventing Death

The second function of the death system is preventing death. If society did not have strategies to prevent death, chaos would result. Professionals who prevent death include police officers, security officers, and emergency and medical personnel.

Death is also prevented through health promotion. For example, dieticians educate individuals about eating a healthy diet to prevent certain diseases that are linked to nutrition. Physicians working with patients with sleep apnea and other sleep conditions can prevent illness and disease that can lead to death by helping patients get regular and adequate amounts of sleep. Gym and health club trainers prevent death by teaching members how to engage in regular physical activity that decreases the risk of cardiovascular disease. Car manufacturers put seatbelts in every vehicle to prevent the deaths of drivers and passengers. In essence, there are many individuals and systems that function to prevent death.

Caring for the Dying

The third function of the death system is caring for the dying in hospitals, long-term care facilities, and at home. Hospice and palliative care have developed as medical specialties to fulfill this function. When caring for the dying, the goal is for a "good" death. Kastenbaum (2004) maintains that some deaths are terrible and dominated by suffering. He suggests that a good death:

- should enact the highest values held by society

- affirms our most significant personal relationships

- transfigures personal experience

- allows people to continue to be themselves as long as possible, preferably to the very end. (p. 518)

Hospice philosophy is based on Dame Cicely Saunders' aim to address the psychosocial and physical suffering of terminally ill patients. Her first visit to the United States in 1963 lasted 8 weeks and, during that time, she met with doctors, psychiatrists, social workers, and chaplains to discuss care of the dying. In 1967, Saunders opened St. Christopher's Hospice in south London, England, with the goal of offering skilled compassionate care for the dying. On July 14, 2005, Saunders died at St. Christopher's Hospice, the same hospice she founded. This hospice became the birthplace of the modern hospice movement, a movement that has made a difference in the lives of thousands of individuals.

Disposing of the Dead

The fourth function of the death system is disposing of the dead. This function includes removal of a body and methods for disposing of it. Disposing of the dead is performed by members of the funeral industry. There are 20,915 funeral homes in the United States (National Funeral Directors Association [NFDA], 2009). Some individuals make their funeral arrangements prior to their deaths. They may choose their caskets and decide whether their bodies will be buried or cremated. For those who didn't preplan, their families make such decisions. According to the NFDA (n.d.), in 2010 the average cost for burials in the United States, with a casket but not including the vault, was $6,195.

Cremation

Cremation comes from the Latin word *cremo*, which means "to burn." Cremation is a process of reducing the human body to bone fragments using high heat and flame. According to the NFDA (2005), 778,025 individuals in the United States were cremated in 2005. No casket is required for a cremation, as a wooden or cardboard container is used and is cremated with the body. In some states, no container or embalming is required. The family may witness the body being placed into the cremation chamber. For an average-size adult, cremation takes approximately 4 hours at a temperature between 1,500° F and 2,000° F.

After the cremation is complete, all organic bone fragments, which are very brittle, as well as unconsumed metal items are "swept" into the back of the cremation chamber and into a stainless steel cooling pan. All unconsumed material is separated from the cremains (ashes). Items such as dental gold and silver are unrecoverable and are comingled with the cremains. Remaining bone fragments, whitish to light gray in color, weighing approximately 5 pounds, are processed in a machine and then placed into a temporary or permanent urn selected by the family. Families have several options regarding what to do with the ashes. They may choose a cremation container. If the cremains will not be buried, the families may choose a rental casket for the service. The cremains are placed in the rented casket only for the service and are then given to the family afterward.

Funerals

Cremation Burial

One nontraditional method of burial is the cremation funeral. According to the Cremation Association of North America (Vargas, 2008), 35% of those who died in the United States in 2007 were cremated. Gadberry (2000) found that single or divorced, wealthy, college-educated individuals who do not live near their families are more apt to choose cremation. He notes that some incentives for cremation include land space conservation, lessened environmental impact, and reduced costs. The average cost for a direct cremation (no funeral or memorial service) with a container provided by the funeral home is $1,792; with a container provided by the family it is $1,692 (NFDA, 2008).

Families can bury the cremains in a cemetery plot or in a cremation garden. It is against the law to scatter cremains on private property. Some families choose to scatter the ashes across the ocean. Another common choice is to place the cremains in an urn that can be kept in a special place. Some religious groups include cremation as part of their funeral custom. Religions that do not allow cremation include orthodox Jewish, Islamic, Eastern Orthodox, and a few fundamentalist Christian faiths. The Catholic Church accepts cremation as long as it is not chosen for reasons that are contrary to Christian teachings. Nearly all Protestant churches allow the urn to be present during the memorial service. Most Catholic churches also allow ashes to be present during the memorial Mass.

Secular, Life-Cycle Funeral

A nontraditional method of burial is the secular, life-cycle funeral, officiated over by a certified funeral celebrant. Celebrants are life-cycle ceremony specialists with a background in the history of ritual, ceremony, and funeral traditions. The Celebrant Foundation & Institute of North America is a member of the International Cemetery, Cremation, and Funeral Association. Many celebrants are interfaith and non-denominational ministers. After spending hours with family members learning about the decedent's wishes, the celebrant composes the eulogy, officiates at the funeral or memorial, and gifts a keepsake ceremony copy to the family. The celebrant creates a ceremony that reflects the beliefs, culture, and religious and nonreligious values of the decedent and family members. The ceremony could take place at the funeral home, crematorium, cemetery, or memorial location.

Fun Funeral

Another nontraditional method of burial is the "fun" funeral. Fun funerals are controversial, even though they show no disrespect to the person who died or the survivors. These funerals are upbeat and celebrate the person's life. Whatever the form of the funeral, memories are shared as people gather together to pay their last respects to the person who died. Through the sharing of memories, the relationships are transformed and the bond is continued. Photographs, mementos, and tributes may solidify and maintain a transformed relationship and bring about positive memories (Gamino, Sewell, & Easterling, 2000).

Personal Insight

Would you consider preplanning your funeral?

If you answered yes, would you do so alone or would you bring someone with you?

As you think about this question, what images come to mind?

Social Consolidation

The fifth function of the death system includes social consolidation after death (Kastenbaum, 2000b). This function includes emotional support, practical assistance, and information. Social consolidation is achieved through spontaneous memorialization, bereavement support groups, and counselors. Professionals who provide social consolidation include nurses, social workers, insurance agents, physicians, and clergy.

Other individuals the bereaved come in contact with are funeral directors and funeral home aftercare staff. These individuals are trained to support the bereaved individually or in a group setting.

Approximately 50% of funeral providers in the United States offer aftercare services (Corr, Nabe, & Corr, 2006). According to Weeks and Johnson (2001),

> Funeral home aftercare may be defined as an organized way to maintain a helpful and caring relationship with clients, offer continuing services to client families beyond the expected body disposition, and accompanying rituals, and provide death, loss, and grief education to both clients and the community. (p. 5)

Making Sense of Death

The sixth function of the death system is making sense of death (Kastenbaum, 2000b). Our explanation of death may be handed down from one generation to another. Religious individuals are more likely to believe in an afterlife, compared to nonreligious people, and that belief can help them find meaning in their loss (Dezutter et al., 2009). Often, people make sense of death by reading poetry. Funerals help people make sense of death and are usually held 1 to 4 days following the death. For those who believe in God, there is usually a religious ceremony at a house of worship or funeral home and a burial ceremony at the gravesite. The religious ceremony can also take place at the gravesite. In special circumstances, a memorial service may be arranged where the body is not present and the focus of the service is on the person's life, not his or her death.

Killing

Examples of killing in the death system include capital punishment, deadly force in times of war, and euthanasia of pets. Capital punishment dates back to the French Revolution when individuals were put to death by the guillotine. Every U.S. state has its own laws regarding capital punishment. Although in recent years there has been a trend to abolish it alltogether, 42 persons in 10 states were executed in 2007: 26 in Texas; 3 each in Alabama and Oklahoma; 2 each in Indiana, Ohio, and Tennessee; and 1 each in South Dakota, Georgia, South Carolina, and Arizona (Fox & Zawitz, 2010). Killing is also justified in times of war. War involves a wide range of violent and traumatic experiences. Another type of killing is euthanizing pets. Society considers it humane for veterinarians to kill pets who are too ill to save.

Physician-Assisted Suicide

Killing in the death system includes euthanasia, which is derived from the Greek words *eu,* meaning "good," and *thanatos,* meaning "death" and is the active form of mercy killing. Euthanasia is defined as the administration of drugs by a physician with the explicit intention of ending a patient's life at his or her request (Rurup, Onwuteaka-Philipsen, & Van Der Wal, 2005).

There are two forms of euthanasia: active and passive. Active euthanasia, otherwise known as assisted suicide or assisted death, involves an intentional act. The patient administers a death-causing agent to end his or her life, with the assistance of someone who provides the means, typically a physician. Passive euthanasia involves withholding or withdrawing life-sustaining treatment, such as turning off a respirator or halting medications. Passive euthanasia has been recognized for decades and usually takes place in hospital nursing homes and other healthcare settings. Oxygen, antibiotics, or intravenous feedings are withheld or withdrawn from those who are terminally ill.

In a poll by the national polling firm Baselice & Associates, of 1,000 registered voters, 48% said physician-assisted suicide should be "legal," 40% said "illegal," and 11% were unsure (Marshall, 2005). Physician-assisted suicide occurs when the physician provides the means, such as giving the patient information on how to end his or her life, prescribing medication, or giving the patient equipment to be used in ending one's life. Active voluntary euthanasia occurs when a clearly competent patient voluntarily requests a physician to administer a lethal dose of medication to end his or her life. Discussed assisted suicide occurs when the physician discusses alternatives and encourages individuals to look at all options. Encouraged assisted suicide occurs when the physician encourages the suicide and may provide the means to end the individual's life.

A consistent finding across studies is that pain and other symptoms are not the most frequent motivations for requests to hasten death, nor are clinical depression and helplessness (Bharucha et al., 2003). The main reasons people choose to hasten death are a desire for control and self-determination, fear of losing control or experiencing an undignified dying process, and not wanting to be a burden to others (Pearlman et al., 2005; Werth, Gordon, & Johnson, 2002). Options other than suicide should be discussed with terminally ill individuals as they communicate their issues and concerns. Nurses should reassure patients that everything possible will be done to facilitate a peaceful, dignified death.

Autonomy is often a key consideration in the assisted suicide debate. Patients fear they will be unable to participate in activities, lose control of bodily functions, and become a burden to family, friends, and caregivers. Physician-assisted suicide is not an autonomous act on the part of terminally ill individuals, as patients relinquish control to physicians and give physicians the right to end their suffering on the physicians' terms. If pain and suffering were relieved first, physician-assisted suicide might not be the chosen option and patients would still maintain their autonomy.

Physician-assisted suicide became a legal option for terminally ill Oregon residents on October 27, 1997. The physician-assisted suicide process includes making two verbal (15 days apart) and one written request to a licensed Oregon physician. To be deemed capable in the opinion of the court, physician, psychiatrist, or psychologist,

patients must have the ability to make and communicate healthcare decisions to healthcare providers and individuals. If patients are considered capable, physicians can then prescribe medications that would end their lives. Between 1998 and 2007, 541 prescriptions for lethal doses of medication were written (almost always secobarbital or pentobarbital), and 341 people died as a result of taking the medications (Steinbrook, 2008).

A review of the literature reveals that terminally ill individuals who die by physician-assisted suicide are suffering in what they believe to be a helpless and hopeless situation. The Oregon Health Council formed Oregon Health Decisions (OHD) as an outreach program that conducts community meetings throughout Oregon to collect residents' views on bioethics and values, and evaluates the issues facing the terminally ill. The findings of the OHD have shown that autonomy and personal control are issues facing the terminally ill that contribute to requests for physician-assisted suicide. Physicians must offer hope that pain will not be ignored, stress and psychological concerns will be treated appropriately, and patients will be cared for in a dignified manner, even though they may lose control of bodily functions.

On March 4, 2009, physician-assisted suicide was legalized for residents of Washington state. Washington state voted 57.82% to 42.18% to allow physician-assisted death for terminally ill patients (Washington Secretary of State Sam Reed, 2009). Initiative 1000, Washington's Death with Dignity Act, is modeled on the Oregon law and is virtually the same. Washington residents must make two separate requests, orally and in writing, more than two weeks apart; must be of sound mind and not suffering from depression; and must have their request approved by two separate doctors. Doctors are not allowed to administer the lethal dose. Washington's Death with Dignity Act uses the phrase "request for medication to end my life in a humane and dignified manner" and not the phrase, "assisted suicide" (Washington's Secretary of State Sam Reed, 2009).

DEATH CERTIFICATES

Another item from the object component of the death system is the death certificate, a unique document that memorializes death. Death certificates include the time and cause of death. After the physician signs the certificate, it is considered a legal proof of death. Each certificate shows the date, time, place, and cause of death. A certified copy of the death certificate is necessary for life insurance and other death benefits. It is also needed for probate, which is the process that transfers legal title of property from the estate of the individual who has died. The U.S. Standard Certificate of Death, last updated in 2003, is divided into three parts: decedent information, cause of death, and disposition of the body (Figure 2-1).

Death certificates are needed for the family to settle financial affairs. Organizations requiring a copy of the death certificate include:

- financial institutions
- probate court
- Social Security Administration
- life insurance companies
- stocks, bonds, and mutual fund companies
- the IRS and state tax agency
- pension administrators
- automobile creditors or other lenders
- organizations governing real estate owned.

Funeral directors can request death certificates for 6 months after the death. If the family needs additional death certificates, they must contact the Health Department or Registrar. The family must substantiate a request with proof of identity (e.g., birth certificate, marriage license, income tax return). Requests for a certified death record should include the decedent's full name, place of death,

relationship to the person who is requesting the record, and the reason for requesting the record. Family members in these cases will be asked certain questions, with the answers recorded on the death certificate. This practice was instituted after the terrorist attacks on September 11th because deceitful individuals were stealing identities of deceased individuals.

CASE STUDY

Wendy is a 29-year-old Hispanic, Catholic woman who is employed by the same company as her husband, Ian. During their lunch hour, Ian and his wife were walking down a steep set of concrete stairs leading to the lunchroom in the office complex. Ian tripped causing him and Wendy to fall to the bottom step. Both were brought to the emergency department by ambulance. Wendy did not sustain any life-threatening injuries. The nurses helped her remain calm as they treated her. Her husband was being treated in another room. One nurse kept going back and forth between Ian's and Wendy's rooms to keep Wendy informed of her husband's condition. At one point, she warned Wendy that her husband was not breathing on his own. Wendy asked the nurse to have the priest give her husband the Sacrament of the Sick and the nurse made the call immediately to pastoral care.

Although everything was done to save him, Ian died from internal injuries soon after being admitted to the hospital. Wendy's nurse remained with her as the emergency department physician notified her that Ian had died.

After the physician left the room, Wendy got up from her wheelchair and sat on the floor weeping uncontrollably. The nurse attempted to comfort her. Although the nurse made several attempts to get Wendy to sit in a chair, she refused. Appearing disoriented, she kept repeating, "I can't believe he's dead."

continued on page 32

FIGURE 2-1: THE U.S. STANDARD CERTIFICATE OF DEATH (1 OF 4)

U.S. STANDARD CERTIFICATE OF DEATH

LOCAL FILE NO.   STATE FILE NO.

NAME OF DECEDENT
For use by physician or institution

To Be Completed/ Verified By:
FUNERAL DIRECTOR:

1. DECEDENT'S LEGAL NAME (Include AKA's if any) (First, Middle, Last) | 2. SEX | 3. SOCIAL SECURITY NUMBER

4a. AGE-Last Birthday (Years) | 4b. UNDER 1 YEAR (Months / Days) | 4c. UNDER 1 DAY (Hours / Minutes) | 5. DATE OF BIRTH (Mo/Day/Yr) | 6. BIRTHPLACE (City and State or Foreign Country)

7a. RESIDENCE-STATE | 7b. COUNTY | 7c. CITY OR TOWN

7d. STREET AND NUMBER | 7e. APT. NO. | 7f. ZIP CODE | 7g. INSIDE CITY LIMITS? ☐ Yes ☐ No

8. EVER IN US ARMED FORCES? ☐ Yes ☐ No | 9. MARITAL STATUS AT TIME OF DEATH ☐ Married ☐ Married, but separated ☐ Widowed ☐ Divorced ☐ Never Married ☐ Unknown | 10. SURVIVING SPOUSE'S NAME (If wife, give name prior to first marriage)

11. FATHER'S NAME (First, Middle, Last) | 12. MOTHER'S NAME PRIOR TO FIRST MARRIAGE (First, Middle, Last)

13a. INFORMANT'S NAME | 13b. RELATIONSHIP TO DECEDENT | 13c. MAILING ADDRESS (Street and Number, City, State, Zip Code)

14. PLACE OF DEATH (Check only one; see instructions)

IF DEATH OCCURRED IN A HOSPITAL: ☐ Inpatient ☐ Emergency Room/Outpatient ☐ Dead on Arrival | IF DEATH OCCURRED SOMEWHERE OTHER THAN A HOSPITAL: ☐ Hospice facility ☐ Nursing home/Long term care facility ☐ Decedent's home ☐ Other (Specify)

15. FACILITY NAME (If not institution, give street & number) | 16. CITY OR TOWN, STATE, AND ZIP CODE | 17. COUNTY OF DEATH

18. METHOD OF DISPOSITION: ☐ Burial ☐ Cremation ☐ Donation ☐ Entombment ☐ Removal from State ☐ Other (Specify): | 19. PLACE OF DISPOSITION (Name of cemetery, crematory, other place)

20. LOCATION-CITY, TOWN, AND STATE | 21. NAME AND COMPLETE ADDRESS OF FUNERAL FACILITY

22. SIGNATURE OF FUNERAL SERVICE LICENSEE OR OTHER AGENT | 23. LICENSE NUMBER (Of Licensee)

ITEMS 24-28 MUST BE COMPLETED BY PERSON WHO PRONOUNCES OR CERTIFIES DEATH | 24. DATE PRONOUNCED DEAD (Mo/Day/Yr) | 25. TIME PRONOUNCED DEAD

26. SIGNATURE OF PERSON PRONOUNCING DEATH (Only when applicable) | 27. LICENSE NUMBER | 28. DATE SIGNED (Mo/Day/Yr)

29. ACTUAL OR PRESUMED DATE OF DEATH (Mo/Day/Yr) (Spell Month) | 30. ACTUAL OR PRESUMED TIME OF DEATH | 31. WAS MEDICAL EXAMINER OR CORONER CONTACTED? ☐ Yes ☐ No

CAUSE OF DEATH (See instructions and examples)

To Be Completed By: MEDICAL CERTIFIER

32. **PART I.** Enter the chain of events--diseases, injuries, or complications--that directly caused the death. DO NOT enter terminal events such as cardiac arrest, respiratory arrest, or ventricular fibrillation without showing the etiology. DO NOT ABBREVIATE. Enter only one cause on a line. Add additional lines if necessary. | Approximate interval: Onset to death

IMMEDIATE CAUSE (Final disease or condition ──→ resulting in death) a. _____ Due to (or as a consequence of): _____

Sequentially list conditions, if any, leading to the cause listed on line a. Enter the **UNDERLYING CAUSE** (disease or injury that initiated the events resulting in death) **LAST** b. _____ Due to (or as a consequence of): _____ c. _____ Due to (or as a consequence of): _____ d. _____

PART II. Enter other significant conditions contributing to death but not resulting in the underlying cause given in PART I | 33. WAS AN AUTOPSY PERFORMED? ☐ Yes ☐ No | 34. WERE AUTOPSY FINDINGS AVAILABLE TO COMPLETE THE CAUSE OF DEATH? ☐ Yes ☐ No

35. DID TOBACCO USE CONTRIBUTE TO DEATH? ☐ Yes ☐ Probably ☐ No ☐ Unknown | 36. IF FEMALE: ☐ Not pregnant within past year ☐ Pregnant at time of death ☐ Not pregnant, but pregnant within 42 days of death ☐ Not pregnant, but pregnant 43 days to 1 year before death ☐ Unknown if pregnant within the past year | 37. MANNER OF DEATH ☐ Natural ☐ Homicide ☐ Accident ☐ Pending Investigation ☐ Suicide ☐ Could not be determined

38. DATE OF INJURY (Mo/Day/Yr) (Spell Month) | 39. TIME OF INJURY | 40. PLACE OF INJURY (e.g., Decedent's home; construction site; restaurant; wooded area) | 41. INJURY AT WORK? ☐ Yes ☐ No

42. LOCATION OF INJURY: State: / City or Town: / Street & Number / Apartment No.: / Zip Code:

43. DESCRIBE HOW INJURY OCCURRED: | 44. IF TRANSPORTATION INJURY, SPECIFY: ☐ Driver/Operator ☐ Passenger ☐ Pedestrian ☐ Other (Specify)

45. CERTIFIER (Check only one):
☐ Certifying physician-To the best of my knowledge, death occurred due to the cause(s) and manner stated.
☐ Pronouncing & Certifying physician-To the best of my knowledge, death occurred at the time, date, and place, and due to the cause(s) and manner stated.
☐ Medical Examiner/Coroner-On the basis of examination, and/or investigation, in my opinion, death occurred at the time, date, and place, and due to the cause(s) and manner stated.

Signature of certifier: _____

46. NAME, ADDRESS, AND ZIP CODE OF PERSON COMPLETING CAUSE OF DEATH (Item 32)

47. TITLE OF CERTIFIER | 48. LICENSE NUMBER | 49. DATE CERTIFIED (Mo/Day/Yr) | 50. **FOR REGISTRAR ONLY**- DATE FILED (Mo/Day/Yr)

To Be Completed By: FUNERAL DIRECTOR

51. DECEDENT'S EDUCATION-Check the box that best describes the highest degree or level of school completed at the time of death.
☐ 8th grade or less
☐ 9th - 12th grade; no diploma
☐ High school graduate or GED completed
☐ Some college credit, but no degree
☐ Associate degree (e.g., AA, AS)
☐ Bachelor's degree (e.g., BA, AB, BS)
☐ Master's degree (e.g., MA, MS, MEng, MEd, MSW, MBA)
☐ Doctorate (e.g., PhD, EdD) or Professional degree (e.g., MD, DDS, DVM, LLB, JD) | 52. DECEDENT OF HISPANIC ORIGIN? Check the box that best describes whether the decedent is Spanish/Hispanic/Latino. Check the 'No' box if decedent is not Spanish/Hispanic/Latino.
☐ No, not Spanish/Hispanic/Latino
☐ Yes, Mexican, Mexican American, Chicano
☐ Yes, Puerto Rican
☐ Yes, Cuban
☐ Yes, other Spanish/Hispanic/Latino (Specify) _____ | 53. DECEDENT'S RACE (Check one or more races to indicate what the decedent considered himself or herself to be)
☐ White
☐ Black or African American
☐ American Indian or Alaska Native (Name of the enrolled or principal tribe) _____
☐ Asian Indian
☐ Chinese
☐ Filipino
☐ Japanese
☐ Korean
☐ Vietnamese
☐ Other Asian (Specify) _____
☐ Native Hawaiian
☐ Guamanian or Chamorro
☐ Samoan
☐ Other Pacific Islander (Specify) _____
☐ Other (Specify) _____

54. DECEDENT'S USUAL OCCUPATION (Indicate type of work done during most of working life. DO NOT USE RETIRED).

55. KIND OF BUSINESS/INDUSTRY

REV. 11/2003

Note. From Center for Disease Control and Prevention (2003). Available at http://www.cdc.gov/nchs/data/dvs/DEATH11-03final-ACC.pdf

continued on next page

FIGURE 2-1: THE U.S. STANDARD CERTIFICATE OF DEATH (2 OF 4)

MEDICAL CERTIFIER INSTRUCTIONS for selected items on U.S. Standard Certificate of Death
(See Physicians' Handbook or Medical Examiner/Coroner Handbook on Death Registration for instructions on all items)

ITEMS ON WHEN DEATH OCCURRED
Items 24-25 and 29-31 should always be completed. If the facility uses a separate pronouncer or other person to indicate that death has taken place with another person more familiar with the case completing the remainder of the medical portion of the death certificate, the pronouncer completes Items 24-28. If a certifier completes Items 24-25 as well as items 29-49, Items 26-28 may be left blank.

ITEMS 24-25, 29-30 – DATE AND TIME OF DEATH
Spell out the name of the month. If the exact date of death is unknown, enter the **approximate** date. If the date cannot be approximated, enter the date the body is found and identify as **date found**. Date pronounced and actual date may be the same. Enter the exact hour and minutes according to a 24-hour clock; estimates may be provided with "Approx." placed before the time.

ITEM 32 – CAUSE OF DEATH (See attached examples)
Take care to make the entry legible. Use a computer printer with high resolution, typewriter with good black ribbon and clean keys, or print legibly using permanent **black** ink in completing the CAUSE OF DEATH Section. **Do not abbreviate** conditions entered in section.

Part I (Chain of events leading directly to death)
•Only **one** cause should be entered on each line. Line (a) **MUST ALWAYS** have an entry. **DO NOT** leave blank. Additional lines may be added if necessary.
•If the condition on Line (a) resulted from an underlying condition, put the underlying condition on Line (b), and so on, until the full sequence is reported. **ALWAYS** enter the **underlying cause of death** on the lowest used line in Part I.
 •For each cause indicate the best estimate of the interval between the presumed onset and the date of death. The terms "unknown" or "approximately" may be used. General terms, such as minutes, hours, or days, are acceptable, if necessary. **DO NOT** leave blank.
 •The terminal event (for example, cardiac arrest or respiratory arrest) should not be used. If a mechanism of death seems most appropriate to you for line (a), then you must always list its cause(s) on the line(s) below it (for example, cardiac arrest **due to** coronary artery atherosclerosis *or* cardiac arrest **due to** blunt impact to chest).
• If an organ system failure such as congestive heart failure, hepatic failure, renal failure, or respiratory failure is listed as a cause of death, always report its etiology on the line(s) beneath it (for example, renal failure **due to** Type I diabetes mellitus).
•When indicating neoplasms as a cause of death, include the following: 1) primary site *or* that the primary site is unknown, 2) benign or malignant, 3) cell type *or* that the cell type is unknown, 4) grade of neoplasm, and 5) part or lobe of organ affected. (For example, a primary well-differentiated squamous cell carcinoma, lung, left upper lobe.)
•Always report the fatal injury (for example, stab wound of chest), the trauma (for example, transection of subclavian vein), and impairment of function (for example, air embolism).

PART II (Other significant conditions)
•Enter all diseases or conditions contributing to death that were not reported in the chain of events in Part I and that did not result in the **underlying cause of death**. See attached examples.
•If two or more possible sequences resulted in death, or if two conditions seem to have added together, report in Part I the one that, in your opinion, most directly caused death. Report in Part II the other conditions or diseases.

CHANGES TO CAUSE OF DEATH
Should additional medical information or autopsy findings become available that would change the cause of death originally reported, the original death certificate should be amended by the certifying physician by **immediately** reporting the revised cause of death to the State Vital Records Office.

ITEMS 33-34 - AUTOPSY
•33 - Enter "Yes" if either a partial or full autopsy was performed. Otherwise enter "No."
•34 - Enter "Yes" if autopsy findings were available to complete the cause of death; otherwise enter "No". Leave item blank if no autopsy was performed.

ITEM 35 - DID TOBACCO USE CONTRIBUTE TO DEATH?
Check "yes" if, in your opinion, the use of tobacco contributed to death. Tobacco use may contribute to deaths due to a wide variety of diseases; for example, tobacco use contributes to many deaths due to emphysema or lung cancer and some heart disease and cancers of the head and neck. Check "no" if, in your clinical judgment, tobacco use did not contribute to this particular death.

ITEM 36 - IF FEMALE, WAS DECEDENT PREGNANT AT TIME OF DEATH OR WITHIN PAST YEAR?
This information is important in determining pregnancy-related mortality.

ITEM 37 - MANNER OF DEATH
•Always check Manner of Death, which is important: 1) in determining accurate causes of death; 2) in processing insurance claims; and 3) in statistical studies of injuries and death.
•Indicate "Pending investigation" if the manner of death cannot be determined whether due to an accident, suicide, or homicide within the statutory time limit for filing the death certificate. This should be changed later to one of the other terms.
•Indicate "Could not be Determined" **ONLY** when it is impossible to determine the manner of death.

ITEMS 38-44 - ACCIDENT OR INJURY – to be filled out in all cases of deaths due to injury or poisoning.
•38 - Enter the exact month, day, and year of injury. Spell out the name of the month. **DO NOT** use a number for the month. (Remember, the date of injury may differ from the date of death.) Estimates may be provided with "Approx." placed before the date.
•39 - Enter the exact hour and minutes of injury or use your best estimate. Use a 24-hour clock.
•40 - Enter the general place (such as restaurant, vacant lot, or home) where the injury occurred. **DO NOT** enter firm or organization names. (For example, enter "factory", **not** "Standard Manufacturing, Inc.")
•41 - Complete if anything other than natural disease is mentioned in Part I or Part II of the medical certification, including homicides, suicides, and accidents. This includes all motor vehicle deaths. The item **must** be completed for decedents ages 14 years or over and may be completed for those less than 14 years of age if warranted. Enter "Yes" if the injury occurred at work. Otherwise enter "No". An injury may occur at work regardless of whether the injury occurred in the course of the decedent's "usual" occupation. Examples of injury at work and injury not at work follow.

Injury at work	Injury not at work
Injury while working or in vocational training on job premises	Injury while engaged in personal recreational activity on job premises
Injury while on break or at lunch or in parking lot on job premises	Injury while a visitor (not on official work business) to job premises
Injury while working for pay or compensation, including at home	Homemaker working at homemaking activities
Injury while working as a volunteer law enforcement official etc.	Student in school
Injury while traveling on business, including to/from business contacts	Working for self for no profit (mowing yard, repairing own roof, hobby)
	Commuting to or from work

•42 - Enter the complete address where the injury occurred including zip code.
•43 - Enter a brief but specific and clear description of how the injury occurred. Explain the circumstances or cause of the injury. Specify **type of gun** or **type of vehicle** (e.g., car, bulldozer, train, etc.) when relevant to circumstances. Indicate if more than one vehicle involved; specify type of vehicle decedent was in.
•44 -Specify role of decedent (e.g. driver, passenger). Driver/operator and passenger should be designated for modes other than motor vehicles such as bicycles. Other applies to watercraft, aircraft, animal, or people attached to outside of vehicles (e.g. surfers).

Rationale: Motor vehicle accidents are a major cause of unintentional deaths; details will help determine effectiveness of current safety features and laws.
REFERENCES
For more information on how to complete the medical certification section of the death certificate, refer to tutorial at http://www.TheNAME.org and resources including instructions and handbooks available by request from NCHS, Room 7318, 3311 Toledo Road, Hyattsville, Maryland 20782-2003 or at www.cdc.gov/nchs/about/major/dvs/handbk.htm

REV. 11/2003

continued on next page

FIGURE 2-1: THE U.S. STANDARD CERTIFICATE OF DEATH (3 OF 4)

Cause-of-death – Background, Examples, and Common Problems

Accurate cause of death information is important
•to the public health community in evaluating and improving the health of all citizens, and
•often to the family, now and in the future, and to the person setting the decedent's estate.

The cause-of-death section consists of two parts. **Part I** is for reporting a chain of events leading directly to death, with the **immediate cause** of death (the final disease, injury, or complication directly causing death) on line a and the **underlying cause** of death (the disease or injury that initiated the chain of events that led directly and inevitably to death) on the lowest used line. **Part II** is for reporting all other significant diseases, conditions, or injuries that contributed to death but which did not result in the underlying cause of death given in Part I. **The cause-of-death information should be YOUR best medical OPINION.** A condition can be listed as "probable" even if it has not been definitively diagnosed.

Examples of properly completed medical certifications

CAUSE OF DEATH (See Instructions and examples)

32. **PART I.** Enter the chain of events--diseases, injuries, or complications--that directly caused the death. DO NOT enter terminal events such as cardiac arrest, respiratory arrest, or ventricular fibrillation without showing the etiology. DO NOT ABBREVIATE. Enter only one cause on a line. Add additional lines if necessary.

		Approximate interval: Onset to death
IMMEDIATE CAUSE (Final disease or condition resulting in death) →	a. Rupture of myocardium Due to (or as a consequence of):	Minutes
Sequentially list conditions, if any, leading to the cause listed on line a. Enter the **UNDERLYING CAUSE** (disease or injury that initiated the events resulting in death) LAST	b. Acute myocardial infarction Due to (or as a consequence of):	6 days
	c. Coronary artery thrombosis Due to (or as a consequence of):	5 years
	d. Atherosclerotic coronary artery disease	7 years

PART II. Enter other significant conditions contributing to death but not resulting in the underlying cause given in PART I

Diabetes, Chronic obstructive pulmonary disease, smoking

33. WAS AN AUTOPSY PERFORMED? ■ Yes ☐ No
34. WERE AUTOPSY FINDINGS AVAILABLE TO COMPLETE THE CAUSE OF DEATH? ■ Yes ☐ No

35. DID TOBACCO USE CONTRIBUTE TO DEATH?	36. IF FEMALE:	37. MANNER OF DEATH
■ Yes ☐ Probably ☐ No ☐ Unknown	■ Not pregnant within past year ☐ Pregnant at time of death ☐ Not pregnant, but pregnant within 42 days of death ☐ Not pregnant, but pregnant 43 days to 1 year before death ☐ Unknown if pregnant within the past year	■ Natural ☐ Homicide ☐ Accident ☐ Pending Investigation ☐ Suicide ☐ Could not be determined

CAUSE OF DEATH (See instructions and examples)

32. **PART I.** Enter the chain of events--diseases, injuries, or complications--that directly caused the death. DO NOT enter terminal events such as cardiac arrest, respiratory arrest, or ventricular fibrillation without showing the etiology. DO NOT ABBREVIATE. Enter only one cause on a line. Add additional lines if necessary.

		Approximate interval: Onset to death
IMMEDIATE CAUSE (Final disease or condition → resulting in death)	a. Aspiration pneumonia Due to (or as a consequence of):	2 Days
Sequentially list conditions, if any, leading to the cause listed on line a. Enter the **UNDERLYING CAUSE** (disease or injury that initiated the events resulting in death) LAST	b. Complications of coma Due to (or as a consequence of):	7 weeks
	c. Blunt force injuries Due to (or as a consequence of):	7 weeks
	d. Motor vehicle accident	7 weeks

PART II. Enter other significant conditions contributing to death but not resulting in the underlying cause given in PART I

33. WAS AN AUTOPSY PERFORMED? ■ Yes ☐ No
34. WERE AUTOPSY FINDINGS AVAILABLE TO COMPLETE THE CAUSE OF DEATH? ■ Yes ☐ No

35. DID TOBACCO USE CONTRIBUTE TO DEATH?	36. IF FEMALE:	37. MANNER OF DEATH
☐ Yes ☐ Probably ■ No ☐ Unknown	☐ Not pregnant within past year ☐ Pregnant at time of death ☐ Not pregnant, but pregnant within 42 days of death ☐ Not pregnant, but pregnant 43 days to 1 year before death ☐ Unknown if pregnant within the past year	☐ Natural ☐ Homicide ■ Accident ☐ Pending Investigation ☐ Suicide ☐ Could not be determined

38. DATE OF INJURY (Mo/Day/Yr) (Spell Month) August 15, 2003	39. TIME OF INJURY Approx. 2320	40. PLACE OF INJURY (e.g., Decedent's home; construction site; restaurant; wooded area) road side near state highway	41. INJURY AT WORK? ☐ Yes ■ No

42. LOCATION OF INJURY: State: Missouri — City or Town: near Alexandria

Street & Number: mile marker 17 on state route 48a — Apartment No.: — Zip Code:

43. DESCRIBE HOW INJURY OCCURRED:

Decedent driver of van, ran off road into tree

44. IF TRANSPORTATION INJURY, SPECIFY:
■ Driver/Operator
☐ Passenger
☐ Pedestrian
☐ Other (Specify)

Common problems in death certification

The **elderly decedent** should have a clear and distinct etiological sequence for cause of death, if possible. Terms such as senescence, infirmity, old age, and advanced age have little value for public health or medical research. Age is recorded elsewhere on the certificate. When a number of conditions resulted in death, the physician should choose the single sequence that, in his or her opinion, best describes the process leading to death, and place any other pertinent conditions in Part II. If after careful consideration the physician cannot determine a sequence that ends in death, then the medical examiner or coroner should be consulted about conducting an investigation or providing assistance in completing the cause of death.

The **infant decedent** should have a clear and distinct etiological sequence for cause of death, if possible. "Prematurity" should not be entered without explaining the etiology of prematurity. Maternal conditions may have initiated or affected the sequence that resulted in infant death, and such maternal causes should be reported in addition to the infant causes on the infant's death certificate (e.g., Hyaline membrane disease **due to** prematurity, 28 weeks **due to** placental abruption **due to** blunt trauma to mother's abdomen).

When **SIDS** is suspected, a complete investigation should be conducted, typically by a medical examiner or coroner. If the infant is under 1 year of age, no cause of death is determined after scene investigation, clinical history is reviewed, and a complete autopsy is performed, then the death can be reported as Sudden Infant Death Syndrome.

When processes such as the following are reported, additional information about the etiology should be reported:

Abscess	Carcinomatosis	Disseminated intra vascular	Hyponatremia	Pulmonary arrest
Abdominal hemorrhage	Cardiac arrest	coagulopathy	Hypotension	Pulmonary edema
Adhesions	Cardiac dysrhythmia	Dysrhythmia	Immunosuppression	Pulmonary embolism
Adult respiratory distress syndrome	Cardiomyopathy	End-stage liver disease	Increased intra cranial pressure	Pulmonary insufficiency
Acute myocardial infarction	Cardiopulmonary arrest	End-stage renal disease	Intra cranial hemorrhage	Renal failure
Altered mental status	Cellulitis	Epidural hematoma	Malnutrition	Respiratory arrest
Anemia	Cerebral edema	Exsanguination	Metabolic encephalopathy	Seizures
Anoxia	Cerebrovascular accident	Failure to thrive	Multi-organ failure	Sepsis
Anoxic encephalopathy	Cerebellar tonsillar herniation	Fracture	Multi-system organ failure	Septic shock
Arrhythmia	Chronic bedridden state	Gangrene	Myocardial infarction	Shock
Ascites	Cirrhosis	Gastrointestinal hemorrhage	Necrotizing soft-tissue infection	Starvation
Aspiration	Coagulopathy	Heart failure	Old age	Subdural hematoma
Atrial fibrillation	Compression fracture	Hemothorax	Open (or closed) head injury	Subarachnoid hemorrhage
Bacteremia	Congestive heart failure	Hepatic failure	Paralysis	Sudden death
Bedridden	Convulsions	Hepatitis	Pancytopenia	Thrombocytopenia
Biliary obstruction	Decubiti	Hepatorenal syndrome	Perforated gallbladder	Uncal herniation
Bowel obstruction	Dehydration	Hyperglycemia	Peritonitis	Urinary tract infection
Brain injury	Dementia (when not	Hyperkalemia	Pleural effusions	Ventricular fibrillation
Brain stem herniation	otherwise specified)	Hypovolemic shock	Pneumonia	Ventricular tachycardia
Carcinogenesis	Diarrhea			Volume depletion

If the certifier is unable to determine the etiology of a process such as those shown above, the process must be qualified as being of an unknown, undetermined, probable, presumed, or unspecified etiology so it is clear that a distinct etiology was not inadvertently or carelessly omitted.

The following conditions and types of death might seem to be specific or natural but when the medical history is examined further may be found to be complications of an injury or poisoning (possibly occurring long ago). Such cases should be reported to the medical examiner/coroner.

Asphyxia	Epidural hematoma	Hip fracture	Pulmonary emboli	Subdural hematoma
Bolus	Exsanguination	Hyperthermia	Seizure disorder	Surgery
Choking	Fall	Hypothermia	Sepsis	Thermal burns/chemical burns
Drug or alcohol overdose/drug or alcohol abuse	Fracture	Open reduction of fracture	Subarachnoid hemorrhage	

REV. 11/2003

FIGURE 2-1: THE U.S. STANDARD CERTIFICATE OF DEATH (4 OF 4)

FUNERAL DIRECTOR INSTRUCTIONS for selected items on U.S.

Standard Certificate of Death (For additional information concerning all items on certificate see Funeral Directors' Handbook on Death Registration)

ITEM 1. DECEDENT'S LEGAL NAME
Include any other names used by decedent, if substantially different from the legal name, after the abbreviation AKA (also known as) e.g. Samuel Langhorne Clemens AKA Mark Twain, **but not** Jonathon Doe AKA John Doe

ITEM 5. DATE OF BIRTH
Enter the full name of the month (January, February, March etc.) Do not use a number or abbreviation to designate the month.

ITEM 7A-G. RESIDENCE OF DECEDENT (information divided into seven categories)
Residence of decedent is the place where the decedent actually resided. The place of residence is not necessarily the same as "home state" or "legal residence". Never enter a temporary residence such as one used during a visit, business trip, or vacation. Place of residence during a tour of military duty or during attendance at college is considered permanent and should be entered as the place of residence. If the decedent had been living in a facility where an individual usually resides for a long period of time, such as a group home, mental institution, nursing home, penitentiary, or hospital for the chronically ill, report the location of that facility in item 7. If the decedent was an infant who never resided at home, the place of residence is that of the parent(s) or legal guardian. **Never** use an acute care hospital's location as the place of residence for any infant. If Canadian residence, please specify Province instead of State.

ITEM 10. SURVIVING SPOUSE'S NAME
If the decedent was married at the time of death, enter the full name of the surviving spouse. If the surviving spouse is the wife, enter her name prior to first marriage. This item is used in establishing proper insurance settlements and other survivor benefits.

ITEM 12. MOTHER'S NAME PRIOR TO FIRST MARRIAGE
Enter the name used prior to first marriage, commonly known as the maiden name. This name is useful because it remains constant throughout life.

ITEM 14. PLACE OF DEATH
The place where death is pronounced should be considered the place where death occurred. If the place of death is unknown but the body is found in your State, the certificate of death should be completed and filed in accordance with the laws of your State. Enter the place where the body is found as the place of death.

ITEM 51. DECEDENT'S EDUCATION *(Check appropriate box on death certificate)*
Check the box that corresponds to the highest level of education the decedent completed. **Information in this section will not appear on the certified copy of the death certificate. This information is used to study the relationship between mortality and education (which roughly corresponds with socioeconomic status). This information is valuable in medical studies of causes of death and in programs to prevent illness and death.**

ITEM 52. WAS DECEDENT OF HISPANIC ORIGIN? *(Check "No" or appropriate "Yes" box)*
Check "No" or check the "Yes" box that best corresponds with the decedent's ethnic Spanish identity as given by the informant. Note that "Hispanic" is not a race and item 53 must also be completed. Do not leave this item blank. With respect to this item, "Hispanic" refers to people whose origins are from Spain, Mexico, or the Spanish-speaking Caribbean Islands or countries of Central or South America. Origin includes ancestry, nationality, and lineage. There is no set rule about how many generations are to be taken into account in determining Hispanic origin; it may be based on the country of origin of a parent, grandparent, or some far-removed ancestor. Although the prompts include the major Hispanic groups, other groups may be specified under "other". "Other" may also be used for decedents of multiple Hispanic origin (e.g. Mexican-Puerto Rican). **Information in this section will not appear on the certified copy of the death certificate. This information is needed to identify health problems in a large minority population in the United States. Identifying health problems will make it possible to target public health resources to this important segment of our population.**

ITEM 53. RACE *(Check appropriate box or boxes on death certificate)*
Enter the race of the decedent as stated by the informant. Hispanic is not a race; information on Hispanic ethnicity is collected separately in item 52. American Indian and Alaska Native refer only to those native to North and South America (including Central America) and does not include Asian Indian. Please specify the name of enrolled or principal tribe (e.g., Navajo, Cheyenne, etc.) for the American Indian or Alaska Native. For Asians check Asian Indian, Chinese, Filipino, Japanese, Korean, Vietnamese, or specify other Asian group; for Pacific Islanders check Guamanian or Chamorro, Samoan, or specify other Pacific Island group. If the decedent was of mixed race, enter each race (e.g., Samoan-Chinese-Filipino or White, American Indian). **Information in this section will not appear on the certified copy of the death certificate. Race is essential for identifying specific mortality patterns and leading causes of death among different racial groups. It is also used to determine if specific health programs are needed in particular areas and to make population estimates.**

ITEMS 54 AND 55. OCCUPATION AND INDUSTRY
Questions concerning occupation and industry must be completed for all decedents 14 years of age or older. This information is useful in studying deaths related to jobs and in identifying any new risks. For example, the link between lung disease and lung cancer and asbestos exposure in jobs such as shipbuilding or construction was made possible by this sort of information on death certificates. **Information in this section will not appear on the certified copy of the death certificate.**

ITEM 54. DECEDENT'S USUAL OCCUPATION
Enter the usual occupation of the decedent. This is not necessarily the last occupation of the decedent. Never enter "retired". Give kind of work decedent did during most of his or her working life, such as claim adjuster, farmhand, coal miner, janitor, store manager, college professor, or civil engineer. If the decedent was a homemaker at the time of death but had worked outside the household during his or her working life, enter that occupation. If the decedent was a homemaker during most of his or her working life, and never worked outside the household, enter "homemaker". Enter "student" if the decedent was a student at the time of death and was never regularly employed or employed full time during his or her working life. **Information in this section will not appear on the certified copy of the death certificate.**

ITEM 55. KIND OF BUSINESS/INDUSTRY
Kind of business to which occupation in item 54 is related, such as insurance, farming, coal mining, hardware store, retail clothing, university, or government. DO NOT enter firm or organization names. If decedent was a homemaker as indicated in item 54, then enter either "own home" or "someone else's home" as appropriate. If decedent was a student as indicated in item 54, then enter type of school, such as high school or college, in item 55. **Information in this section will not appear on the certified copy of the death certificate.**

NOTE: This recommended standard death certificate is the result of an extensive evaluation process. Information on the process and resulting recommendations as well as plans for future activities is available on the Internet at: http://www.cdc.gov/nchs/vital_certs_rev.htm.

REV. 11/2003

Another nurse standing nearby responded, "He is resting in peace," but Wendy's nurse told her, "I'm sorry Ian died."

Wendy showed the nurse a picture from her wallet. It was a picture of Ian, Wendy, and their three small children. As the nurse looked at the picture, she found it difficult to make sense of his death and wondered how the family would cope with such a loss.

Wendy said, "Please take me to him." After gently handing the picture back to Wendy, the nurse went to the room to prepare the body for viewing. She wanted to make sure the room and body were presentable before bringing Wendy into the room.

Questions

1. What persons in the death system were in contact with the patient and her husband?

2. Who will Wendy need to contact?

3. What places in the death system will Wendy be reminded of years after the death?

4. Why will seeing ambulances or wheelchairs in the future remind Wendy of the loss?

5. What could the nurse have said instead of using a death euphemism?

6. What functions of the death system did the nurse perform?

7. In what way will the nurse attempt to make sense of the death?

Discussion

Nurses make up a component of the death system. The nurse was present when Wendy was brought into the hospital, a place in the death system. An important component of the death system is time. The nurse assisted Wendy during the time when her husband was being treated and immediately after his death. As the nurse went from one room to another, she also provided the warning and prediction function of the death system. Because Wendy was brought into the hospital by ambulance and was told of her husband's death while sitting in a wheelchair, these two objects may always remind her of his death. Although euphemisms should not be used, the nurse standing nearby simply wanted to comfort her and said, "He is resting in peace." Wendy's nurse, realizing that the correct terms should be used, then said, "I'm sorry Ian died." Nurses can listen to the terms and phrases the bereaved are using and use similar phrasing. The nurse understood the significance of culture and religion and contacted the hospital clergy. Lastly, one of the most notable things the nurse did was to check the condition of the body and room prior to bringing in the next of kin. This protected Wendy from a scene that could have been traumatizing.

SUMMARY

Nurses are a part of the American death system. Their roles may include preventing death, caring for the dying, or disposing of the dead. Social consolidation is important after a death. Nurses should be aware of physician-assisted suicide as a legal option in Oregon and Washington, and understand the needs and feelings that lead patients to request such assistance and other options at the end of life.

WEB RESOURCES

Cremation Association of North America
http://www.cremationassociation.org

Hospice Foundation of America
http://www.hospicefoundation.org

National Funeral Directors Association
http://www.nfda.org

Celebrant Foundation & Institute
http://www.celebrantusa.org

National Cremation
http://www.nationalcreamation.com

EXAM QUESTIONS

CHAPTER 2
Questions 10-19

Note: Choose the one option that BEST answers each question.

10. The five components of Kastenbaum's model of the Contemporary American Death System are

    a. people, places, times, culture, and society.
    b. people, places, times, objects, and symbols.
    c. people, places, death, symbols, and media.
    d. people, places, objects, healing, and symbols.

11. Funeral homes are required by law to have

    a. an area for the family to meet privately.
    b. the ability to cremate the body.
    c. a list of goods and services including prices.
    d. bereavement care for survivors.

12. The *times* component of the death system refers to

    a. the time of death.
    b. the age of the person who has died.
    c. holidays or seasons when the dead are remembered.
    d. the time of the funeral service.

13. Two common symbols of death include

    a. culture and the media.
    b. anxiety and the media.
    c. traditional figures and anxiety.
    d. crows and the grim reaper.

14. Two common euphemisms used for death in the United States are

    a. warning and expired.
    b. cremation and passed on.
    c. skeleton and tombs.
    d. expired and passed on.

15. One of the functions of the death system is to

    a. prevent death.
    b. document death.
    c. honor death.
    d. symbolize death.

16. The warning and predicting function of the death system includes

    a. storm warnings and warning labels on harmful substances.
    b. emergency personnel and spontaneous memorialization.
    c. social consolidation after death.
    d. emergency personnel and body disposal.

17. Social consolidation after death includes

    a. cremation.
    b. bereavement support groups.
    c. weather forecasting.
    d. choice of caskets.

18. The type of euthanasia that involves withholding or withdrawing life-sustaining treatment is

    a. active euthanasia.

    b. passive euthanasia.

    c. killing euthanasia.

    d. active voluntary euthanasia.

19. In order to file for life insurance benefits, other death benefits, and probate, the following document is needed:

    a. marriage certificate.

    b. funeral director certificate.

    c. death certificate.

    d. statement of Social Security certificate.

CHAPTER 3

COPING WITH DYING

CHAPTER OBJECTIVE

After completing this chapter, the reader will be able to describe the ways that individuals and family members cope with dying.

LEARNING OBJECTIVES

After studying this chapter, the reader will be able to

1. explain the importance of "meaning making" as one approaches death.

2. describe theoretical models that focus on patient, family, and caregiver responses to death and dying.

3. discuss the nurse's role in supporting terminally ill patients and their caregivers.

4. describe care at the time of death.

INTRODUCTION

Learning about the meaning of death trajectories, development of death awareness, and theoretical models of the dying process enables nurses to better understand and help those who are terminally ill. The key to learning what dying patients and family members want lies within the word, "meaning." When nurses know what dying means to their patients, they will learn what it means to have lived; relationships, friendships, belief sys-tems, culture, and history are melded together to form the meaning of a person's life and death.

MAKING SENSE OF DYING

Life transitions force individuals to move from one place in their lives to another. Although some are positive, such as getting married or giving birth to a child, people typically feel vulnerable and challenged to deal with the losses that come with every transition. Parents experience the loss of their roles when children leave for college, friends experience the loss of having a confidant when friends move away, retirees experience the loss of their place in the workplace when they retire, older adults experience the loss of their family homes when they decide to move to an adult community, and, most significantly, people experience loss of themselves when they are dying. What links these experiences is the meaning individuals give to them. Whether having friends move away, leaving behind a home where children were raised, or knowing that life is ebbing away, the key point is that meaning can be found in each life transition. As individuals face dying, they may attempt to find meaning in their losses, their lives, their dying and, most importantly, in their own deaths.

The loss experience can have an effect on how dying individuals adjust to previously held beliefs about themselves and their world (Breitbart,

Gibson, Poppito, & Berg, 2004). Nurses often find themselves journeying with terminally ill patients and bereaved families on a profound and sometimes painful search for understanding (Currier, Holland, & Neimeyer, 2008). An explanation of meaning involves "sense-making" or the ability to develop a subjective sense of understanding the loss (Gillies & Neimeyer, 2006). Most theories identify cognitive processing as an underlying mechanism of positive transformation to deal with loss, whether it is called meaning making or sense making (Park & Helgeson, 2006).

> ### *Personal Insight*
> *What is the meaning of your life...and your death?*

Nurses are often present as terminally ill patients and family members attempt to find meaning in their prognosis, dying, and death and may be called upon to provide support. In a recent study, 33% of nurses reported referring dying patients and their families to other helping professionals who could focus more explicitly on the dying or bereaved individual's grief needs. This is not to say that the majority of nurses do not attend directly to issues of meaning-making in their work (Currier et al., 2008). One of the nurses in this study stated:

> I try to be a supportive presence in their personal search to make sense of loss. I reflect back what I hear being said and ask for clarity to help the patient and their family find clarity themselves. In addition to listening, I also suggest alternative possibilities in conversation. Depending on the person, I validate what I hear being said when the person appears to be coping or not. I also offer or suggest ongoing therapy if needed. (p. 130)

When nurses talk with their patients about dying, the focus should be on maintaining dignity and increasing their sense of purpose and meaning. Chochinov et al. (2005) studied the impact of giving 100 terminally ill patients the opportunity to discuss issues that mattered most or that they most wanted remembered by others. The four queries asked of the patients were:

1. Tell me a little about your life history, particularly the parts that you either remember most or think are most important.

2. Are there specific things that you would want your family to know about you, and are there particular things that you would want them to remember?

3. What are your hopes and dreams for your loved ones?

4. What have you learned about life that you would want to pass along to others?

The responses were recorded and transcribed into a written document, which was then read to the patients. After they made revisions, the patients shared it with others. A large majority of patients (91%) reported being satisfied with the intervention, and 81% thought it would help their family. A majority of patients indicated the intervention gave them a heightened sense of dignity, an increased sense of purpose, and a deeper sense of meaning (Chochinov et al., 2005).

Dying persons can be distressed at the thought of leaving their loved ones (Yang & Rosenblatt, 2007). The reality of children growing up unobserved and spouses managing houses alone transforms thinking about the meaning of relationships. Because couples assign meaning to their bonds and the things they do, dying partners can feel enraged that their loved ones will live on after they are dead.

With a dying patient's permission, the nurse may talk with dying persons about these issues in the presence of their loved ones. Nurses can ask about their feelings of rage, their fears, and meaningful connections that have happened since becoming ill. When these questions are explored, patients and family members are given an opportunity to identify how their loved ones are coping.

When patients talk about death it can make family members feel depressed (Hinton, 2003). It is difficult to listen to a terminally ill loved one discuss his or her dying and impending death. It is therefore important for family members to find ways to cope with their own feelings. Allowing a range of emotions to be expressed, can help the patient cope. It can also bring the terminally ill person closer to his or her loved ones. Nurses must be mindful that although a terminally ill person talking about his dying and death may cause depression in family members, it is not unhealthy for patients to do so. Richman (2006-2007) maintains,

> At the beginning of therapy he said, "I am not afraid of dying, but I worry about what will happen to my wife." Eventually, his illness advanced, and he had to discontinue treatment. At the end of therapy I asked him, "Can you see anything good coming out of having a terminal illness?" It was a genuine question, and he gave a genuine answer, "Yes. My wife and I have never been so close." (p. 46)

Personal Insight
Imagine your death bed scene. Are you alone or with someone? Where are you? How old are you? Describe your last moments.

Dying and Living to Talk About It

Near-death experiences occur when the pulse and breathing have stopped and individuals are very close to death or clinically dead. Those who have had near-death experiences believed they were going to die. Many people reveal they had a near-death experience during surgery, when they were physically ill, or when they had an accident. These individuals report an out-of-body experience where they are observing their physical existance from a distance. The person returns to life with memories of what occurred during the time of death (Long, 2003).

Although no two near-death experiences are the same, there are similar patterns reported, such as moving through dark tunnels, experiencing intense emotions that range from happiness to anguish, and seeing lights or deceased loved ones. Those who go through near-death experiences may review their lives or reexperience milestones from their pasts. Their perceptions of those experiences help them to make changes in their lives. Near-death experiences have been reported for thousands of years and are common in all cultures; nurses may encounter patients who have experienced such phenomena (Laszlo & Currivan, 2008). Some believe near-death experiences result from neurophysical processes. Regardless of personal explanations for the phenomenon, it is important for nurses and others to acknowledge patients' beliefs and perceptions about their experiences. These experiences may be life-altering.

Personal Insight
If you were to undergo a near-death experience, do you think you would feel terror and anger? Would your thoughts be resigned to death? Would you pray and remain calm?

Dying Awareness Contexts

Awareness is based on information and how that information is perceived by significant others. A study found that 84.9% of patients with palliative care plans and 89% of other patients want as much information as possible, good or bad (Fallowfield, Jenkins, & Beveridge, 2002).

For decades, the Glaser and Strauss (1968) Awareness of Dying Model has guided research on patients' awareness of their conditions. The model describes four types of awareness contexts: closed awareness, suspected awareness, mutual pretense, and open awareness.

In *closed awareness,* the patient does not know he or she is dying, but everyone else is aware. Often, family members keep the news from the patient.

In *suspected awareness,* the patient suspects what others know and attempts to find out more information about the prognosis. The patient becomes suspicious as he or she becomes increasingly ill. Although the patient may want to know how sick he or she really is, the patient is not told that he or she is dying.

 In *mutual pretense,* the patient, family members, and professionals pretend they do not know the prognosis. Unless the patient initiates the conversation about impending death, no one talks about it. Everyone involved acts as though the patient is going to live.

In *open awareness,* the patient is aware of impending death, both preparing for it and discussing it. During open awareness, the patient can openly talk about forgiveness, gratitude, and love.

When individuals are aware they are dying, they can address unfinished business. Byock (2004) maintains that these patients can improve relationships in their lives by saying: Please forgive me, I forgive you, thank you, I love you, and good-bye. Imagine these as last words and the effect the words can have for the dying person as well as for the individuals privileged to hear such words spoken.

> *Personal Insight*
> *Which awareness would you prefer if you*
>   *were dying?*

Valentine (2007) interviewed bereaved individuals and found that final moments may be highly significant in relation to the dying trajectory, as a whole, and to making sense of the bereavement experience. For family members, the experience of a loved one's dying becomes a profound and memorable occasion (Valentine, 2007). A participant in Valentine's study reported the following after a loved one's death:

Of course she'd come from a nursing background and she knew exactly what was happening to her and from September she stopped eating and she stopped eating on purpose because she didn't want to extend her life, so although she was still quite hungry, her mind

was quite hungry, there was still a part that she just didn't want to extend her life (p. 225)...I kept pushing the nurses, the doctors, is she gonna live longer – how long can she live because her body was just shrinking and you know to me it was like surely to God she's gonna die soon?...I just became obsessed with knowing, just trying to get some certainty over this very uncertain process (p. 228)...that was just an amazing moment – I mean it was just absolutely amazing because as I say she died looking straight into my eyes with her hands on my cheek and I knew she knew it was me and I knew it was just that moment of recognition...of connection, absolutely nonverbal you know incredible. (p. 229)

THEORETICAL MODELS OF THE DYING PROCESS

Theoretical models help us understand the dying process, but it is important to remember that each patient deals with the process in a unique way. Should patients go through stages in order to achieve a good death? Should they become spiritually minded and reflect upon the meaning of their deaths? Do they need to accomplish tasks or achieve landmarks as their lives ebb away? The more important question is, what do nurses need to know about the various theoretical models of the dying process that will help them intervene appropriately and offer the best quality of life for their dying patients?

Theoretical models of the dying process date back to 1969, and include stage-based, task-based, phase-based, landmarks-based, and spiritually-based models. When responding to patient's symptoms and monitoring coping skills, nurses can broadly think about the approaches and how they apply to each patient.

Stage-Based Approach to Coping With Dying

In her groundbreaking work, *On Death and Dying,* Elizabeth Kübler-Ross (1969) outlined the emotional stages of the dying patient. This five-stage model was created to help professionals understand the needs of the dying. Although many professionals and grieving individuals have taken the Kübler-Ross stage-based model and applied it to grieving after a loss, it was not intended to be applied to the survivor's grief.

Based on her many conversations with dying persons, Kübler-Ross delineated five stages of dying: denial, anger, bargaining, depression, and acceptance. When confronted by death, individuals will first deny it is happening. This serves as a coping mechanism. Denial acts as a buffer. Unable to take in the information, patients may seek out other physicians for second opinions or act as if they aren't aware of their prognoses. Kübler-Ross maintains that once individuals acknowledge death is inevitable, reactions change to anger. The patient may attempt to blame others or become hostile or enraged about his or her condition. The third stage is bargaining. At this point, dying persons want to postpone the inevitable and attempt to make a deal with God or others in order to prolong their lives. They may bargain to live until a goal is reached. For instance:

- A terminally ill patient promises to quit smoking if only God will let her live long enough to attend her granddaughter's wedding.

- A dying person tells her physician that she will donate her body to science if only she can have more time.

Kübler-Ross contends that, eventually, people move into the fourth stage, depression. They realize they are dying and feel sad about leaving behind all that is significant to them. They may withdraw from others and have little to say. According to Kübler-Ross, the fifth and last stage is acceptance, in which people come to terms with dying; mourn the loss of self, others, and possessions; and resign themselves to the inevitable. Hope is not abandoned, as persons may still have realistic goals, such as being pain free or having a last visit with a dear friend.

Nurses can look at the stages as a means for understanding a person's transitions as death approaches. The underlying philosophy of the stage-based model is not to manipulate and move those who are terminally ill through milestones. The stages do not occur in a fixed sequence. In fact, acceptance may never be achieved.

For many years, this popular paradigm of the dying process was recognized by nurses as a model to understand the emotional changes of the dying person. Critics of Kübler-Ross have argued that her theory focuses too much on stages that don't always occur and not enough on those things that need to be done to cope with dying. Kastenbaum (2000b) maintains there is no evidence for the establishment of stages or that people actually do move from stage 1 through stage 5. According to Bregman (2006):

> This theory may never have tested out empirically. Its status as 'scientific' was always dubious. The model of psychology used by Kübler-Ross seemed to start out psychoanalytic, but became humanistic, echoing the themes of the human potential movement which flourished during that same post-Vietnam era. (An anthology Kübler-Ross edited, entitled *Death: The Final Stage of Growth,* makes this explicit.) In an intriguing recent remark made by a chaplain at a conference, reminiscing about Kübler-Ross and her work, the speaker declared "She worked within psychology, but if she were working now, she'd be doing spirituality." The implication was not that she would have changed her approach drastically, but that the kind of psychology she used as a vehicle was actually closer to what

now is called 'spirituality,' than to the empirical psychological research tradition. (p. 21)

Task-Based Model for Living with Life-Threatening Illness

As the years passed, theorists moved from the stage-based model to the task-based model. In 1992, Corr created a model that focuses on terminally ill individuals coping with dying by completing four areas of task work. These areas include physical, psychological, social, and spiritual tasks. Physical tasks involve managing bodily needs and minimizing physical distress, such as controlling pain and constipation. Psychological tasks maximize psychological security, autonomy, and richness in living. Social tasks enhance significant attachments and address the social implications of dying. To foster hope while coping with dying, spiritual tasks address meaningfulness, connectedness, and transcendence.

Phase-Based Approach to Coping with Dying

Doka (1995-1996) describes phases of life-threatening illness that include prediagnostic, acute, chronic, terminal, and recovery phases. The tasks of coping change at the various phases of the illness. In the *prediagnostic phase,* individuals suspect an illness and seek out medical attention. The *acute phase* is initiated by the diagnosis. Individuals attempt to understand the disease, maximize health, develop coping strategies, explore the effect of the diagnosis, express feelings, and integrate the present reality into their sense of past and future. The *chronic phase* involves managing the symptoms and side effects, while carrying out health regimes, normalizing life, and maximizing social support, at the same time as expressing feelings and finding meaning in the suffering. Terminally ill individuals can inform their spouses of the location of insurance documents and important papers, make contact with everyone in their address books, renew old friendships, and express their love to others. By addressing unfinished busi-

ness, whether practical or emotional, dying individuals feel in control. In the *terminal phase,* individuals cope with dying by managing pain, symptoms, health procedures, and related stress. Dying persons prepare for death by saying goodbye and finding meaning in life and death. Some individuals experience a *recovery phase* during which their disease is cured or in remission.

Landmarks and Taskwork for Coping with Dying

Today, nurses help terminally ill patients review their lives, find meaning, complete important tasks, and accept the reality of death. This approach is based on the work of Ira Byock (1996) who identified the importance of terminally ill patients attaining certain landmarks prior to death (Table 3-1). At each landmark, individuals have taskwork to complete. These landmarks include completing one's affairs, resolving relationships, finding a sense of meaning in one's life, experiencing love of self and others, acknowledging the finality of life and a sense of a new self, and letting go.

Spirituality-Based Approach to Coping with Dying

When supporting dying patients, nurses can enhance a patient's quality of life by addressing spiritual needs. Patients with cancer in an urban hospital who reported their spiritual needs were not being met rated their quality of care lower and reported lower satisfaction with care than those who felt such needs were met (Astrow, Wexler, Texeira, He, & Sulmasy, 2007).

Wallace and O'Shea (2007) investigated perceptions of spirituality and spiritual care among older nursing home residents at the end of life. The participants reported moderately high views of aspects of spirituality and spiritual care, supporting spirituality as a framework for life. The sample reported on several nursing interventions that support the expression of spirituality:

TABLE 3-1: A WORKING SET OF DEVELOPMENTAL LANDMARKS AND TASKWORK FOR THE END OF LIFE

Landmarks	Taskwork
Sense of completion of worldly affairs	Transfer of fiscal, legal, and formal social responsibilities
Sense of completion in relationships with community	Closure of multiple social relationships (employment, commerce, organizational, congregational) Components include: expressions of regret, expressions of forgiveness, acceptance of gratitude and appreciation Leave taking; the saying of good-bye
Sense of meaning about one's individual life	Life review The telling of one's stories Transmission of knowledge and wisdom
Experienced love of self	Self-acknowledgment Self-forgiveness
Experienced love of others	Acceptance of worthiness
Sense of completion in relationships with family and friends	Reconciliation, fullness of communication, and closure in each of one's important relationships Component tasks include expressing regret, forgiveness, acceptance, gratitude, appreciation, and affection and accepting gratitude and appreciation Leave-taking; the saying of goodbye
Acceptance of the finality of life – of one's existence as an individual	Acknowledgment of the totality of personal loss represented by one's dying and experience of personal pain of existential loss Expression of the depth of personal tragedy that dying represents Decathexis (emotional withdrawal) from worldly affairs and cathexis (emotional connection) with an enduring construct Acceptance of dependency
Sense of a new self (personhood) beyond personal loss	Developing self-awareness in the present
Sense of meaning about life in general	Achieving a sense of awe Recognition of a transcendent realm Developing/achieving a sense of comfort with chaos
Surrender to the transcendent, to the unknown – "letting go"	In pursuit of this landmark, the doer and "taskwork" are one; here, little remains of the ego except the volition to surrender

Note. From "The Nature of Suffering and the Nature of Opportunity at the End of Life" by Ira Byock, May 1996. *Clinics in Geriatric Medicine,* Vol.12, No.2, pp 237-251. Reprinted with permission.

- arranging visits with religious personnel
- showing kindness
- spending time listening to residents (presence)
- showing respect for resident's needs.

Spiritual care of dying patients is within the scope of nursing practice. Tan, Braunack-Mayer, and Beilby (2005) studied the impact of the hospice environment on patient spiritual expression and found nurses are significant in assisting in patients' spiritual expression. Nurses' needs for training in listening skills, confidence in talking about spiritual issues, and time to provide individualized spiritual care should be assessed to ensure optimal patient spiritual expression (Tan et al., 2005).

COMPASSIONATE COMMUNICATION

Effective communication is an essential element in establishing rapport and maintaining any type of interpersonal relationship. Communication can be defined as the ability to understand and to be understood, and it occurs when information is transferred in a meaningful way.

Being a good listener is the most important communication skill. Good communicators appreciate the significance of listening to the whole story and understand the feelings and perceptions being expressed.

To communicate effectively, an opportunity and time should be provided for patients and their caregivers to discuss choices, share information, offer support, and share their fears. This can be accomplished by using open-ended questions such as:

• How did you decide that?

• Can you tell me more about how you came to that conclusion?

• Can you explain what you just said to me once again?

• What other alternatives have you thought about?

Improving conversations about the end of life is an important part of improving care of the dying patient and family (Larson & Tobin, 2000). However, Lowey (2008) reviewed the literature on communication between nurses and family caregivers and found that no studies focused specifically on the nature of nurse-family communication during the final days or hours of patient's lives.

The belief that death and dying is often seen as a failure of the healthcare system, rather than a natural part of life, affects nurses. Despite their undisputed technical and interpersonal skills, they may not be entirely comfortable with the knowledge and skills they need to give their patients quality end-of-life care (American Association of Colleges of Nursing [AACN], 2009). How do nurses respond when patients ask how long they have to live or whether they are dying? Loprinzi, Johnson, and Steer (2000) suggest that the use of the word *dying* is life-changing information that must be sensitively shared. Berry (2008) maintains that using the words "death" or "dying" may not be the right words for every patient, but these words could help improve discussions about death with many patients:

> The next time you must let someone know they are dying, the best way of doing this may be to say, "you are dying." It's more than just semantics. Using the word "die" will clarify conversations with patients and let them know that death doesn't need to be considered unnatural or a failure. Reintroducing words like "death" and "dying" into those conversations will allow us to take better care of our patients as they live, and as they die. (p. 159)

Nurses may feel extremely uncomfortable speaking with terminally ill patients about the upcoming death. Nurses who are uneasy may interrupt their patients as they talk about dying and may attempt to change the subject, rather than patiently listen. If a patient tells her nurse she just wants to die and the nurse responds by saying, "Oh, you really don't mean that," the response will negate the patient's feelings. If a patient says, "I think that I am going to die soon," or "I just want this over," the nurse can effectively communicate by asking, "What happened today that makes you say this?" An attempt should not be made to have the patient think about something else. Rather, the patient should be encouraged to discuss his or her thoughts and feelings.

> **Personal Insight**
> *How comfortable are you using the word "dying?"*

Reflecting the patient's content and emotion encourages the patient to share his or her feelings.

If a patient says, "No one visits me anymore," the nurse might say, "You sound as if you are feeling lonely." A response to the statement "No one is listening to me," might be, "I really hear you saying that you are frustrated." The patient's emotions can be reflected in statements such as:

- "I'm picking up that you are scared of dying."

- "It sounds as if you are most concerned with how your family is coping with your dying."

- "I gather this is hard for you."

- "I wonder if you are saying that you want to speak to the clergy."

- "If I am hearing you correctly, you are afraid of being left alone."

- "You sound as if you really do not want any aggressive treatment."

Such facilitative listening using reflections helps patients to label their emotions.

Nonverbal messages are just as important as what is said. Such messages include body language, posture, eye contact, facial expressions, and tone of voice (Carter, 2008). Because such messages are often subtle, it is important to be a good observer.

As patients communicate their needs, they take control of their dying. This begins with devising a plan of action and having an advance directive. The advance directive will enable their wishes to be known when they are no longer capable of communicating those wishes. Communicating one's needs to one's family and nurses includes discussing issues regarding dying at home or in the hospital, the use of hospice, experiences of anticipatory grief, and the generalized fear of one's own suffering.

To be compassionate communicators at the end of life, nurses must identify their own feelings about dying and recognize ways they might cope with their own deaths. Such self-awareness is essential because focusing on a patient's feelings requires comfort with such topics.

ANTICIPATORY GRIEF

The concept of anticipatory grief was first introduced by Eric Lindemann in 1944 (Tomer, Eliason, & Wong, 2007). Anticipatory grief occurs before the actual death in the anticipation of a future loss, and it can begin any time after a diagnosis. Both the dying patient and families experience anticipatory grief. When death is expected, individuals experience pre-death mourning and may complete unfinished business, prepare for the loss, and gradually grasp the certainty of the impending death (Straub & Roberts, 2001).

The current understanding of anticipatory grief stems from research dating back to 1971, when Fulton and Fulton described four components of anticipatory grief for the patient's family: depression, heightened concern for the terminally ill person, rehearsal of the death, and attempts to adjust to the consequences of the death.

The Family of the Dying Patient

Cultural beliefs, customs, and rituals bring comfort to the entire family. As the patient's condition deteriorates, the entire family is affected. Nurses can provide families with education and offer options, while respecting their beliefs and choices.

Lack of experience with dying, sleep deprivation, and physical exhaustion are factors that influence the way family members cope with their loved ones being terminally ill. Family members may feel:

- guilt about the lack of time spent with the patient.

- a need to blame someone for their loved one's sickness.

- anger at God for allowing the illness to happen.

- fear and worry that the situation will become more than they can bear.

These feelings are normal and nurses can help caregivers express such emotions in a healthy way.

Technical language should not be used when educating patients and families. Because family members might not always be up-front about what they do and do not understand, the nurse should ask about their understanding of the patient's condition and encourage them to ask questions.

McConnell Lewis (2007) offers ways nurses can paraphrase and help persons feel they are understood. Using such phrasing as "You mean…," or "Let me see if I understand you" helps the listener feel listened to (p. 74). The simple technique of echoing opens up discussion. Caregivers may say, "I feel so sad." By repeating the word in question form – "Sad?" – caregivers are encouraged to talk and can then expound on the feelings.

Kim and Choi (2000) maintain that individuals who care for their terminally ill partners may feel as though the terminally ill person is demanding and unappreciative of the caregiver's fatigue, anxiety, and loneliness. Family caregivers live with high levels of stress. Furman (2001) points out stress-taming tips that nurses can recommend to family members or caregivers:

- Stop negative thoughts about inadequacy as a caregiver by mentally repeating positive thoughts.

- Practice deep-breathing exercises before and after stressful activities.

- Express feelings by talking, crying, screaming, beating a pillow, or writing.

- Stop setting standards of perfection.

- Resist self-judgment.

- Ask for help.

- Take breaks.

- Write things down to help with memory (p. 41).

Caregivers may also cope with a loved one's terminal illness using humor. Richman (2006-2007) maintains that shared humor reduces stress and affirms life for individuals who are terminally ill and their caregivers.

DIAGNOSING DYING

The Dying Process

Patients and family members are reassured when nurses share information about what they might expect as the disease takes its natural course. Such conversations should begin early in the death trajectory. Nurses need to become knowledgeable and comfortable talking about what happens to the body during the dying process.

Months Prior to Death

Months prior to their deaths, patients may acknowledge their dying and begin to withdraw and communicate less with those around them. They may lose interest in watching TV or reading the paper, sleep more than usual, and take naps throughout the day. Physical distress and suffering is common, but often it can be prevented or relieved.

Weeks Prior to Death

Weeks prior to death, patients will often sleep for most of the day and night. Anorexia and marked weight loss are common among dying patients. Sometimes there is a physical reason for the lack of appetite, such as constipation, gastritis, nausea, or oral lesions that should be treated. However, anorexia is often an unavoidable consequence of an end-stage disease process. It is also common for patients to spontaneously ask for a meal or be alert, oriented, and ready for a conversation, when previously they were withdrawn or lethargic. This "rally" is usually short-lived.

Days Prior to Death

Days prior to death, terminally ill patients are usually bed bound. Common symptoms at the end of their lives include pain, constipation, fatigue, depression, and delirium (Lee & Washington, 2008). Frequently, terminally ill individuals experience nausea, vomiting, and confusion, which can lead to disorientation to time (von Gunten, 2005). Shortness of breath, which can include labored and noisy breathing, is common in the days prior to death. Very little or no nutritional or fluid intake, respiratory symptoms, generalized weakness, somnolence, fever, cachexia/anorexia, difficulty swallowing, dehydration, and extreme tiredness are also common symptoms (Brandt et al., 2005).

Pain should be aggressively treated throughout the dying process. It is very difficult for family members to watch their loved ones die in physical agony. Opioid therapy should be prescribed in adequate doses on a continuous basis to alleviate pain at the end of life, and adjuvant medications should be available for breakthrough pain. Although addictive behaviors are rare and easily controllable at the end of life, fears of side effects and addiction are the greatest barriers to effective pain management (Miller, 2008).

Nurses can speak with patients and their families about their beliefs about pain management and help patients and family members overcome fears about using narcotics. Any misconceptions about pain medications, especially opioids, can be addressed.

Last Words

The words and stories that dying patients speak to nurses and others give meaning and substance to the end of life. Kenyon, Clark and de Vries (2001) note, "It is important to listen to stories not as irrelevant ramblings that waste high-priced healthcare time, but as essential sources of information" (p. 48).

Brain Candy Celebrity Quotes lists several of the last words spoken by famous individuals. President Woodrow Wilson seemed prepared for death when he said, "I am ready." Edward VII, King of the United Kingdom, however, was not ready: "No, I shall not give in. I shall go on. I shall work to the end." Last words can focus on being fearless: President George Washington said, "I die hard but am not afraid to go;" and Charles Darwin

said, "I am not the least afraid to die." Acceptance can also be found as in the case of the playwright George Bernard Shaw, whose last words to his nurse were, "Sister, you're trying to keep me alive as an old curiosity, but I'm done, I'm finished, I'm going to die." Louis XIV, King of France, also focused on acceptance and being ready for death when he said at the time of his death, "Why do you weep. Did you think I was immortal?"

Words spoken at the end of life can be directed at friends and family members. Dying individuals may reflect on those they are leaving behind. President Andrew Jackson said, "Oh, do not cry – be good children and we will all meet in heaven." Ethel Barrymore, the actress, said, "Is everybody happy? I want everybody to be happy. I know I'm happy."

Whether or not patients are famous, their last words have an impact on those privileged to hear them. Last spoken words are often unique and influenced by the dying person's age, occupation, circumstances (whether the death was sudden or anticipated), religion, and culture. Family members may benefit from hearing last words. Sometimes words spoken in the last moments of a person's life will forever change a relationship.

Personal Insight
Think about what you might say before you die. What are your last words? To whom are you speaking?

CARE AT THE TIME OF DEATH

The Pronouncement

In *The Wizard of Oz,* the Coroner of Munchkin Land made a most entertaining death pronouncement:

As coroner, I must aver
I thoroughly examined her
And she's not only merely dead
She's really, most sincerely dead!

In reality, the pronouncement of death is a moving and profound time for the family members and staff. Pronouncement of death is defined as the opinion or determination that, based on a physical assessment, life has ceased. In Dyer's (2001) definition, a death pronouncement includes the actual declaration of death, the patient examination to determine death, notification of the family, and proper documentation of the death.

In most instances, physicians are responsible for death pronouncement. If the patient's physician is unable to be present within a reasonable time and the death is due to natural causes, nurses employed by agencies can pronounce death. Also, hospice nurses can pronounce the death of a hospice patient dying at home. Although nurses cannot determine the cause of death, they can record the time at which the assessment was completed, which is the official time of death. The physical examination and death are then documented in the medical record and can include the following: date, time of death, autopsy request, notification of family, attending physician, donor services, and coroner. An example of such documentation follows:

> No pulse or breathing noted at 12:00 p.m. Dr. Williams notified and at 12:15 p.m. she pronounced death and called the patient's spouse. Foster's funeral home was notified. Mortuary personnel unavailable until 6:00 p.m. Postmortem care was provided and the body was transported to the morgue after family departed. (Kuhn Timby, 2009)

Death pronouncement is the final medical act. Every hospital and facility may have their own policies regarding the death pronouncement.

First, the patient is identified (i.e., hospital ID tag) and the general appearance of the body is noted. It is ascertained whether the patient rouses to verbal or tactile stimuli. It is unnecessary to use painful stimuli such as skin twisting or rubbing knuckles into the sternum to verify that there is no response (Heidenrach & Weissman, 2000). The person verifying the death listens for the absence of apical and carotid pulses and breath sounds. The position of the pupils and the absence of pupillary light reflex are noted and recorded. Pupils should be fixed and dilated. The eyes may or may not remain open. Skin turns pale, waxen, and cool to the touch, and the muscles become relaxed. The jaw falls open, and the sphincters release stool and urine. The face stiffens prior to the hands and feet and the body is stiffest between 12 and 48 hours after the death (Holland, Jenkins, Solomon, & Whittam, 2008).

Postmortem Care

Postmortem care is usually performed by nursing staff, sometimes with the assistance of bereaved family members. Cultural and religious beliefs often dictate how the body will be handled after death. Some families want to particpate in postmortem care and all should be invited to do so. Some religious communities have designated members who wash the body after death.

Postmortem care should be done as soon as possible as rigor mortis can set in anytime from 2 to 6 hours after the death. During rigor mortis, the skeletal muscles partially contract and the joints stiffen. Rigor mortis starts with the eyelids, neck, and jaw (Encyclopedia of Death and Dying, n.d.b).

Nurses need to wash their hands before and after providing postmortem care. Hospitals and other facilities often have postmortem kits containing gauze squares, bed protector, wash basin, soap, bath towel, dressings (if necessary), washcloths, comb, envelope for jewelry, body cover, safety pins, tape, plastic bags for clothing, and disposable gloves.

Postmortem care begins by positioning the patient in a supine position, elevating the head about 30 degrees, placing a washcloth under the chin to keep the mouth closed, straightening the limbs, and gently closing the eyes. If the body has a wristband identification, it should be kept in place. IV lines, tubes, and catheters are capped or clamped rather than removed (unless facility policy requires removal). Leaving the lines intact facilitates the autopsy and embalming processes and prevents leaking of fluids and tissue swelling that might occur if pulled. Prior to washing patients, pads should be placed under the patient's buttocks as well as any areas that are draining.

Nurses should allow family members to care for the deceased. They can comb the loved one's hair, wash the hands and face, stroke the head, apply lotions to arms, wash the entire body, and/or dress the loved one in fresh pajamas or clothing before the body is sent to the morgue or funeral home.

If family members chose the nightgown, pajamas, shroud, or other type of garment, gently ask why that particular one was chosen. This is the time to talk to family members about rituals, beliefs, clothing, and objects of signifance. If no night garments are chosen, a hospital gown, sheet, or body bag can be used to cover the body. The body is left on the bed for the funeral director or is transported to the morgue. If the patient died from an infectious disease, nurses should label the body according to their hospital or facility policies. All jewelry should be removed, placed in an envelope, and documented. Sometimes the wedding ring remains on the body. After identifying information about the deceased is written on ID tags, they are placed on toes or ankles. Postmortem care includes giving the patient's clothing and jewelry to the families. If families are not present, personal belongings should be bagged and labeled and may be stored or given to the funeral director for later retrieval by the family.

CASE STUDY

*M*rs. Baker is a 64-year-old African American Christian woman with heart disease. Her husband has been caring for her at home with the help of his two daughters who visit daily. Mrs. Baker had open heart surgery 2 years ago. She was hospitalized several times before discharge to hospice care 7 months ago. During the past week,

she has been sleeping most of the day and night. Her food and beverage intake has decreased dramatically.

Sharon, Mrs. Baker's hospice nurse, received a call from Mr. Baker that his wife was not responsive. He told her that he attempted to wake her for breakfast but she appeared lethargic and did not want to eat. Upon arrival at the home, Sharon examined Mrs. Baker and informed her husband that Mrs. Baker did not appear to be in any pain and was actively dying. He became anxious and told the nurse, "Do something. Save her!" The nurse explained that she would focus on making his wife's last hours comfortable. The nurse recommended that he call their two daughters. Within the hour, they arrived and were extremely distraught.

The family declined hospice pastoral care and called their own pastor. The nurse made several recommendations to support the patient and family members. She knew that Mrs. Baker loved gospel music and suggested to her daughter that she put on a tape of one of her mother's favorite gospel CDs. The Bible was always on Mrs. Baker's bedside table. The nurse asked if anyone wanted to read to Mrs. Baker. Her husband immediately picked up the Bible and read several passages. He appeared comforted in doing so. Later, he thanked the nurse for giving him something to do to care for his dying wife. During her last hour, Mrs. Baker sweated profusely and the nurse told the husband that he could gently wipe her brow with a cool rag. The nurse assured him that this was normal and explained what might occur during the dying process. He told her that he read about what to expect in a booklet the nurse gave him a few months ago. The nurse assured the family members that the symptoms would be controlled and Mrs. Baker would die with dignity, feeling loved. Mrs. Baker died within the hour.

After Mrs. Baker was pronounced dead and the funeral home was contacted, the nurse asked Mr. Baker and his daughters if they wanted to assist *with postmortem care. He declined but the two daughters accepted. The daughters combed their mother's hair and gently rubbed lotion on her hands and feet. With the nurse's assistance, they placed a clean gown on the body and waited for the funeral director to arrive. During this time, the daughters called several family members and friends. The hospice nurse stayed with them until the body was removed from the home. She called the next day to inquire about funeral arrangements and planned to attend the services. The nurse attended the patient's wake and shared her own memories of Mrs. Baker.*

Questions

1. What type of dying trajectory did this patient experience?

2. What was the patient's death awareness?

3. How could the spiritual-based approach help the patient cope with dying?

4. In what way did providing postmortem care help the daughters cope with their mother's death?

5. Do you think it was appropriate for the nurse to attend the funeral?

Discussion

From the very start, the nurse made sure the patient and family member's needs were met. Mrs. Baker was a dignified woman who loved her family and her faith. The nurse wanted to make sure that she died in the same manner in which she lived. The nurse focused on the patient's comfort level and availability of pastoral care. The patient did not appear to be in any pain and there were no signs of dyspnea. The nurse explained to the family members what was happening during the dying process. The family members were assured that everything was being done to keep their loved one comfortable.

Beyond teaching the family about what to expect at the end of life, the nurse met the needs of family members by allowing them to take part in caring for the dying patient. It is a good idea to offer a booklet about the dying process months before the death to prepare the family for what may occur at various times throughout the dying process. It appears as though the spouse had read the material, but it would have been helpful for the nurse to review it with him and answer any related questions. The nurse should have followed up with him to see if he had any questions about what he had read in the book.

The family's experience was enhanced by giving them the opportunity to participate in postmortem care. The daughters lovingly cared for their mother before the funeral director's arrival. Because the nurse felt close to this patient, she attended the wake. Prior to attending, it is important to call and ask if outsiders can attend. Most families appreciate the presence of the hospice nurse during these rituals.

SUMMARY

This chapter began by considering what it means to die. Typically the response is a medical one. However, this chapter explored the deeper significance of dying for patients, families, and nurses who care for them. Dying is a process with various trajectories and degrees of awareness that make the experience unique for each person. Dying is not an easy experience for those going through it and those who watch it happen. While patients are dying, they and their families rely on nurses to help them through the process.

WEB RESOURCES

Americans for Better Care of the Dying
 http://www.abcd-caring.org

Compassion and Choices
 http://www.compassionandchoices.org

Finding Our Way
 http://www.findingourway.net

My Care Community
 http://www.mycarecommunity.org

EXAM QUESTIONS

CHAPTER 3
Questions 20-29

Note: Choose the one option that BEST answers each question.

20. Cognitive processing of a loss, which enables understanding and a positive transformation, is referred to as

    a. meaning or sense making.

    b. near death experience.

    c. anticipatory grief.

    d. closed awareness.

21. Experiences commonly described by persons who have been near death include

    a. fear of punishment.

    b. physical pain.

    c. seeing lights or deceased loved ones.

    d. air hunger.

22. When patients, families, and staff pretend they don't know the prognosis of a dying patient, this would be referred to in Glaser and Strauss' Awareness of Dying Model as

    a. closed awareness.

    b. mutual pretense.

    c. suspected awareness.

    b. open awareness.

23. If patients are aware of their prognoses and impending deaths, they are more likely to

    a. experience increased physical pain.

    b. give up all hope.

    c. ask for a second opinion.

    d. improve relationships and resolve unfinished business.

24. The five stages of dying in Kübler-Ross' model are

    a. denial, anger, anxiety, depression, and acceptance.

    b. denial, anger, bargaining, depression, and acceptance.

    c. denial, anger, hope, sadness, and acceptance.

    d. denial, anger, hope, depression, and anxiety.

25. According to Corr, terminally ill individuals cope with dying by completing four areas of task work that include

    a. physical, psychological, social, and spiritual tasks.

    b. physical, behavioral, social, and spiritual tasks.

    c. physical, chronic, religious, and spiritual tasks.

    d. physical, psychological, recovery, and spiritual tasks.

26. Ira Byock hypothesized that terminally ill persons need to complete

    a. a living will.

    b. specific phases of awareness.

    c. a period of depression followed by acceptance.

    d. task work related to achieving important landmarks.

27. Spiritual care of dying patients is

    a. beyond the scope of nursing practice.

    b. only provided by a chaplain or clergy person.

    c. supported by listening and showing respect.

    d. only provided to patients who belong to a religious community of faith.

28. A normal form of grief that may arise before the actual death, in anticipation of a future loss, is called

    a. normal grief.

    b. anticipatory grief.

    c. actual grief.

    d. future grief.

29. When providing postmortem care it is important to

    a. totally remove all catheters and IV lines.

    b. ask the family if they would like to assist in washing and preparing the body.

    c. request that the family leave the room as quickly as possible.

    d. lie the body flat with arms folded over it.

CHAPTER 4

PALLIATIVE AND HOSPICE CARE

CHAPTER OBJECTIVE

After completing this chapter, the reader will be able to define and describe hospice and palliative care as treatment approaches for end-of-life care.

LEARNING OBJECTIVES

After studying this chapter, the reader will be able to

1. describe palliative care and hospice care.

2. discuss eligibility requirements, services, and members of the interdisciplinary team as related to the Medicare Hospice Benefit.

3. identify settings in which hospice and palliative care is provided.

INTRODUCTION

"You matter to the last moment of life and we will do all we can, not only to help you die peacefully, but to live until you die."

– Dame Cicely Saunders

Many individuals are not aware of palliative and hospice care as treatment options for patients and families experiencing life-limiting illnesses. Too often, such care is delayed until the patient is within days of death. Why wait until the last days of life to initiate palliative care? Why not access the best quality of care as soon as possible that sup-

ports the patient as well as the family members? One does not have to be a hospice or palliative care nurse to appreciate the significance of such care and services. All nurses will be involved with seriously ill and dying patients and should therefore become educated and empowered to obtain the most effective care indicated as death approaches. This chapter describes palliative care services for patients and families dealing with life-threatening illness and hospice care for those in the last months of life.

In the United States, funding mechanisms, reimbursement issues, and regulatory requirements have delineated hospice as appropriate care for patients anticipated to be in the last months of life, whereas palliative care can be offered much earlier in the trajectory of a life-threatening illness. The average length of stay for hospice patients was 69.0 days in 2010, decreasing from 69.5 days in 2009. (National Hospice and Palliative Care Organization [NHPCO], 2010), demonstrating the fact that hospice is most often provided only at the very end of the terminal illness.

PALLIATIVE CARE

What is Palliative Care?

Palliative care helps individuals improve their quality of life by providing prevention and relief of suffering, early identification, holistic assessment and treatment of pain, and support for physical, psychosocial, spiritual, and bereavement issues (World Health Organization [WHO], 2008) (Table 4-1). Palliative care can and should be initiated early in the trajectory of a life-threatening illness.

TABLE 4-1: HOW PALLIATIVE CARE IMPROVES QUALITY OF LIFE

- Provides relief from pain and other distressing symptoms
- Affirms life and regards dying as a normal process
- Intends neither to hasten nor postpone death
- Integrates the psychological and spiritual aspects of patient care
- Offers a support system to help patients live as actively as possible until death
- Offers a support system to help the family cope during the patient's illness and in their own bereavement
- Uses a team approach to address the needs of patients and families, including bereavement counseling, if indicated
- Enhances quality of life and may also positively influence the course of illness
- Is applicable early in the course of illness, in conjunction with other therapies that are intended to prolong life, such as chemotherapy or radiation therapy, and includes those investigations needed to better understand and manage distressing clinical complications.

Note. From "Cancer: Palliative Care," by World Health Organization (WHO), 2008. Retrieved on August 28, 2008, from http://www.who.int/cancer/palliative/definition/en

Similar to hospice care, palliative care focuses on expert symptom management provided by an interdisciplinary team. The patient and the family compose the unit of care. Care is comprehensive and holistic; focuses on physical, psychosocial, and spiritual issues; and continues into the bereavement period.

In 1997, the Institute of Medicine made seven recommendations regarding the care of patients at the end of life approaching death (Table 4-2).

These recommendations challenged the nation to provide improved supportive care to the dying, effectively treat pain and other symptoms, improve preparatory education, develop the specialty of palliative care, and strengthen the knowledge base via research.

Nursing education and preparation in palliative care has historically been lacking, but recent efforts have contributed to better training in this area of practice. Dickenson (2007) found that topics most frequently addressed are advance directives, grief and bereavement, attitudes toward death and dying, communication with dying patients, and communication with family members. Since 2000, the End-of-Life Nursing Education Consortium (ELNEC), a joint project of the City of Hope and the American Association of Colleges of Nurses (AACN), has offered end-of-life training to nurse educators and nurses in practice (AACN, 2009). The Hospice and Palliative Nurses Organization exists to support nurses and advance the practice of this specialty care, and nurses can now be certified as specialists in hospice and palliative care by the National Board for Certification of Hospice and Palliative Nurses.

Education, coupled with programs to improve care, has been shown to have the best result. Ersek and Wilson (2003) found that nursing home staff education alone will not improve end-of-life care in nursing homes. It has been reported that a combination of palliative care education and quality improvement programs focusing on pain management has resulted in reduction of pain prevalence in the nursing home (Baier et al., 2004).

Palliative care research is crucial if such care is to be improved and evidence based. Gelfman and Morrison (2008) found "research funding, particularly federal funding, for palliative medicine research is inadequate to support improvements in care for the most seriously ill patients and their families" (p. 36). Although there have been recent efforts by major funders, such as the Robert Wood

TABLE 4-2: INSTITUTE OF MEDICINE RECOMMENDATIONS ON THE CARE OF PATIENTS AT THE END OF LIFE

Recommendation 1: People with advanced, potentially fatal illnesses and those close to them should be able to expect and receive reliable, skillful, and supportive care.

Recommendation 2: Physicians, nurses, social workers, and other health professionals must commit themselves to improving care for dying patients and to using existing knowledge effectively to prevent and relieve pain and other symptoms.

Recommendation 3: Because many problems in care stem from system problems, policy-makers, consumer groups, and purchasers of health care should work with healthcare practitioners, organizations, and researchers to strengthen methods for measuring the quality of life and other outcomes of care for dying patients and those close to them; develop better tools and strategies for improving the quality of care and holding health care organizations accountable for care at the end-of-life; revise mechanisms for financing care so that they encourage, rather than impede, good end-of-life care and sustain, rather than frustrate, coordinated systems of excellent care; and reform drug prescription laws, burdensome regulations, and state medical board policies and practices that impede the effective use of opioids to relieve pain and suffering.

Recommendation 4: Educators and other health professionals should initiate changes in undergraduate, graduate, and continuing education to ensure that practitioners have relevant attitudes, knowledge, and skills to care well for dying patients.

Recommendation 5: Palliative care should become, if not a medical specialty, at least a defined area of expertise, education, and research.

Recommendation 6: The nation's research establishment should define and implement priorities for strengthening the knowledge base for end-of-life care.

Recommendation 7: A continuing public discussion is essential to develop a better understanding of the modern experience of dying, the options available to patients and families, and the obligations of communities to those approaching death.

Note. From *Approaching Death, Improving care at the end of life,* by M.J. Field & C.K. Cassel (Eds.), 1997, Committee on care at the end of life, Division of Health Care Services, Institute of Medicine National Academy Press, Washington D.C. Retrieved on August 15, 2009, from http://www.nap.edu/openbook.php?record_id=5801. Reprinted with permission from the National Academies Press ©1997, National Academy of Sciences.

Johnson Foundation, the National Institutes of Health, the National Institute of Nursing Research, the American Cancer Society, and the National Palliative Care Research Center, palliative care research funding pales in relation to the amounts directed toward curative efforts.

HOSPICE CARE

> *Personal Insight*
> *How familiar are you with hospice? Based on what you know about hospice, would you recommend it to your terminally ill patients?*

What is Hospice?

The term 'hospice' dates back to medieval times and refers to a place where travelers and those who were sick found a comforting setting for rest. In

1974, Hospice, Inc., the first hospice in the United States, opened its doors; it was later renamed Connecticut Hospice. Over 30 years later, as of 2009, more than 1.55 million patients had received care from the nation's hospice providers, a number that continues to rise (NHPCO, 2010). There has been a more than 100% increase in hospice care in the last 10 years (NHPCO, 2001; NHPCO, 2008). NHPCO estimates that approximately 41.6% of all persons who died in the United States in 2009 were under the care of a hospice program (NHPCO, 2010).

Hospice care is a program of palliative and supportive care services providing physical, psychological, social, and spiritual care for dying persons and their families (Hospice Foundation of America, n.d.). Table 4-3 compares hospice and palliative care programs. The National Quality Forum Consensus Report, *A National Framework and Preferred Practices for Palliative and Hospice Care Quality,* provides guidance and sets quality standards for both palliative care and hospice programs in the United States (see Appendix).

SIMILARITIES BETWEEN HOSPICE AND PALLIATIVE CARE

Symptom Management

Alleviation of physical and psychosocial symptoms is the major focus of both palliative and hospice care. Pain management is a central concern. The seriously ill should have frequent, comprehensive pain assessments followed by aggressive nursing interventions to manage the pain. In combination with pain medication, physical and emotional suffering can be treated with biofeedback, relaxation techniques, transcutaneous electrical nerve stimulation (TENS), complementary therapies, supportive counseling, and spiritual care. Treatments for pain may also include radiation therapy, nerve blocks, and surgery. It is particularly important to inform

patients that pain can ultimately be controlled because this information can significantly relieve patients' anxieties.

Other physical symptoms that may evolve as the disease takes its natural course are ascites, anorexia, dyspnea, alterations in bowel and bladder functioning, hiccups, dry mouth, nausea and vomiting, skin breakdown, and altered breathing patterns. Hospice and palliative nurses must become experts in the management of such symptoms and the dying process.

Hospice care includes management of psychological as well as physical symptoms.

The terminally ill need nurses to be effective listeners as patients express their concerns and fears, which may include changes in body image, loss of bodily functions, unfinished business, relationship issues, loss of independence, and the need to know the truth about their illnesses and prognoses.

Interdisciplinary Care

Hospice and palliative care are provided by interdisciplinary teams working in coordination to provide patient- and family-centered care. The Hospice Medicare Benefit requires that hospices have a physician, nurse, social worker, spiritual care provider or counselor, and nursing assistant available, as well as team members from other disciplines, such as physical, respiratory, and speech therapy as needed for the patient's individualized plan of care. Palliative care teams usually have a similar composition. Depending on the setting in which the care is provided, care teams most often operate within inpatient or clinic settings. Team members work together to assess and plan for the patient's and family's care.

The Patient and the Family as the Unit of Care

Hospice and palliative care include the family as well as the patient in communications and care planning. Family members are often taught to pro-

Characteristic	Hospice	Palliative Care
TABLE 4-3: COMPARISON OF HOSPICE AND PALLIATIVE CARE (1 OF 2)		
Definition	Service delivery system with an interdisciplinary approach to caring for terminally ill individuals. Provides supportive care rather than traditional medical care and curative treatment. Hospice care allows the patient to remain at home as long as possible by providing support to the patient and family, and by keeping the patient as comfortable as possible while maintaining his or her dignity and quality of life.	Active total treatment of patients dealing with a life-threatening illness. Improves quality of life of individuals and their families facing problems associated with life-threatening illness. Focuses on the prevention and relief of suffering by means of early identification, assessment and treatment of pain, and physical, intellectual, emotional, social, and spiritual concerns.
Time frame	Hospice care is a very specific type of care provided within a defined time frame at the end of life.	Palliative care can be provided at any time of life when there is a need to anticipate, prevent, and treat suffering to optimize a patient's quality of life.
Similarities	Offers relief from pain and other symptoms. Affirms life and regards dying as normal. Intends neither to hasten nor postpone death. Integrates psychological and spiritual aspects.	Offers relief from pain and other symptoms. Affirms life and regards dying as normal. Intends neither to hasten nor postpone death. Integrates psychological and spiritual aspects.
Differences	Focused on terminally ill patients who no longer seek curative treatments.	Appropriate at any point in an illness and provided at the same time as treatment that is meant to cure the patient.
Evolution of Program	Program began in Great Britain.	Program began in Great Britain.
Eligibility	Individual with an illness having a prognosis (life expectancy) < 6 months is eligible.	Individual who has a physician's order and diagnosis of a serious illness is eligible, regardless of life expectancy. Determined by program.
Age requirement	All patients from time of diagnosis with a life-threatening or debilitating condition, *regardless* of age are eligible.	All patients from time of diagnosis with a life-threatening or debilitating condition, *regardless* of age, are eligible.
Professional Services	Interdisciplinary team approach: physician, nurse, social worker, pastoral counselor, certified nursing assistant, others as needed.	Interdisciplinary or multidisciplinary team approach: physician, nurse, social worker, others as needed.
Medications, Supplies, Equipment, and Treatment	Medications and treatment are aimed at relieving symptoms; durable medical equipment may be needed.	No required services; palliative care and curative care are provided at the same time as determined by the program.

continued on next page

TABLE 4-3: COMPARISON OF HOSPICE AND PALLIATIVE CARE (2 OF 2)

Characteristic	Hospice	Palliative Care
Location of Services	Comprehensive: Home care, long-term care facility (LTCF), inpatient care as needed.	Location based on program: some comprehensive, some inpatient only, some LTCF based. Some programs require networking between hospital and hospice, nursing facilities, healthcare clinics, or home-based home health programs.
Funding	Medicare Hospice Benefit. State Medicaid programs. Health maintenance organizations (HMOs). Commercial insurers. Charity (not-for-profit hospices).	Traditional hospital coverage. Traditional home care coverage. Private insurance or private pay. Support from hospitals and hospice partner organizations, grants, charity. Community support for individuals with limited resources.
Duration of Services	Service continues as long as individual meets hospice criteria of an illness with life expectancy of months, not years.	Duration depends upon individual's care needs and coverage individual has through Medicare, Medicaid, or private insurance.
Complementary Therapies	Massage therapy, aroma therapy, pet therapy, hair and makeup therapy, and music therapy may be provided.	Massage therapy, aroma therapy, pet therapy, hair and makeup therapy, and music therapy may be provided.

(Kinzbrunner, 2002; National Consensus Project for Quality Palliative Care, 2009; World Health Organiztion [WHO] 2007 and 2008)

vide care to the patient and are educated about the disease process and what to expect as the disease progresses. Family meetings are often held to ensure that the patient and family are knowledgeable about the patient's condition and aware of the treatment plan. Usually the patient is central to decision making, but in some cultures, other members of the family may be designated to make decisions about the patient's care.

Bereavement Care

Hospice and palliative care offer support to bereaved family members as they anticipate the patient's death and in its aftermath. Hospice programs providing care to Medicare beneficiaries must offer bereavement care for 12 months after the death, whereas palliative care teams may have shorter periods of follow up and refer those needing more bereavement care to other community resources.

Complementary Therapies

Many hospice and palliative care programs incorporate complementary therapies into their programs, and the popularity and acceptance of such modalities is increasing (Demmer, 2003). Examples of complementary therapies are:

- yoga
- Reiki
- hypnotherapy
- pet therapy
- hair and makeup therapy
- relaxation therapy including guided imagery
- healing touch
- massage
- biofeedback
- TENS
- aromatherapy

- reflexology

- acupuncture.

Complementary therapies such as acupuncture, mind-body techniques, and massage have been shown to relieve symptoms and improve the physical and mental well-being of patients (Deng & Cassileth, 2005). Patients often benefit from incorporating massage therapy and the use of touch into their total symptom management plan. Nurses can educate family members as to the importance of touch, as they may be hesitant to touch their loved ones, afraid of causing them additional pain. Music therapy has been found to reduce anxiety in seriously ill patients (Horne-Thompson & Grocke, 2008).

Reimbursement

Table 4-4 shows the sources of payment for hospice care, such as private insurance, own income or family support, Medicare, or Medicaid. The Hospice Medicare Benefit reimburses the hospice providing care on a per diem basis and the hospice must manage this payment to cover all required services. According to an independent 2007 Duke University study, hospice saves Medicare an average of $2,300 per patient, for a total savings of approximately $2 billion per year (NHPCO, 2009).

Hospice Services as Defined by the Hospice Medicare Benefit

The Hospice Medicare Benefit specifies the services to be provided to Medicare beneficiaries who choose to receive hospice care. The following section describes the requirements of the benefit.

Patient Eligibility

Hospice care is available to Medicare beneficiaries if:

- the patient is eligible for Medicare Hospital Insurance (Part A).

- the patient's doctor and the hospice medical director certify that the patient is terminally ill.

TABLE 4-4: PRIMARY SOURCES OF PAYMENT FOR HOSPICE

- Private insurance, own income, or family support – includes private health insurance (health maintenance organization (HMO), independent practice association, or preferred provider organization), family income, Social Security (including Supplemental Security Income), retirement funds, or welfare. It does not include Veterans Administration (VA) contracts, pensions, or other VA compensation.

- Medicare – money received under the Medicare program for home health or hospice care, obtained through fee-for-service Medicare or Medicare HMO. Medicare is a health insurance program for people 65 years of age and older, some disabled people younger than 65 years of age, and people with end-stage renal disease (permanent kidney failure treated with dialysis or a transplant).

- Medicaid – money received under the Medicaid program for home health or hospice care, obtained through fee-for-service Medicaid or Medicaid HMO. Medicaid provides medical assistance for certain individuals and families with low incomes and resources. Medicaid eligibility is limited to individuals who fall into specific categories. Although the federal government establishes general guidelines for the program, Medicaid requirements are established by each state. Whether a person is eligible for Medicaid will depend on the state of residence.

- All other sources – includes religious organizations, foundations, Veterans Administration contracts, pensions or other VA compensation, and other military medicine. The category also includes no charges for care, payment sources not yet determined, and unknown sources.

Note. From "National Home and Hospice Care Data, Hospice Care Definitions of Terms," by Centers for Disease Control and Prevention, National Center for Health Statistics (NCHS), August 2007. Retrieved on December 14, 2008, from http://www.cdc.gov/nchs/about/major/nhhcsd/nhhcsdefhospicecare.htm

- the patient signs a statement choosing hospice care instead of standard Medicare benefits for the terminal illness (Department of Health and Human Services [HHS], 2008).

The Medicare hospice benefit limits eligibility to those who have a medical prognosis with a life expectancy of 6 months or less if the illness runs its normal course (Carlson, Morrison, & Bradley, 2008). The prognosis is based on the clinical judgment of the patient's attending physician and the hospice medical director or hospice physician.

Although patients with cancer made up most of hospice admissions in the past, this has changed in recent years. Less than 25% of hospice deaths in the United States are now caused by cancer, with the majority of deaths due to chronic conditions (Minino, Heron, Murphy, & Kochanek, 2007). Hospice-appropriate diagnoses besides cancer include:

- amyotrophic lateral sclerosis
- motor neuron diseases
- dementia including Alzheimer's/dementia
- cardiac disease
- debility
- endstage HIV/AIDS disease
- endstage liver disease
- endstage renal disease
- lung disease such as chronic obstructive lung disease
- stroke or coma

The National Hospice and Palliative Care Organization reports that despite the growth in the number of hospice agencies and beneficiaries of hospice, the Medicare hospice benefit remains one of Medicare's smallest programs and is used by only one third of Medicare beneficiaries prior to death (NHPCO, 2009).

Interdisciplinary Team

The Hospice Medicare Benefit stipulates that members of the hospice team will include members of specific disciplines with roles defined as follows:

The *medical director* oversees patients' medical care and is instrumental in helping the entire team plan each patient's care plan. The medical director can be a hospice employee or may contract with the hospice. This physician supervises any other hospice physicians and consults with the patient's primary care physician regarding pain and control of symptoms. Another medical director responsibility is to review clinical information and determine hospice eligibility and recertification.

Registered nurses coordinate patients' care and assess and manage symptoms. They provide patient and family education, collaborate with the physician and other team members, initiate and administer treatments, provide physical care, and offer emotional support.

Social workers seek out community resources, evaluate and support caregiving resources, assist patients and families with any legal or insurance concerns, and offer supportive counseling. The significance of social workers on hospice teams was noted in a study by Reese and Raymer (2004). The study found higher patient and family member satisfaction and fewer nights of hospice inpatient care when there was frequent social work intervention on hospice teams. Social workers are effective communicators who are prepared to intervene in family dynamics, and advocate for clients' self-determination (Reese & Raymer, 2004).

Chaplains or *pastoral counselors* offer spiritual support to patients and family members. Studies indicate that spirituality receives slightly less emphasis than the biopsychosocial dimensions of care in the current healthcare system, even though the majority of patients want to discuss spiritual issues (Puchalski, 2007-2008). Although patients' spiritual needs may not be met in our current healthcare system, they are clearly met in hospice, where the spiritual dimension of care is directed by the patient's belief system. Patients and families may choose to garner support from the hospice chaplain or clergy of their own community of faith.

Chaplains are also available to the staff as a resource to address their spiritual concerns. Daaleman, Usher, Williams, Rawlings, and Hanson (2008) found three aspects of spiritual care in palliative care:

1. *Being present:* Physical proximity and intentionality expressed a purposeful action to provide care that went beyond medical treatment.

2. *Opening eyes:* Caregivers became aware of their patient's life course and the individualized experience of their patient's current illness.

3. *Co-creating:* A mutual, fluid activity between patients and those who care for them affirmed their life experiences and led to a holistic care plan that focused on humanity and dignity.

Some hospices assign spiritual care to *bereavement counselors* rather than pastoral counselors, whereas other hospices are able to employ both pastoral counselors and bereavement counselors. Bereavement counselors facilitate support groups, train bereavement volunteers, and design and distribute bereavement material to families. Bereavement support begins before the death to help the patients and family members with anticipatory grief. After patients die, bereavement support is made available to family members for one year. Support can include telephone calls, cards sent on significant days (birthdays, anniversaries), newsletters, bereavement support groups, educational groups, individual counseling, and home visits.

Integral members of the team are *hospice nursing assistants* or *aides.* Aides work under the direction of the hospice nurses to provide personal care and light housekeeping for the patient and family. Hospice aides must have completed a state approved hospice or nurse's aide training and

competency evaluation and receive 12 hours of inservice education yearly. The National Board for Certification of Hospice and Palliative Nurses offers certification to aides with hospice experience who pass a test verifying their competency.

Volunteer coordinators administer and develop the volunteer programs for each hospice. The coordinators recruit, train, and assign volunteers to hospice patients. Lectures, group discussions, and reading materials prepare volunteers for their important role in providing inpatient or home care as well as bereavement support. Family caregivers may receive peer comfort from volunteers, essential members of the hospice team who provide a multitude of services, including transportation, companionship, and respite care.

Services 35

Medicare requires that the following services are provided by Medicare-approved hospice programs:

- durable medical equipment (e.g., wheelchairs or walkers)

- medical supplies (e.g., bandages and catheters)

- laboratory and diagnostic studies

- medications for symptom control or pain relief

- services of the interdisciplinary team

- on-call availability 24 hours a day

- short-term inpatient care

- short-term respite care in a Medicare-approved facility, such as a hospice inpatient facility, hospital, or nursing home.

According to Brazil et al. (2005), family caregivers report the five most valuable hospice services are:

1. in-home nursing care

2. continued care and supervision by their family physician

3. involvement of medical specialists trained in providing end-of-life care

4. housekeeping and personal care assistance

5. religious/spiritual support.

The Initial Assessment

At the time of admission, the patient and family members meet with a hospice nurse for an initial assessment. "The hospice registered nurse must complete an initial assessment within 48 hours after the election of hospice care" (HHS, 2008, p. 32102). After introducing patients and families to the hospice philosophy, the nurse conducts a careful assessment, beginning with the presenting problem and moving through the individual's history. During this time, the most prevalent issues facing the patient and family members are identified and direct the development of the initial plan of care. Often, a second member of the interdisciplinary (e.g., social worker or chaplain) will also be involved in the initial assessment.

The initial care plan is then developed and will guide the care provided during the first days of hospice care. This plan will be updated based on the more comprehensive assessments of the full interdisciplinary team.

Comprehensive Assessments

Hospice team members complete a comprehensive assessment no later than 5 calendar days after the election of hospice. A comprehensive assessments recognizes the patient's need for hospice services; the need for physical, psychosocial, emotional, and spiritual care; palliation; and terminal illness management (HHS, 2008). The content of the comprehensive assessment includes identification of the physical, psychosocial, emotional, and spiritual needs related to the terminal illness that will be addressed in promoting the patient's well-being, comfort, and dignity throughout the dying process.

Areas covered by the comprehensive assessment include: medical history; current medications and treatments; pain and other distressing symptoms; cognitive and functional status; nutritional status; social and caregiving support; legal preparation, including wills, advance directives, and funeral planning; identification of significant family members and friends; spiritual assessment; communication styles; need for supportive equipment and supplies; financial situation; and anticipated bereavement needs.

Issues faced by terminally ill patients include losing independence, maintaining self-determination and a sense of control, decision making related to how and where to die, declining functions and related concerns of being a burden, and fearing pain and other distressing symptoms. Such issues are identified during the comprehensive assessment that will subsequently guide the plan of care.

After the assessments, the hospice team creates an interdisciplinary plan of care. The plan of care identifies the patient- and family-specific needs, related goals, and an appropriate plan. It should be updated as frequently as necessary based on the patient's changing status and needs but no less frequently than every 15 calendar days (HHS, 2008, p. 32096).

Bereavement Plan of Care

A bereavement assessment is included in the comprehensive plan of care. Bereavement assessments will change and be updated according to the specific needs of patients and families, but it is important to do this assessment early so that the family and patient can be assisted with anticipatory grief. Bereavement counseling offers emotional, psychosocial, and spiritual support and services to patients and families while patients are still alive and after their death (HHS, 2008). Counseling helps bereaved families cope with grief, loss, and adjustment. Approximately two family members per hospice death receive bereavement support (e.g., phone calls, visits, mailings, cards) through the post-death year (NHPCO, 2009).

In smaller hospices, 20% of the nurses play a role in providing bereavement support, and 1% of the nurses provide bereavement support in large hospices (Foliart, Clausen, & Siljestrom, 2001). Spiritual counselors or bereavement counselors play a bigger role in larger hospices. However, every member of the hospice team can provide some type of bereavement support.

Foliart et al. (2001) found that 98% of all hospices offered telephone support, 96% had scheduled mailings, 95% gave brochures about grief, 90% had pastoral visits, and 82% had volunteer visits. The results of this study underscore the value of providing support to the bereaved. Grieving individuals feel supported when professionals call them to see how they are coping. Families appreciate receiving mailings that invite them to support groups or memorial services, as it gives them an opportunity to share their pain of loss with others.

SETTINGS FOR PALLIATIVE AND HOSPICE CARE

Hospice Home Care

Muramatsu, Hoyem, Yin, and Campbell (2008) noted that although most Americans prefer to die at home, the majority of individuals who are terminally ill die in institutions. It is not easy for family members to take care of their dying loved ones without outside support. Home-based hospice services enable patients to remain at home by providing supportive care and equipment, teaching family members and friends to provide care at home, and offering on-call services around the clock. The patient may receive acute care in a hospital or inpatient hospice setting for symptom management, respite, or situations that the family cannot effectively handle in the home. In the United States, hospice care is most often provided in the home setting, but some hospices do operate residential facilities for those without families or adequate support to stay in their own residences.

Palliative Care and Hospice in Long-Term Care and Similar Facilities

Many of those who are chronically ill or dying reside in nursing homes and depend on the facility staff to relieve their suffering. Teno, Bird, and Mor (2002) note that 67% of older persons die in either hospitals or nursing homes and by the year 2020, 40% of older individuals who die of nontraumatic causes will live in nursing homes at the time of their deaths. Long-term care institutions are home to the frailest, oldest patients and it's those individuals who may not want aggressive medical interventions (Gillick, 2004). These older residents of nursing homes usually have multiple medical problems and are more likely than any other subgroup of the population to develop acute, potentially fatal illnesses.

Hospice care can be provided in nursing homes, extended care, and assisted-living facilities. Such facilities can contract with a hospice program, and the hospice team will work with residents providing the same services available to patients living in their own homes. The Hospice Medicare Benefit covers hospice services provided in such facilities. The hospice team works with the facility staff to implement a hospice plan of care for those residents who consent to hospice.

To achieve partnership success between nursing homes and hospices, Miller (2007) reported three key collaborative solutions:

1. Systematic processes facilitate communication between nursing homes and hospice staff and between all levels of staff.

2. Hospice chief executive officers are well-versed in nursing home regulations and care environments, are skilled leaders, and convey a consistent vision for hospice nursing home care.

3. Nursing homes share their care expectations with their hospice partners (within regulatory guidelines and as practical) and provide feedback to hospices (p. 3).

Table 4-5 outlines collaborative solutions that can enable hospices and nursing homes to join together in providing quality hospice care to residents (Miller, 2007).

Hospital-Based Palliative Care Programs

Palliative care programs provide intense symptom management and support for the seriously ill in many hospitals. Patients who have advanced life-limiting illnesses or chronic, incurable, debilitating illnesses are treated by an interdisciplinary team in hospital-based palliative care programs. Although early palliative care programs were initiated by oncology services for cancer patients, currently these services are for patients with any diagnosis in a hospital or hospice setting (Santa-Emma, Roach, Gill, Spayde, & Taylor, 2002; Smith, 2003).

According to the Center to Advance Palliative Care (CAPC) analysis of the latest data released from the 2008 American Hospital Association (AHA) Annual Survey of Hospitals, 1,299 hospitals (31%) of the 4,136 hospitals appropriate for palliative care nationwide have such programs compared to 632 programs in 2000 (Center to Advance Palliative Care [CAPC], 2008). Forty-seven percent of hospitals with over 50 beds have a program and 77% with over 250 beds (large hospitals) have a program (Morgan, 2008). As stated by Diane Meier, director of CAPC:

> Palliative care represents a paradigm shift in how we treat serious illness in America. Ten years ago there were almost no hospital palliative care programs in the U.S. But if we're going to meet the needs of an aging population, it's going to be necessary for every hospital to have a program. (CAPC, 2008)

In a study of early palliative care alongside trauma care in intensive care units, it was reported that 10% to 20% of trauma patients admitted to the ICU will die of their injuries (Mosenthal et al., 2008). The findings indicate that early family

bereavement support, discussions regarding patient preferences, interdisciplinary family meetings, care discussions regarding do-not-resuscitate (DNR) orders and withdrawal of life support should occur as soon as possible to ensure the best quality of care for the seriously ill patient receiving critical care (Mosenthal et al., 2008).

Hospital/Hospice Partnerships in Hospital-Based Palliative Care

Older individuals may have health problems that cause frequent trips to the hospital. Many individuals fear trips to the hospital, believing that is the place where they will die. Although they may recover from each of the numerous trips, their capacity diminishes when they do not have enough reserve or resiliency to bounce back from illness. They may ultimately welcome death, which becomes an avenue to see long-lost loved ones, go to heaven, or be free from suffering (Amella, 2003). Hospice care provided in a hospital setting can alleviate suffering as patients approach death. Although ultimately patients are the ones who get the most benefit from the programs, hospitals and hospices also can benefit from such partnerships.

Hospitals benefit from such partnerships in the following ways:

- The hospice interdisciplinary team provides the hospital with daily palliative care expertise.

- The hospice team assists the hospital in providing patients with pain and symptom management and counseling.

- The hospice medical director can serve as the hospital's palliative medicine consultant, extending pain management to hospital patients not on hospice.

- Hospice staff can provide end-of-life education to patients, families, and staff.

- An inpatient unit's presence within the facility demonstrates to the community the hospital's

TABLE 4-5: NOTABLE COLLABORATIVE SOLUTIONS FOR HOSPICE/NURSING HOME PARTNERSHIPS

Resources/Inputs

- Nursing homes and hospices share similar philosophies of care; and
- Nursing homes openly acknowledge the occurrence of death in nursing homes and have practices in place to provide special care and/or services to dying residents/families.

Activities – Infrastructure

- Partnership and staff relationships (at all levels) result from planned systems and activities – they are not dependent on individual, time, and not left "to chance;"
- Hospices cultivate collaborative relationships with nursing homes' managed care providers to promote the providers' recognition and use of the value-added care/support provided by hospices;
- Mechanisms are in place to facilitate regular assessment of the partnership;
- Education addresses relationship building and conflict resolution, the unique aspects of care provided by nursing home and hospice staff, and nursing home and hospice regulatory and care environments;
- Dedicated hospice teams provide care focusing exclusively on nursing home residents (as feasible per hospice size); and
- Hospice presence is high in nursing homes.

Activities – Processes

- Regular meetings and/or dialogue occur between nursing home and hospice chief executive officers;
- Hospices respond promptly to nursing home requests;
- Hospice visits are purposefully structured – hospice staff check in with like discipline upon arrival and departure and ask for input;
- Dialogue on care planning and provision is frequent;
- Nursing home Medicaid per diem payment is prompt (even when state Medicaid payment is slow) and 100% of per diem is paid by hospices; and
- Hospices provide support to nursing homes during Medicare/Medicaid surveys as well as with bureaucracy such as Medicaid applications/follow-up for hospice residents.

Note. From *Nursing Home/Hospice Partnerships: A Model for Collaborative Success – Through Collaborative Solutions,* by S.C. Miller, Brown Medical School Center for Gerontology and Health Care Research, 2007, a report funded by the Robert Wood Johnson Foundation Grant #49891,p. 4. Retrieved August 23, 2010, http://www.nhpco.org/files/public/nhhp-final-report.pdf. Copyright 2007. Reprinted with permission from the Robert Wood Johnson Foundation.

commitment to provide end-of-life care (Kuebler, Davis, & Moore, 2005).

Hospices benefit from partnerships with hospitals in the following ways:

- Hospice identity in the community linked to the inpatient facility increases the hospice's credibility.
- Medical and hospital staff education on the benefits of hospice services results in earlier referral and increased patient utilization of hospice.

- Hospices receive exposure to a broader continuum of palliative care needs, which patients who are not yet ready for hospice services may require in the future.

(Kuebler et al., 2005).

Palliative and Hospice Care Programs for Children Living with Life-Threatening Conditions

Palliative and hospice care are appropriate for children and their families. Palliative care for children is:

...the active total care of the child's body, mind and spirit, and involves giving support to the family which begins when illness is diagnosed, and continues regardless of whether or not a child receives treatment directed at the disease. Health providers must evaluate and alleviate a child's physical, psychological, and social distress. Effective palliative care requires a broad multidisciplinary approach that includes the family and makes use of available community resources; it can be successfully implemented even if resources are limited. It can be provided in tertiary care facilities, in community health centers and even in children's homes. (WHO, 1998)

Treating children living with life-threatening conditions is particularly difficult for nurses, as very few are highly experienced in caring for dying children. Palliative care programs across the United States must be created to address the needs of terminally ill children and their families as well as provide education to meet the needs of professionals who will work with this population. A group of experts in palliative care created a document, "A Call for Change: Recommendations for Improving the Care of Children Living with Life-Threatening Conditions." This document highlights challenges of pediatric palliative care. (See Table 4-6.)

Children need qualified professionals to help them live with their life-threatening conditions. Families depend upon nurses to ease children's suffering and apply their wisdom and intelligence. Although parents often ask nurses what to say to their terminally ill children, children can be effective communicators and are often more knowledgeable about their illnesses than one might think. Caring Connections, a Program of the National Hospice and Palliative Care Association, recommends that parents trust their instincts, discuss things in smaller bits, and be patient. Table 4-7 provides a list of communication tips to share with parents of terminally ill children.

CASE STUDY

*M*rs. Young is an alert and oriented 88-year-old Caucasian diagnosed with congestive heart failure with an ejection fraction of 20. Ten years have passed since the death of her beloved husband, and both of her children are deceased. Most of her friends are deceased or living in nursing homes. Her best friend has Alzheimer's disease. Mrs. Young lives in her own home and is cared for by a live-in assistant, Marina. Mrs. Young has been Dr. Smithson's patient for the past 4 years.

With Marina by her side, Dr. Smithson informs Mrs. Young that her heart failure is not curable and her life expectancy is limited. With a compassionate tone and in a language the patient understands, the doctor explains that she probably has less than 6 months to live. Dr. Smithson tells her about hospice care and she agrees to an introductory meeting, which is arranged for the next day.

The next day, Mrs. Young and Marina meet with the hospice nurse, Ann Marie, and social worker, Tim. They spend the next 2 hours discussing the philosophy of hospice care and services that can be provided through the Hospice Medicare Benefit. Ann Marie explains the guidelines for determination of appropriateness for hospice services. After Ann Marie does a patient assessment, she explains how hospice can provide care in Mrs. Young's home. Marina explains that she is fearful that hospice wants to take her job away. The hospice social worker makes it clear that Marina will still be the primary caregiver and the hospice team will support her as she cares for Mrs. Young.

Mrs. Young appears anxious and asks what the nurse will do to her during visits. Ann Marie attempts to alleviate any fears and explains that during each visit she will perform a physical assessment, discuss any problems, and update the plan of care according to the patient's wishes. In very simple language, the nurse explains what the physical assessment will entail. She discusses the

TABLE 4-6: WHAT MAKES PEDIATRIC PALLIATIVE CARE CHALLENGING?

1. Our society does not expect children to die.

2. Families often believe medicine can currently or imminently cure all ills.

3. There is a huge disparity in Western countries in resource allocation, favoring "cure-oriented" acute care interventions over palliative care.

4. Death is inherently a social/community event, not a medical event.

5. At the present time, it is placed in the hands of a medical community ill-prepared to meet these unique needs, particularly for children who frequently die in the hospital.

6. Determining prognosis and estimating time of death for children with neurological compromise, rare diagnoses, and other common causes of pediatric death is an inherently uncertain process, representing a barrier to palliative care if estimated survival time is a criterion for eligibility to receive palliative or hospice services.

7. There is a misperception among healthcare professionals, legislators, administrators, and the general public that palliative care is only of use when all curative efforts have been exhausted and is mutually exclusive with life-prolonging care.

8. Variation in the cognitive, emotional, and social development of the child affects communication and decisional capacities. Determining the best interests of a child with unknown current and future values is difficult for families and professionals.

9. Very few individual practitioners are highly experienced in guiding decision making with or caring for dying children and their families.

10. Poor communication, guilt, and societal expectations often force children to endure therapies that adults, given the choice, reject for themselves. Families willing to forgo life-prolonging therapy are at risk of being accused of not caring about their children.

11. Obligations to the child patient and family may be conflicting and difficult for healthcare professionals to resolve.

12. Current regulations may interfere with family/patient centered decision making.

Note. From "A Call for Change: Recommendations to Improve the Care of Children Living With Life-Threatening Conditions," by M. Levetown et al., 2001, Alexandria, VA: The Children's International Project on Palliative/Hospice Services (ChIPPS) Administrative/Policy Workgroup of the National Hospice And Palliative Care Organization, pp. 9-10. Retrieved on August 23, 2010, from http://www.nhpco.org/files/public/ChIPPSCallforChange.pdf. Reprinted with permission.

questions she will ask about expected symptoms such as pain, changes in appetite, and bowel and bladder function. Ann Marie offers a detailed explanation about respiratory issues that will be addressed as well as alterations in skin integrity, urinary elimination, and cardiac/circulatory function. The nurse explains everything in non-medical language and continually asks Mrs. Young and Marina if they understand or have questions. Ann Marie discusses the hospice nurse's role in managing medications and consulting with the patient's physician. She describes a symptom management comfort pack that will be kept in the home with medications for pain or other distressing symptoms

that may arise. Ann Marie explains that she will visit weekly to oversee Mrs. Young's care but Marina will remain her primary caregiver. If Marina wants help, hospice can provide an aide several times a week to assist with Mrs. Young's care. Marina thinks that is a great idea as it would give her a much-needed break.

Tim recommends certain safety measures, including the removal of area rugs to prevent falls, adequate lighting, adequate phone access, and oxygen precautions. Tim tells Mrs. Young and Marina that if either of them has any problems coping he, along with the bereavement and spiritual counselors, can provide support. Tim explains

TABLE 4-7: TIPS FOR TALKING WITH YOUR CHILD ABOUT HIS OR HER ILLNESS

- Let your child know you will always love him or her no matter what he or she might say or think. Repeat this often.

- If you don't feel completely comfortable talking about goals and hopes, take a few moments to think about how you have talked about other difficult issues with your child and draw upon that experience. Try to use those same ways to engage your child so he or she will feel safe.

- Rather than trying to cover everything all at once, try discussing things in smaller bits, giving your child time to take in the information.

- Trust your instincts to help you determine how much to say and when. The right moments will appear and, when they do, you can talk with your child lovingly and confidently.

- If your timing is off, just be patient. Your child will let you in when he or she is both able to talk and needs to do so.

- Young children naturally focus on more concrete information. Make sure your child understands the plan for today and what's going to happen in the next few hours or next couple of days.

- Older kids often try to go it alone. They may find it easier to talk to peers with similar medical conditions. Talk to your child's medical team about appropriate chat rooms and making contact with other children with similar experiences.

- Reassure your child that you will do whatever you can to prevent pain and help him or her cope with any changes.

- Ask to meet with a child life specialist (at the hospital or clinic) who can help your child talk about feelings and fears through conversation and/or play therapy.

- Be kind to yourself and to other family members who may be involved. This is a challenging time for all of you and each of you will have your "difficult moments" along the way.

- Keep communication open during healthcare visits. How much and when to share information regarding your child's condition is an important topic.

- Ask your doctor and the team caring for your child for guidance as they begin to know and understand your child.

- Discuss ways to help your child feel in control at a time when so much seems beyond control.

- Use comforting language and a tone of voice that expresses confidence and warmth.

- Be sure your child understands everything that is discussed during doctors' appointments or treatments.

- Don't be afraid to give the healthcare team feedback if they are not getting through or are confusing or frightening your child. "Medical talk" confuses most adults, let alone children who may be scared by their doctor and other healthcare workers.

- Help your child prepare a list of questions for the healthcare team before visits and practice going through the questions to help your child become confident about speaking up when something is not understood.

- Remember, you know and understand your child better than anyone else.

Note. From "Talking With Your Child About His or Her Illness," by Caring Connections, a Program of the National Hospice and Palliative Care Organization, 2007. Retrieved on August 23, 2010 from, http://caringinfo.org/CaringForSomeone/pediatrics/TalkingWithYourChildAboutHisOrHerIllness.htm. Reprinted with permission.

to Mrs. Young that he will order a hospital bed, oxygen, and a wheelchair. Mrs. Young asks for a walker instead. Tim informs her that he could get her both a wheelchair and a walker, and she is very pleased. When Tim asks about advance directives, Mrs. Young gives him a copy of her living will and states that her neighbor and close friend is her healthcare surrogate and understands her wishes.

Mrs. Young expresses concerns about the role of her family physician. She says that she trusts him and, although she wants to go on hospice, she does not want to lose the doctor she has seen for the past 4 years. Tim assures her that Dr. Smithson can remain her primary care physician, and Ann Marie explains that she will make frequent reports to the physician and he will continue to provide medical orders.

At the end of the meeting, Tim mentions setting up a meeting with the bereavement coordinator for next week. Ann Marie gives Marina a magnet with the hospice telephone numbers and she places it on the refrigerator for easy access. They ask if Mrs. Young or Marina have any further questions. Before leaving, they each schedule follow-up home visits.

Questions

1. Is hospice the best choice for Mrs. Young?

2. Do you think the nurse and the social worker did an adequate job of explaining hospice services? Why or why not?

3. Were Mrs. Young's major concerns adequately addressed during this visit?

Discussion

Dr. Smithson informed Mrs. Young that she was dying. It did not appear as though he felt uncomfortable informing her of her terminal illness, nor did he neglect to mention hospice. Hospice can only be offered to patients when the attending physician determines that the patient has a time-limited prognosis and curative care is no longer appropriate. During the initial meeting, the

hospice nurse and social worker spent 2 hours discussing hospice care with the patient and her caregiver. It was paramount that the caregiver understood that hospice is not going to take over care of the patient. Although an aide can come in several hours a week and a nurse will oversee the patient's care, the primary responsibility remains with the live-in caretaker.

When Mrs. Young appeared worried, Ann Marie took the time to clearly alleviate any fears and explain in detail what would be done each week. This dialogue encouraged the patient's trust in the hospice team.

Although Tim recommended certain safety measures, he neglected to discuss her many losses. It did not sound as though either the nurse or social worker addressed the patient's emotional concerns. Her husband and both children have died, she has lost many friends, and her best friend has Alzheimer's disease. Clearly, she may have bereavement issues as a result of past losses. Being that Marina cares deeply for Mrs. Young, her anticipatory grief needs should be examined as well. Although it is not the social worker's job to address bereavement issues, he could have taken the time to see how much of a concern these losses were to the patient and if they are compounding any other losses she may be experiencing due to her terminal illness. Although he did recommend an initial visit with the bereavement and spiritual counselor, he did not take the time to discuss his or her role.

SUMMARY

The goal of hospice and palliative care is to reduce the patient's distressful symptoms (physical, emotional, and spiritual) and improve his or her quality of life. When nurses are familiar with palliative care and hospice, they can be instrumental in helping patients and their family members understand and become comfortable with this type of care. Making appropriate and timely referrals for hospice and palliative care is one way that nurses can prevent needless suffering for patients with life-threatening conditions.

WEB RESOURCES

American Academy of Hospice and Palliative Medicine
http://www.aahpm.org

Hospice Association of America
http://www.nahc.org/haa

Hospice Foundation of America
http://www.hospicefoundation.org

National Hospice and Palliative Care Organization (NHPCO)
http://www.nhpco.org

Hospice and Palliative Nurses Association (HPNA)
http://www.hpna.org

EXAM QUESTIONS

CHAPTER 4
Questions 30-38

Note: Choose the one option that BEST answers each question.

30. Palliative care is best initiated

    a. early during the trajectory of a life-threatening illness.

    b. when death is imminent.

    c. only in the last 6 months of life.

    d. when patients have stopped all other treatments.

31. Care that is focused on a terminally ill patient determined to have a prognosis of approximately 6 months, who is no longer seeking curative treatment, is

    a. palliative care.

    b. curative care.

    c. hospice care.

    d. interdisciplinary care.

32. To be eligible for hospice care under the Hospice Medicare Benefit, individuals must be eligible for

    a. Medicare Part B and have two doctors certify that they are terminally ill.

    b. Medicare Part A and have two doctors certify that they are terminally ill.

    c. Medicare Part A and have one doctor certify that they still want their regular Medicare benefits.

    d. Medicare Part B and have one doctor certify that they are terminally ill.

33. The two persons who must verify that the hospice patient's prognosis is 6 months or less are

    a. the team nurse and social worker.

    b. the hospice medical director and the registered nurse.

    c. the hospice medical director and the patient's attending physician.

    d. the hospice administrator and the medical director.

34. The team member responsible for supportive counseling, resource referrals, and assisting with legal or insurance concerns is

    a. the chaplain.

    b. the bereavement counselor.

    c. the registered nurse.

    d. the social worker.

35. Which of the following does Medicare require when the care is provided by a Medicare-approved hospice program?

    a. Durable medical equipment and drugs to hasten death.

    b. Durable medical equipment and short-term inpatient care.

    c. Transportation to medical appointments and long-term inpatient care.

    d. Short-term inpatient care and long-term respite care in a Medicare-approved facility.

36. The setting where hospice services are most commonly provided in the United States is

    a. nursing homes.

    b. hospice facilities.

    c. hospital settings.

    d. patients' homes.

37. Hospital based palliative care programs are

    a. only for patients with a terminal cancer diagnosis.

    b. found primarily in small community hospitals.

    c. increasing in numbers nationwide.

    d. exclusively used for elderly patients.

38. Palliative care for children is

    a. never appropriate because children should not be expected to deal with issues of death and dying.

    b. unnecessary because most children recover from their illnesses.

    c. beneficial to many children who are facing life-threatening illness.

    d. never covered by health insurance or Medicaid.

CHAPTER 5

ADVANCE CARE PLANNING

CHAPTER OBJECTIVE

After completing this chapter, the reader will be able to describe the significance of advance care planning and various methods for conveying one's wishes for end-of-life care.

LEARNING OBJECTIVES

After studying this chapter, the reader will be able to

1. describe various formats used to convey end-of-life wishes, including living wills, medical powers of attorney, and advance care planning discussions.

2. discuss ethical issues related to end-of-life care, such as informed consent, self-determination, and sedation and pain management.

3. explain the purpose and meaning of a do not resuscitate (DNR) order.

INTRODUCTION

Advance care planning is essential if a person's preferences for end-of-life care are to be communicated and honored. Advance care planning involves decision making, expressing treatment preferences, and completing documents that communicate the patient's values and beliefs for health care when he or she can no longer speak for himself or herself. Compassionate nurses recognize that advanced illness conversations should address the patient's emotional and physical needs and include language that is positive and hopeful. This chapter will focus on what nurses need to know to help patients understand and communicate their healthcare choices at the end of life. It is important for nurses to consider quality of life and support decision making in culturally sensitive ways (Berzoff & Silverman, 2004).

ADVANCE DIRECTIVES

Most Americans (88%) feel comfortable discussing issues relating to death and dying, yet only 42% have a living will (VITAS Innovative Healthcare, 2004). Living wills and medical powers of attorney for health care are types of advance directives recognized under state law that can direct the provision of healthcare when the individual is incapacitated. In order to execute an advance directive, individuals must be at least 18 years old.

A Living Will

Living wills, otherwise known as instruction directives, are legal documents indicating the types of medical treatments a person would accept or reject in different situations. Living wills are a type of written advance directive that states a person's wishes about the medical care to be implemented should the person become unable to communicate at the end of life.

Although every state has its own advance directive laws and related forms, Pennsylvania's advance directives are typical of other states. This state's declaration notes the individual's preferences for life-prolonging treatments (such as cardiac resuscitation, mechanical respiration, tube feedings, blood or blood products) should the person become terminally ill and be unable to communicate his or her own wishes (Pennsylvania Department of Aging, n.d.). By law, each state defines when the living will becomes effective and may limit the treatments addressed by the document. A living will can also specify that an individual wants all possible medical treatment to prolong life. State-specific advance directive forms can be obtained at www.caringinfo.org.

> **Personal Insight**
> *Do you have a completed advance directive? If you do not have an advance directive, why not?*

Medical Power of Attorney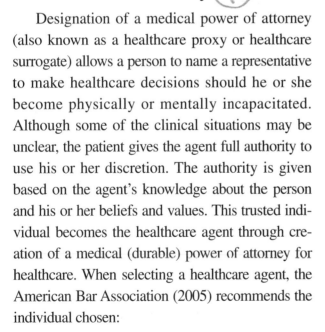

Designation of a medical power of attorney (also known as a healthcare proxy or healthcare surrogate) allows a person to name a representative to make healthcare decisions should he or she become physically or mentally incapacitated. Although some of the clinical situations may be unclear, the patient gives the agent full authority to use his or her discretion. The authority is given based on the agent's knowledge about the person and his or her beliefs and values. This trusted individual becomes the healthcare agent through creation of a medical (durable) power of attorney for healthcare. When selecting a healthcare agent, the American Bar Association (2005) recommends the individual chosen:

1. meet the legal criteria in your state for acting as agent or proxy or representative.

2. would be willing to speak on your behalf.

3. would be able to act on your wishes and separate his/her own feelings from yours.

4. live close by or could travel to be at your side if needed.

5. knows you well and understands what is important to you.

6. is someone you trust with your life.

7. will talk with you now about sensitive issues and listen to your wishes.

8. will likely be available long into the future.

9. would be able to handle conflicting opinions between family members, friends, and medical personnel.

10. can be a strong advocate in the face of an unresponsive doctor or institution. (p. 1)

What Laws Govern the Use of Advance Directives?

Federal and state laws govern the use of advance directives. All 50 states and the District of Columbia have laws honoring advance directives. Passed by Congress in 1990, the Patient Self-Determination Act requires a health agency, hospital, skilled nursing facility, or hospice program to inform all adult patients about their rights to accept or refuse treatment and execute an advance directive. Written policies should be in place that guarantee patients will be given written information on advance directives.

Upon admission to a healthcare agency, hospital, skilled nursing facility, or hospice program, patients should be made aware of the provider's willingness to comply with their wishes. If providers refuse to comply with directives, it pits the patients' rights to have their wishes honored against providers' rights to refuse care for reasons of conscience (Hosay, 2003).

Nurses need to make sure they understand their state guidelines and their facility policies regarding how advance directives are to be communicated and honored (Herrin Allen, 2008). Each state regulates advance directives differently. Although many states honor out-of-state advance directives, there must be no conflict with that state's law. Unfortunately, advance directives may be overlooked in a crisis situation, as there is no time in an emergency either to consult the advance directive or to determine a person's underlying medical condition.

Informed Consent 41

Ethically and legally, patients have the right to be included in any decision-making process regarding their healthcare. Informed consent is a legal doctrine requiring physicians to inform patients about their conditions and the potential benefits and risks involved in treatments. The informed consent documents the fact that communication – a dialogue and process – between the practitioner and patient has occurred. It is not uncommon for patients to feel intimidated by professionals who ask them to sign forms regarding their healthcare. Throughout the dialogue and process of informed consent, nurses should assess the patient's understanding of what is being said.

During the informed consent process, nurses can discuss all possibilities in lay terms so patients understand their options. Competent patients should be offered reasonable choices about the proposed intervention and be allowed to independently (without coercion from clinicians or family) accept or reject the intervention based upon an honest representation of the facts. Although competence is a legal term, with the determination of a patient's competence sometimes made by a court of law, routine assessment of competence is generally made by the patient's attending physician.

FACTORS THAT INFLUENCE THE DECISION-MAKING PROCESS

Winter, Parker, and Schneider (2007) asked 40 elderly individuals questions about dying without life-prolonging treatments, eliciting beliefs about duration, pain, loneliness, and palliative care.

Little consensus was found about how long it would take to die. A few of the respondents spontaneously mentioned palliative care and more than three quarters believed comfort care would be available when needed. They also believed that comfort care would be effective. A prevalent finding was that participants thought dying would be a lonely experience. The participants reported that death without antibiotics was rated the worst. About one quarter of the participants reported they were not aware of death without tube feedings (Winter et al., 2007).

The ability to discuss advance directives may be influenced by patients' personal death attitudes and experiences that cause them to fail to act objectively (Black, 2007). Taking patients' past histories of death experiences is an important part of understanding their wants and needs at the end of life. One's personal preferences for end-of-life care are influenced by past experiences with dying family members. Race, ethnicity, gender, age, and family values are also factors that may influence the decision-making process.

Patients' treatment decisions may be influenced by race and ethnicity. Although the Chinese acknowledge that death and dying is a part of the life span, they won't talk about it because they believe it's a taboo. In order to postpone bad luck, they will try to prolong the patient's life as long as possible (Hsu, O'Connor, & Lee, 2009). African Americans express greater acceptance of life in worse health (Winter, Dennis, & Parker, 2007-2008). They also express stronger preferences for tube feeding and are more likely to receive these services than Caucasians (Phipps et al., 2003). However, a recent study revealed no significant differences in the preferences to continue dialysis based on race on the part of Black and White patients (Pruchno, Cartwright, & Wilson-Genderson, 2009). The study found treatment decisions at end of life for both races were based on fear of death and religion. Due to deep cultural values, African Americans are less interested in advance directives, are more likely to choose life-prolonging and aggressive treatments, and associate treatment limitations and hospice care with "giving up" (Hopp & Duffy, 2000; Jenkins, Lapelle, Zapka, & Kurent, 2005; Phipps et al., 2003; Torke, Garas, Sexson, & Branch, 2005).

Winter et al. (2007-2008) examined the "will of God" as a potential mediator of racial differences in treatment preferences at end of life. The five items on the God's Will Scale that have been shown to affect the decision-making process are:

1. I feel guided by God in the midst of daily activities.

2. God plays a role in how I choose my path in life.

3. I try to make sense of the situation and decide what to do without relying on God.

4. I work together with God as partners to get through hard times.

5. I look to God for strength, support, and guidance in crises. (p. 274)

Nurses need to be aware of the significance of God's will when discussing advance directives with African American patients. Many African Americans believe their terminal illnesses are the will of God and the acceptance of God's will guides their medical decision making at the end of their lives (Duffy, Jackson, Schim, Ronis, & Fowler, 2006; Johnson, Elbert-Avila, & Tulsky, 2005). In a review of the literature on spiritual beliefs and practices of African Americans, Johnson et al. (2005) found the following recurrent themes:

- Spiritual beliefs and practices are a source of comfort, coping, and support and are the most effective ways to influence healing;

- God is responsible for physical and spiritual health;

- The doctor is God's instrument. (p. 711)

Attitudes about death have a direct bearing on the decisions made about end-of-life wishes, which are different between the sexes. Older men express a stronger preference for life-sustaining treatment than older women, whereas older women express a greater desire to have a dignified death than men. Gender differences may be due to women not wanting to be a burden and putting others before themselves (Arber, Vandrevala, Daly, & Hampson, 2008).

Older individuals want personal control and independence to be maintained as they take part in decisions about their lives and their deaths. When older persons become too ill to make decisions about their healthcare, families can assume the roles of surrogate decision makers.

Advances in medical technology have made health care options more complex as older adults and their families are confronted with difficult decisions about how aggressively to pursue medical treatments capable of prolonging existence in states characterized by a very low quality of life. (Zettel-Watson, Ditto, Danks, & Smucker, 2008, p. 273)

Individuals differ in their decision-making style. As end-of-life decisions are discussed, nurses will need to know if patients tend to make decisions on their own or if they usually defer to others. It is important to consider how individual decisions may be affected by the opinions of family members. Professionals may initiate discussions with their patients regarding advance directives to determine their preferences, or patients may discuss their wishes on their own accord with family caregivers (Pickett, Barg, & Lynch, 2001).

An individual's values and the values of their family members are the most important influences on end-of-life decisions. Patients and their family members can complete a values exercise with their healthcare professionals to clarify their expectations and fears in clinical circumstances (see Figure 5-1).

Family plays a significant role in end-of-life discussions and choices. A VITAS survey (2004) found:

FIGURE 5-1: END-OF-LIFE DECISION MAKING: WORKSHEET 1: VALUES QUESTIONNAIRE

The following questions can help you think about your values as they relate to medical care decisions. You may use the questions to discuss your views with your health care agent and others, or you may write answers to the questions as a help to your agent and health care team. (If you fill out this worksheet and want it to be part of your DPA/HC, sign it in the presence of witnesses and attach it to your DPA/HC form.)

1. What do you value most about your life? (For example: living a long life, living an active life, enjoying the company of family and friends, etc.)

2. How do you feel about death and dying? (Do you fear death and dying? Have you experienced the loss of a loved one? Did that person's illness or medical treatment influence your thinking about death and dying?)

3. Do you believe life should always be preserved as long as possible?

4. If not, what kinds of mental or physical conditions would make you think that life-prolonging treatment should no longer be used? Being:
    *   unaware of my life and surroundings;
    *   unable to appreciate and continue the important relationships in my life;
    *   unable to think well enough to make every-day decisions;
    *   in severe pain or discomfort;
    *   other (describe)

5. Could you image reasons for temporarily accepting medical treatment for the conditions you have described? What might they be?

6. How much pain and risk would you be willing to accept if your chances of recovery from an illness or injury were good (50-50 or better)?

7. What if your chances of recovery were poor (less than one in 10)?

8. Would your approach to accepting or rejecting care depend on how old you were at the time of treatment? Why?

9. Do you hold any religious or moral views about medicine or particular medical treatments? What are they?

10. Should financial considerations influence decisions about your medical care? Explain.

11. What other beliefs or values do you hold that should be considered by those making medical care decisions for you if you become unable to speak for yourself?

12. Most people have heard of difficult end-of-life situations involving family members or neighbors or people in the news. Have you had any reactions to these situations If so, describe:

Date: _____ *Signature:* _____ *Date of birth:* _____

Address: _____

Witness: _____ *Witness:* _____

Note. From Vermont Ethics Network, (n.d.-a). Available from http://www.vtethicsnetwork.org/WorkSheet1.htm. Reprinted with permission.

• Nine out of ten people who have discussed death and dying have done so with a family member.

• An overwhelming majority of Americans – 83% – would rather be at home with family than in a hospital or medical facility if they were dying from a terminal illness.

• Even when they are faced with conditions such as Alzheimer's or Parkinson's disease, the majority – 58% – still would prefer to be at home.

• When asked to choose what a "good death" means, for many Americans it means dying with family members around (27%).

ADVANCE CARE PLANNING DISCUSSIONS

Advance care planning takes time. The questions and answers do not need to be decided in one visit. As patients become more comfortable in discussing their own desires, they also become more comfortable addressing these wishes with their physicians. Individuals should be informed that they can always change their mind and either change or revoke their advance directives as conditions change.

Physicians and nurses need to use the right terminology in end-of-life discussions as patients and their family members may negatively react to certain words (Pellegrino, DeJonge, Crawley, Cohen-Almagor, & Connolly, 2008). Rather than using words and phrases such as "terminal" or "persistent vegetative state," Raphael Cohen-Almagor, a speaker at the "Ethical Decision-Making at the End of Life" program organized by the Division of United States Studies and the Global Health Initiative, suggested that terminology such as "prolonged unawareness" or "post-coma unawareness" would be more neutral and less frightening (Pellegrino et al., 2008). It is helpful to focus on the impact of treatments on quality of life. Zamperetti,

Bellomo, and Ronco (2008) maintain that artificial organ support can delay death temporarily while failing to restore a quality of life acceptable to the patient.

Artificial organ support can also be a temporary positive measure. A patient may say, "I never want to be put on a ventilator. A ventilator is never an option no matter what." The nurse might respond by asking, "What if you were able to come off the dependency of the machine in a few days or weeks? Under those circumstances, would you still not want a breathing machine?" The patient might then respond, "In that case, I would definitely want to be on a ventilator." If the nurse did not explore "what if" circumstances, the patient's true wishes would not have been known. When persons complete advance directives, they cannot predict what will happen to them. Because actual clinical circumstances may not follow the situations written in advance directives, physicians can better interpret what patients want based on discussions of various scenarios (see Figure 5-2).

Linda Norlander, Project Manager for the Allina End of Life Project, helped develop an advance care planning discussion model, The Kitchen Table Discussion, for professionals. The model focuses is on the discussion that takes place between professionals, patients, and family members. The discussion includes patients' understanding of their illnesses, their personal death experiences, and their goals and values.

Although nurses may be effective communicators, they can learn much from the work of Norlander and McSteen (2000) who suggest excellent questions to ask patients when facilitating discussions about the end of life. They note that only asking whether patients want to be resuscitated if their hearts stop ignores "the larger context and history of the person's illness and life" (p. 533) and suggest these reflection questions be used to identify patient's perspectives on their illness:

FIGURE 5-2: END-OF-LIFE DECISION MAKING: WORKSHEET 2: MEDICAL SITUATIONS AND THEIR TREATMENT PLANS

This worksheet presents possible treatment plans for a variety of common medical situations. You may use these examples to discuss your views with your health care agent and others, or you may write down your choices as a help to your agent and health care team. (If you fill out this worksheet and want it to be part of your DPA/HC, sign it in the presence of witnesses and attach it to your DPA/HC form.)

Possible Treatment Plans:

A. I would want all possible efforts to preserve life as long as possible.

B. I would want comfort care only, and would not want medical treatment, including tube-feeding, to prolong my life.

C. I would want comfort care and tube-feeding, but would not want other types of medical treatment to prolong my life.

D. My agent should consider the possible benefits and burdens of disease-fighting treatment, and consent only to treatment that he or she believes is in my best interests, as we have discussed them. My agent may refuse any active treatment or may consent to a trial of treatment and then stop treatment if it is not beneficial.

E. Treatment plan D, as described above, except that I would always want tube-feeding.

Possible Medical Situations:

1. Suppose you have a fatal ("terminal") condition. You are unconscious and death is expected soon, with or without treatment. What treatment plan would you want? (Select from above, or write your own.)

2. Suppose you are permanently unconscious from an accident or severe illness. There is no reasonable hope of recovering awareness, but life support could keep your body alive for years. (This is called "persistent vegetative state" or "permanent coma.") What treatment plan would you want? (Select from above, or write your own.)

3. Suppose you are in a state of very advanced loss of mental capability, due perhaps to stroke or Alzheimer's disease. You cannot recognize or communicate with those close to you, and can do almost nothing for yourself. You could survive in this state for some time with medical treatment. What treatment plan would you want? (Select from above, or write you own.)

4. Suppose you are in a state of permanent but not total confusion, perhaps from stroke or Alzheimer's disease. You are legally "incompetent" and cannot recognize people and interact with them in a meaningful way, but you are up and around and people are taking care of you. You are not in distress and seem to be able to experience some satisfactions in daily life, such as in eating or hearing music. Then you get an illness that might be fatal. What treatment plan would you want? (Select from above, or write your own.)

5. Suppose you are frail, chronically ill and uncomfortable, with a limited rage of activities available to you. Then you become unconscious, at least temporarily, due to an acute illness. The illness is likely to be fatal unless vigorously treated in a hospital, but even intensive care offers only a small chance of recovery to your former condition. It's much more likely that you will end up worse off than before, or will die in spite of all heroic measures. What treatment plan would you want. (Select from above, or write your own.)

6. Suppose you unexpectedly suffer a serious injury or illness. You have less than a 5 percent chance of good recovery and, if you survive, will have serious brain damage. What treatment plan would you want? (Select from above, or write your own.)

7. Use this space to describe any other medical situations you'd like to address:

Date: _____ *Signature:* _____ *Date of birth:* _____

Address: _____

Witness: _____ *Witness:* _____

Note. From Vermont Ethics Network, (n.d.-b). Available from http://www.vtethicsnetwork.org/Worksheet2.htm. Reprinted with permission.

- "It appears your condition is changing. What has the doctor told you?"

- "You've been hospitalized three times in the last 2 months. Tell me how this has been for you."

- "Have you talked with your family about your health?"

- "How are you coping with all of this?"

- "What is your understanding of your treatment options and your prognosis?"

- "Do you have any fears about your illness getting worse?" (p. 538)

The discussion also explores how family members can support the goals and values of the patients and includes exploration of other personal resources (Norlander & McSteen, 2000).

Advance care planning discussions with patients are made easier when prepared documents can be used as a guide. Two of these documents are Five Wishes and Physician Orders for Life-Sustaining Treatment (POLST).

> ***Personal Insight***
> *Are you comfortable asking patients if they have an advance directive? Explore the reason for your feelings.*

Five Wishes

Although many years have passed since Five Wishes was created by Jim Towey, the founder of Aging with Dignity, it is often used today with the assistance of physicians, nurses, lawyers, and experts in end-of-life care. This easy-to-understand form helps individuals express how they would like to be treated if seriously ill and unable to speak for themselves. Simply stated, Five Wishes is a document that addresses the person's medical, personal, emotional, and spiritual needs and encourages discussing wishes with family and physicians. Five Wishes lets a patient tell family members and healthcare providers:

1. the person I want to make care decisions for me when I can't.

2. the kind of medical treatment I want or don't want.

3. how comfortable I want to be.

4. how I want people to treat me.

5. what I want my loved ones to know.

Organizations, such as churches, synagogues, hospices, hospitals, medical and legal offices, and social service agencies, distribute this document in 40 states and the District of Columbia. Five Wishes speaks in plain language and is easily understood by those who are not lawyers or physicians. Patients should be advised to complete a document similar to Five Wishes before they become seriously ill. In case of a health crisis rendering them unable to speak, their doctors, and families will then know exactly what their wishes are, as the completed documents will speak for them.

Physician Orders for Life-Sustaining Treatment

Advance care planning discussion can also include the POLST document (see Figure 5-3). To improve the quality of end-of-life care, the POLST Paradigm Program was founded in Oregon. Other states currently have POLST programs in place or are developing programs at this time (Center for Ethics in Health Care, Oregon Health & Science University, 2008). On August 4, 2008, Governor Schwarzenegger of California signed a new law that ensures that when patients have completed POLST forms, their treatment preferences regarding life-sustaining treatments, resuscitation, nutrition, pain management, cardiopulmonary resuscitation (CPR), medical interventions, antibiotics, and artificially administered nutrition will be honored. The POLST form complements, but does not replace, advance directives. Although this form is voluntary and not required by law, it must be honored by all healthcare providers. The POLST form is a physician's order for a plan of care reflecting the patient's wishes.

continued on page 83

FIGURE 5-3: POLST FORM (1 OF 2)

HIPAA PERMITS DISCLOSURE TO HEALTH CARE PROFESSIONALS AS NECESSARY FOR TREATMENT

Physician Orders
for Life-Sustaining Treatment (POLST)

<u>First</u> follow these orders, <u>then</u> contact physician, NP, or PA. These medical orders are based on the person's current medical condition and preferences. Any section not completed does not invalidate the form and implies full treatment for that section.

Last Name / First / Middle Initial	
Address	
City / State / Zip	
Date of Birth (mm/dd/yyyy) ___ , ___ , ___	Last 4 SSN	Gender ☐M ☐F

A
Check One

CARDIOPULMONARY RESUSCITATION (CPR): Person has no pulse **and** is not breathing.

☐ Attempt Resuscitation/CPR   ☐ Do Not Attempt Resuscitation/DNR (<u>A</u>llow <u>N</u>atural <u>D</u>eath)

When not in cardiopulmonary arrest, follow orders in **B**, **C** and **D**.

B
Check One

MEDICAL INTERVENTIONS: Person has pulse and/**or** is breathing.

☐ **Comfort Measures Only** Use medication by any route, positioning, wound care and other measures to relieve pain and suffering. Use oxygen, suction and manual treatment of airway obstruction as needed for comfort. *Do not transfer to hospital for life-sustaining treatment. **Transfer** if comfort needs cannot be met in current location.*

☐ **Limited Additional Interventions** Includes care described above. Use medical treatment, IV fluids and cardiac monitor as indicated. Do not use intubation, advanced airway interventions, or mechanical ventilation. May consider less invasive airway support (e.g. CPAP, BiPAP). ***Transfer** to hospital if indicated. Avoid intensive care.*

☐ **Full Treatment** Includes care described above. Use intubation, advanced airway interventions, mechanical ventilation, and cardioversion as indicated. ***Transfer** to hospital if indicated. Includes intensive care.*

Additional Orders: _____

C
Check One

ANTIBIOTICS

☐ No antibiotics. Use other measures to relieve symptoms.
☐ Determine use or limitation of antibiotics when infection occurs.
☐ Use antibiotics if medically indicated.

Additional Orders: _____

D
Check One

ARTIFICIALLY ADMINISTERED NUTRITION: Always offer food by mouth if feasible.

☐ No artificial nutrition by tube.
☐ Defined trial period of artificial nutrition by tube.
☐ Long-term artificial nutrition by tube.

Additional Orders: _____

E

REASON FOR ORDERS AND SIGNATURES

My signature below indicates to the best of my knowledge that these orders are consistent with the person's current medical condition and preferences as indicated by the **discussion with**:

☐ Patient   ☐ Health Care Representative   ☐ Parent of Minor

☐ Court-Appointed Guardian   ☐ Other _____

Print Primary Care Professional Name	Office Use Only
Print Signing Physician / NP / PA Name and Phone Number ( )	
Physician / NP / PA Signature (mandatory)	Date

SEND FORM WITH PERSON WHENEVER TRANSFERRED OR DISCHARGED

continued on next page

FIGURE 5-3: POLST FORM (2 OF 2)

HIPAA PERMITS DISCLOSURE TO HEALTH CARE PROFESSIONALS AS NECESSARY FOR TREATMENT

Information for Person Named on this Form

This form records your preferences for life-sustaining treatment in your **current** state of health. It can be reviewed and updated by your health care professional at any time if your preferences change. If you are unable to make your own health care decisions, the orders should reflect your preferences as best understood by your surrogate.

Signature of Person or Surrogate

Signature	Name (print)	Relationship (write "self" if patient)

Contact Information

Surrogate (optional)	Relationship	Phone Number	Address	
Health Care Professional Preparing Form (optional)	Preparer Title		Phone Number	Date Prepared
PA's Supervising Physician			Phone Number	

Directions for Health Care Professionals

Completing POLST

- Should reflect person's current preferences. Encourage completion of an advance directive.
- POLST must be signed by a physician/NP/PA to be valid. Verbal orders are acceptable with follow-up signature by physician/NP/PA in accordance with facility/community policy.
- Use of original form is encouraged. Photocopies and FAXes are legal and valid.

Using POLST

Section A:
- No defibrillator (including AEDs) should be used on a person who has chosen "Do Not Attempt Resuscitation."

Section B:
- When comfort cannot be achieved in the current setting, the person, including someone with "Comfort Measures Only," should be transferred to a setting able to provide comfort (e.g., treatment of a hip fracture).
- IV medication to enhance comfort may be appropriate for a person who has chosen "Comfort Measures Only."
- Treatment of dehydration is a measure which prolongs life. A person who desires IV fluids should indicate "Limited Additional Interventions" or "Full Treatment."

Section D:
- Oral fluids and nutrition <u>must</u> always be offered if medically feasible.
- A person with capacity, or the surrogate of a person without capacity, can void the form and request alternative treatment.

Reviewing POLST

This POLST should be reviewed periodically and if:
- The person is transferred from one care setting or care level to another, or
- There is a substantial change in the person's health status, or
- The person's treatment preferences change.

Draw line through sections A through E and write "VOID" in large letters if POLST is replaced or becomes invalid.

Example of a POLST Paradigm form. The POLST program was developed by the Oregon POLST Task Force and is housed at OHSU's Center for Ethics in Health Care. For permission to use the copyrighted form contact the Center. Information on the POLST program is available online at **www.polst.org** or at polst@ohsu.edu. Reprinted with permission.

SEND FORM WITH PERSON WHENEVER TRANSFERRED OR DISCHARGED

Note. From "Physicians Orders for Life Sustaining Treatment (POLST)," by Center for Ethics in Health Care, Oregon Health & Science University, 2008. Retrieved on August 23, 2010, from http://www.ohsu.edu/polst/programs/documents/POLST.August.2008.sample.pdf

ETHICAL ISSUES IN END-OF-LIFE DECISIONS

Ethics is a branch of philosophy that helps nurses understand the moral dimension of conduct in the healthcare system. Ethics are systems of moral values that guide professionals in their conduct and treatment of patients. Simply stated, ethical practice is knowing and doing what is right. An established set of moral standards is known as a code of ethics.

In addressing the choices patients have regarding their end-of-life care, the significance of ethical issues and the fundamental rights of patients must be recognized. Acknowledging and respecting patient goals, preferences, and choices can cause personal ethical dilemmas for nurses. Such dilemmas *are* dilemmas because of a discord between the rightness or wrongness of actions and the goodness or badness of the cost of those actions (Ross, 2008).

Nurses must respect patient self-determination, which encompasses the active inclusion of patients in decisions regarding their care (American College of Obstetrics & Gynecologists, 2008). Patients should be informed, as studies show informed patients and family members will make the right choices and participate in decision making if they are well-informed about the terminal illnesses (Yeolekar, Mehta, & Yeolekar, 2008). Nurses must provide honest and factual information and then respect their patients' wishes while preventing harm when possible.

Do Not Resuscitate Orders

Nurses are often key resources for providing support and comfort to patients as their terminal illnesses are discussed. Patients generally would rather have at least partial disclosure of the fact they are terminally ill rather than nondisclosure, and they also prefer to be told of their prognoses in the presence of loved ones (Marwit & Datson, 2002). Once the difficult task of delivering bad news to patients is complete, healthcare professionals can assist patients and families to consider advance directives and in particular, do not resuscitate (DNR) orders.

A DNR is a written physician's order not to conduct CPR in the event of cardiac arrest. If the patient or surrogate decision maker and physician are in agreement, the physician writes the order in the patient's medical record. For terminally ill patients, CPR can be viewed as an assault that, if successful, prolongs the dying process and related suffering. For most terminally ill patients, CPR and other aggressive medical interventions are most often without benefit. Patients need to be informed that if they choose DNR, other treatments will still be made available to them, such as treatment for pain and other distressing symptoms. For those who are terminally ill, a DNR order is a valuable tool for avoiding needless invasive treatment.

Emanuel (2008) found that more than 85% of Americans die without CPR, and more than 90% of decedents in intensive care units (ICUs) do not receive CPR. Of the ICU decedents, 90% died after medical treatments were withheld or withdrawn – an average of 2.6 interventions per person (Emanuel, 2008). These interventions could include blood transfusions, antibiotics, respirators, artificial hydration, and nutrition.

Although these advance care conversations are important and professionals need to be comfortable having them, many physicians are uncomfortable talking about DNR orders with patients. There is a conflict today between discussing end-of-life issues openly and attempting to spare individuals the pain of knowing they are dying. Nurses can play an active role in the DNR discussion with patients. Studies show that staff nurses, when compared with their physician colleagues, are more likely to believe they should be allowed to initiate DNR discussions, are more confident in their ability to discuss DNR than physician house officers, and have more positive attitudes toward this patient option (Sulmasy, He, McAuley, & Ury, 2008).

Terminal Sedation

After a terminally ill patient refuses treatment to prolong his or her life, nurses no longer have a duty to do so. Issues regarding DNR, withdrawing of treatment, withholding food and fluids, and administering terminal sedation can cause stress for nurses who are not comfortable with care rather than cure. Although some nurses look at palliative care as a moral dilemma, palliative care benefits nurses, who receive great satisfaction in relieving the pain and suffering of their patients and improving the quality of their lives.

Palliative sedation is the intentional sedation of patients, rendering them unconscious, when aggressive management of pain and symptoms associated with terminal disease is not effective and patients continue to suffer from underlying symptoms that will shortly end their lives (Chochinov, 2006; Cohen et al., 2005; de Graeff & Dean, 2007; Lo & Rubenfeld, 2005). Boyle (2004) notes that the use of terminal sedation to control the intense discomfort of dying patients appears to be an established practice in palliative care and runs counter to the moral and legal norm that forbids healthcare professionals from intentionally killing patients. Simon, Kar, Hinz, and Beck (2007) found that terminal sedation in dying patients with uncontrollable physical symptoms was considered morally acceptable by virtually all respondents (98% with a medical background and 97% without a medical background).

Rietjens, Hauser, van der Heide, and Emanual (2007) studied nursing attitudes regarding the use of palliative sedation to address physical suffering in severely ill patients and found that nurses fell into three groups. The first group of nurses thought palliative sedation did not accelerate death. The second group of nurses thought it may accelerate death but was justified when there was no other way of relieving discomfort in patients. A third group thought

palliative sedation was similar to euthanasia and found it difficult to be involved in its use. However, all of the nurses surveyed considered palliative sedation to positively contribute to the patient's quality of dying (Rietjens et al., 2007).

Engstrom, Bruno, Holm, and Hellzen's (2007) literature review of articles published between 1990 and 2005 to describe the phenomenon of palliative sedation found palliative sedation was given to fewer than 40% of dying patients during their last 4 days of life. The sedation was given to patients to relieve pain, agitation, and/or dyspnea. Although professionals usually have positive attitudes toward palliative sedation, the public considers it as being close to euthanasia. Its intent, however, is not to cause death (Cowan & Walsh, 2001). Few studies have focused on nursing care during palliative sedation. Further research describing the nurses' roles during palliative sedation is needed (Engstrom et al., 2007).

Personal Insight
What is most significant to you: the quality or the length of your life?

Pain Management

Barriers that contribute to the undertreatment of pain at the end of life include lack of pain education and system-wide accountability, poor pain assessment, and exaggerated fears of addiction and respiratory depression (Cuvala, 2008). The Pain and Policy Studies Group (2008) found that a frequent negative provision remaining in state policy is confusion of the terms *physical dependence* and *addiction* (Table 5-1).

Pain management should be a top priority for the physician treating patients at the end of life. Some physicians fear they are hastening death when aggressively managing pain at this stage. The ethical principle of double effect evaluates the permissibility of performing an action to achieve a good outcome (such as relieving pain) when the action can also cause an undesirable impact (such as contributing to a patient's early death). If the pri-

TABLE 5-1: ACHIEVING BALANCE IN STATE PAIN POLICY

Although 37 states have adopted language that clarifies the distinction between these clinical phenomena, which usually is contained in healthcare regulatory guidelines or policy statements, the statutes of 14 states and the healthcare regulations of two states continue to classify physical dependence as synonymous with addiction. Consequently, 12 states have conflicting standards about what constitutes addiction, which are present in different policies and can create confusion for practitioners. Also, a definition of addiction (or drug dependence) in law, which can be established solely by the presence of physical dependence, can legally classify as an "addict" a patient who is being treated with chronic opioid therapy. When such an archaic standard is applied in practice, it has the potential to stigmatize pain patients and restrict prescribing practices, leading to inadequate pain management. Most states' statutory definitions of addiction were modeled after the definition found in the federal Public Health and Welfare Act (42 USCS § 201), which is still present and was created almost 40 years ago. Special attention should be given to repealing this prevalent state statutory or regulatory definition that no longer conforms to the current medical and scientific understanding of addiction.

Note. From *Achieving Balance in State Pain Policy. A progress report card* (4th Edition), by Pain & Policy Studies Group, University of Wisconsin School of Medicine and Public Health. Paul P. Carbone Comprehensive Cancer Center, 2008, page 19. Retrieved on August 23, 2010, from http://www.painpolicy.wisc.edu/Achieving_Balance/PRC2008.pdf

mary intention is to relieve pain, an unavoidable secondary effect is seen as ethically acceptable. The Pain and Policy Studies Group (2008) reports that state pain policies are becoming more balanced. According to their grading system, positive changes since 2007 include:

- 13 states adopted new policies containing language that fulfilled at least one evaluation criterion, and in seven of those states the policy change was sufficient to improve their grade.

- Oregon achieved an A in 2008 and joins Kansas, Michigan, Virginia, and Wisconsin as having the most balanced pain policies in the country.

- Georgia showed the largest grade improvement, increasing from a D+ to a B.

- 88% of states now have a grade above the average C.

- No state's grade decreased in the last year or even since 2000. (p. 3)

Tissue, Organ, and Body Donation

The U.S. Department of Health and Human Services maintains that transplantation saves lives. Approximately 56 people each day receive organ transplants because an individual said "yes" to organ and tissue donation on a donor card and/or on a dri-

ver's license (Organ Procurement and Transplantation Network [OPTN], 2010). There were 28,462 transplants from January to December 2009, and more than 28,000 patients had healthier lives due to organ transplants that year (OPTN, 2010). As of March 19, 2010, there were 106,593 people on waiting lists for organ donation (OPTN, 2010).

Individuals must express their willingness to donate their organs by informing their families about their decisions, signing donor cards, and carrying them with them (Wu & Tang, 2009). Anyone over the age of 18 can agree to be a donor; those under 18 must have a parent's consent. When individuals die who have not filled out donor cards, their next of kin can donate their organs and tissues at the time of death. Newborns as well as senior citizens can become donors. After the death of someone under the age of 18, parents or legal guardians make the decision about donation. This is called nonliving donation.

At the time of death, medical suitability for donation is determined. Through the United Network for Organ Sharing (UNOS), organ donors are matched to waiting recipients 24 hours a day, 365 days a year across the United States (UNOS, 2009). Recipients are matched to organs ranked by tissue match, blood type, length of time on waiting list, immune status, and geographical distance between the recipient and donor (UNOS, 2009).

Truog and Miller (2008) note that organ transplantation has been guided by the ethical requirement termed the *dead donor rule,* which maintains patients must be declared dead before the removal of any vital organs for transplantation. There is almost always some brief time lapse between the actual trauma and the declaration of brain death. During this period, patients are supported with ventilators – initially in an attempt to save their lives and eventually to maintain the organs for transplantation.

Being able to renew the lives of others through donation can bring comfort to survivors and victims. In some circumstances, such as advanced age or medical condition, patients may not be eligible for donation. If family members want to donate their loved one's organs or tissues and are told they cannot do so, they may feel disappointed and saddened.

Donors should carry their donor cards with them to make their wishes known immediately. It is also important to discuss such a decision with family. Nurses and social workers may have to provide grief support to family members as they decide whether to donate their loved one's organs. Even in cases in which individuals have requested that their organs be donated, organ retrieval is not allowed without the family's consent, as shown in the following example:

Sally and Frank arrived at the hospital and were told that their 21-year-old daughter, Anne, was in critical condition following a car accident. Anne was being kept alive by a ventilator and was considered brain dead. The nurse prepared them for what they would see and explained the reasons for the machines, tubes, and equipment. The hospital had a system in place to discuss organ donation with family members. The hospital staff introduced the subject of organ and tissue donation in a caring and compassionate manner. Although

Anne had checked the back of her driver's license to indicate she was a donor, her parents were against organ donation. Her father said, "I won't have them cut her up. She won't even be able to have an open casket." Sensing his fear and need for guidance, the hospital staff addressed his concerns and discussed that the appearance of Anne's body would not be changed. He was assured that his daughter's body would be treated with respect and dignity. The casket could remain open and no one would know that she was an organ donor unless they were told. Although the parents did not believe in organ donation and felt torn between their own beliefs and their daughter's, they respected their daughter's wishes. They allowed the donation to take place, and Frank signed the consent form. Although they were not interested in keeping track of Anne's gifts, the organ procurement coordinator told them that this was an option as well as being able to communicate with the recipient through anonymous letters forwarded by the coordinator. The hospital staff recommended that Sally and Frank attend a donor family support group, a place to tell their story and discuss Anne's life. They attended several meetings, where they asked questions and shared their feelings with other grieving families.

Personal Insight
Are you an organ donor? What factors influenced your decision to be or not be a donor?

CASE STUDY

Mr. Gold, a 75-year-old Jewish man living with advanced hypertension, diabetes, and severe heart failure, was no longer able to care for himself. He had difficulty breathing and the pain from his headaches was unbearable. He lived with his wife who was compromised because of intense arthritis. Their son, daughter, and grandchildren lived far away. One night, Mr. Gold got out of bed to go to the bathroom. He fell and broke his hip. After hip replacement surgery, he spent 4 weeks in rehabilitation. Before he was discharged, his blood pressure was uncontrolled and he was diagnosed with pulmonary edema. As a side effect of the medication that was prescribed for him, his blood sugar remained consistently high. He was readmitted to acute care and during his hospitalization, the family met his physician and nurse to discuss his terminal illness and advance directives.

The physician explained, "Living wills are a type of advance directive in which a person's wishes about medical care are written, in case the person is unable to communicate at the end of life." Mr. Gold seemed very confused and told the physician to speak to his wife as she knows what's best. The nurse explained how his wife could become his healthcare proxy.

In a joint meeting, the physician and nurse explained the legal forms in a way Mr. Gold and his wife could comprehend. The physician and nurse helped the couple clarify how the patient would like to die. Mr. Gold deferred to his wife throughout the conversation. Mrs. Gold wanted him to die at home and hospice was recommended.

The nurse reviewed with Mrs. Gold what she felt her husband would want regarding CPR and medical interventions. Although she wanted him to have comfort measures only to relieve pain and suffering, she wanted to discuss the options with her children. She did not want him to be intubated and chose no artificial nutrition. Although Mr. Gold was present through the conversation, he offered no input and trusted his wife to make the decisions for him.

Terminal sedation was explained in terms they could both understand. When the nurse asked Mrs. Gold about what her husband thought about it, Mr. Gold looked at his wife and said, "I don't want to suffer and I want to die at home. Don't let them make me suffer like my parents suffered in the hospital." He talked about his parents' painful deaths

from cancer during the 1960s. The physician and nurse assured him they would make him comfortable.

Questions

1. What alternative care options might be considered?

2. What are the priority care issues to consider in the care of Mr. Gold?

3. How involved should the children be in the decision as they live far away and are not involved in the care?

4. Is the language used to describe the options easy for Mrs. Gold to understand?

Discussion

Discussing advance directives is not an easy task. At first, both Mr. and Mrs. Gold seemed confused with the terminology. Although Mr. Gold was competent, he trusted his wife to make his healthcare decisions for him. Family support is important. The nurse realized Mrs. Gold's role in his care. Although Mr. Gold appeared competent to make decisions regarding his health care, he chose not to. The physician and nurse respected his wishes and addressed options with his wife, even though he was present. The nurse could have spent some time discussing what she believed his children and grandchildren would feel about the decisions Mrs. Gold was making regarding his care. Informing the children of the couple's decisions should be encouraged. Mrs. Gold was given medical power of attorney as she was willing to speak on his behalf, was trusted, and would act on his wishes and separate her own feelings from his. Mr. Gold's parents' painful deaths impacted him. Mr. Gold informed the nurse that he feared that his death might be similarly painful. By discussing these past experiences, the physician and nurse were able to reassure him. A full explanation of the option of palliative care should have been offered.

SUMMARY

End-of-life conversations are often distressful. If physicians and patients are uncomfortable talking about advance directives, it may prevent the patient's wants and desires from being acknowledged, understood, and respected. All patients need to become comfortable talking in advance about the kind of care they desire, especially to address circumstances when they are no longer able to communicate. They can only be comfortable if the professionals helping them are comfortable. Nurses must be aware that patients need their expertise and guidance to make intelligent decisions regarding their directives.

WEB RESOURCES

Aging with Dignity
    http//:www.AgingWithDignity.org

Caring Connections
    http//:www.caringinfo.org

United Network for Organ Sharing (UNOS)
    http//:www.unos.org

EXAM QUESTIONS

CHAPTER 5
Questions 39-44

Note: Choose the one option that BEST answers each question.

39. The type of advance directive in which a person's wishes about medical care are documented is

    a. medical power of attorney.

    b. informed consent.

    c. do not resuscitate.

    d. living will.

40. The advance directive that allows individuals to name a representative to make healthcare decisions if they are incapacitated is called

    a. medical power of attorney.

    b. informed consent.

    c. do not resuscitate.

    d. living will.

41. A legal doctrine requiring physicians to inform patients about their conditions and any risks involved in treatments is

    a. medical power of attorney.

    b. informed consent.

    c. do not resuscitate.

    d. living will.

42. Two types of physician orders related to treatment at the end of life are

    a. Five Wishes and living wills.

    b. DNR and POLST.

    c. informed consent and DNR.

    d. POLST and advance directives.

43. The intentional sedation of terminal patients, rendering them unconscious following other ineffective pain management efforts is

    a. palliative sedation.

    b. opioid rotation.

    c. DNR.

    d. conscious sedation.

44. The ethical principle that allows the nurse to perform an action to achieve a good outcome (such as relieving pain), even if the action can also cause an undesirable effect (such as contributing to a patient's early death), is called the principle of

    a. autonomy.

    b. nonmaleficence.

    c. double effect.

    d. justice.

CHAPTER 6

PALETTE OF GRIEF®

CHAPTER OBJECTIVE

After completing this chapter, the reader will be able to describe how individuals grieve after experiencing a loss.

LEARNING OBJECTIVES

After studying this chapter, the reader will be able to

1. recognize examples of emotional, physical, cognitive, and behavioral reactions to grief.

2. identify four determinants of grief.

3. differentiate between intuitive and instrumental grieving patterns.

4. describe disenfranchised and complicated grief.

INTRODUCTION

Individuals are attached to their loved ones. When that attachment is severed through death, whether anticipated or sudden, they experience grief. Grief is a blending of reactions directly due to loss. In order to better understand how the grief process is perceived by patients, family members, and significant others, nurses need to use terms grieving people use, understand their realities, and be sensitive to that diversity (Rosenblatt, 2008). In this chapter, nurses will learn about the Palette of Grief® concept

and the factors that affect how people cope with loss and influence the way they grieve. Although there is enormous diversity in the emotional responses of grieving individuals (Bonanno, 2004), this chapter will focus on commonalities of the grieving process and what nurses need to know about the way people express their grief.

PALETTE OF GRIEF®

Metaphors

Many individuals refer to their grief process as a "journey of grief." This common phrase is a part of figurative language that expresses what individuals experience after loss. Metaphors are the use of rhetorical expression that help the bereaved fully grasp their story of loss (Rubel, 2011. In Press). Rosenblatt (2008) maintains that metaphors assist individuals to transfer important meanings from a primary, already known domain to a new domain.

Metaphors work because they highlight aspects of the situation to which they are applied. They help to focus attention, organize thinking, and aid perception of certain aspects of the situation. The use of metaphors can capture the individual's point of view and painful emotional experience of grief (Young, 2007-2008). The participants in Young's study reported using the following metaphors to describe their grief:

*   Quicksand, whirlwinds, storms

- The process of glass becoming sand on the beach

- A sand sculpture washed out to sea in the tide

- A bird singing as it flew into the sky

- A ripped page

- Empty chairs

- Fading clouds

- Spider webs and cobwebs.

Arnold and Gemma (2008) maintain that parental grief is complex, ongoing, and non-linear. Parents may use metaphors to describe their grief. Images that metaphorically described their feelings included a volcano that could possibly erupt, falling into a well, and a tree of life without a limb. Three fourths of the parents in this study described a hollow or empty space inside as the most fitting metaphor to describe their grief.

For the metaphor *palette of grief,* the primary concept is a palette. A palette is literally a thin and usually oval flat tablet with a thumb hole at one end that painters hold and use to blend a range of paint colors. When the palette is metaphorically applied to a new domain of loss, it becomes that which holds and blends grief. The Palette of Grief® can include a blending of reactions that are seen as colors of loss (Rubel & McCown, 2007). This metaphor captures the blending of physical, emotional, cognitive, behavioral, and spiritual grief reactions after a final separation.

> *Personal Insight*
> *Have you ever used a metaphor to describe your grief? If so, identify and describe the metaphor.*

Physical Sensations

Grieving individuals may experience physical reactions, such as sensitivity to noise, changes in appetite, headaches, dry mouth, neck and shoulder pain, and tightness in the chest. Females can experience menstrual irregularities. Both men and women may experience an increase in colds and infections. Other physical responses include tiredness or exhaustion. Temporary slowing of reactions, muscular aches, rashes, breathlessness, tension, and exaggeration of allergies are also common. Bereaved persons may also experience bowel and bladder disturbances, feelings of hollowness in the stomach, ulcers, and nausea.

Many newly bereaved individuals experience sleep disturbances, including an inability to fall asleep or sudden awakening from a deep sleep. They may not want to go to sleep for fear of having nightmares or dreams about the deceased. If grieving individuals are having problems sleeping, it might be due to an underlying fear of mortality. They may fear that they will not wake up. If their loved ones died, they recognize that they, too, can die, and this fear can manifest itself in their sleeping patterns. In time, most grieving persons return to their regular sleeping patterns.

Dreams can provide information and insight to the bereaved. During the dream, the deceased may attempt to tell or teach them something. In exploring the meaning of the dream and what transpired, the bereaved may attempt to figure out what a loved one was trying to tell them. This advice can clarify a problem the bereaved person was having and even help to resolve it.

Although dreams can be comforting, they can also be heartbreaking. Upon awaking, dreams make individuals painfully aware that their loved ones are really dead. Imagine a widow, having slept with her spouse for 65 years, faced with sleeping in a bed alone after his death. During a dream, she may see her spouse walking along a beach, his favorite pastime. In seeing him, she is made aware that he is safe and content, but she wakes up alone.

Emotional Reactions

Physical reactions can blend together with emotional reactions, making the separation or loss a difficult process. Emotional factors include shock, numbness, sadness, and fear. Loneliness is especially difficult for those individuals living alone. Emotional reactions are stressful; apathy, crying, and anxiety may be blended with aggression, guilt, withdrawal, rejection, jealousy, pining, yearning, and anger. Anger and rage can be directed at physicians, nurses, God, the deceased, and themselves. Although grieving individuals may be preoccupied with thoughts of the deceased, they may also find relief in their deaths as in the cases of:

- widows who are no longer caretakers of their terminally ill husbands.

- children brought to their dying grandmother's home every day and told to play quietly, who can now run around and make noise.

- daughters who moved into their parents' homes to help their fathers care for their dying mothers and can now move back home with their husbands.

- neighbors with busy schedules who no longer shop for their terminally ill friends.

Bereaved individuals may initially find relief after a death because they no longer watch the person suffer. However, attempts to return to life as it was before the death can bring about guilt feelings. Even though the individuals may have provided excellent care to their loved ones, after the loss the focus can shift to regret over things not done. It is not uncommon to hear "If only I had taken him to the doctor sooner;" "If only I had been to see her that morning;" "If only I had forced him to take his medication and stick to his diet." As the bereaved share their "if onlys" with nurses, it is best to comfort them by listening; it is not necessary to make them see how they are not at fault.

Dos and don'ts of nursing interventions with the bereaved include:

Do:

- Give them an opportunity to voice their concerns.

- Encourage them to express their feelings.

- Offer them an opportunity to test their reality and issues of responsibility.

- Teach them about the grief process.

Don't:

- attempt to make them see why they should not feel that way.

- attempt to change their minds.

Cognitive Reactions

Physical and emotional grief reactions may become blended with cognitions. Alterations in thought processes or cognitive changes may include an inability to concentrate, disorientation, and confusion. Grieving persons may become absent-minded, obsessive in their thinking, and overly critical of their own actions. In addition, individuals may attempt to avoid reminders of the loss, may not want to think about the deceased, or may continually review the circumstances of the death. Certain thoughts help the bereaved find meaning in their experiences. Positive cognitive processing that happens after a death is one of the most important factors in determining likely growth (Tedeschi & Calhoun, 2004).

Behavioral Reactions

Behavioral reactions do not follow a set pattern or sequence. Often the grieving person is reacting to a particular event or trigger. Many grieving individuals experience searching, where they look for their loved ones in a crowd or experience events that remind them of their special persons. They may cry and demonstrate absentminded behavior such as placing keys in the refrigerator, not recalling where their car is parked, or forgetting often-called phone numbers. It is not unusual for a grieving person to become aggressive, hoard, increase their drug use, increase sexual activity, become hyperactive, or talk nonstop. Behavioral reactions may also include changes in eating habits, which can result in weight changes and health problems. Many people retreat into a private world of grief; although this is a normal response, it is during this time that persons need the most support.

Spiritual Reactions

It is not uncommon to hear grieving individuals say, "Life seems empty," or "Something died within me when my loved one died." Grieving individuals may raise questions about their right to be alive, the reason for living, or the reason for dying. They often ask, "Who am I now without you?" They may sense the presence of their loved ones and these post-death encounters may have a healing effect on the bereaved (LaGrand, 2005; Nowatzki & Kalischuk, 2009). Bereaved individuals report that after their post-death encounters with the dead, they feel warmth, love, peace, hope, happiness, and comfort (Nowatzki & Kalischuk, 2009). One participant in the study reported,

> Comforted, I was not afraid. I thought I'd be terrified to stay in the house that he had died in after all the company was gone. I always say to people and even now, "I'm alone but I'm not lonely"…it's like he's…it's a good feeling, it's …almost protection, comforting, I don't know… (Nowatzki & Kalischuk, 2009, p. 96)

Spiritual reactions may revolve around hope. For some bereaved, there is no hope, whereas for others, hope springs eternal. They may spend time in reflection and be hopeful that the meaning and purpose of their lives is found in completing the work of the deceased. Some individuals may struggle with loss and experience distress (e.g., intrusion, avoidance, and hyperarousal), whereas others experience posttraumatic growth at the same time. Posttraumatic growth is a lifelong process (Tedeschi & Calhoun, 2004) that evolves as the bereaved relates to others, considers new possibilities, gains a sense of personal strength, and experiences spiritual changes and appreciation for life (Taku, Calhoun, Cann, & Tedeschi, 2008).

> **_Personal Insight_**
> *Describe a time when you experienced a death of a significant person in your life. What grief reactions did you have to the death?*

DETERMINANTS OF GRIEF

In order to determine why individuals grieve in a certain way, the focus shifts from grief reactions to determinants of grief. In brief, determinants are the things that influence the way individuals grieve after a loss. Let's take a closer look at the metaphor *palette of grief* as it applies to the determinants of grief. In one domain, the palette, a tablet, holds the paint and is where the paint is blended together. When the palette is used metaphorically in a new domain, it becomes that which holds and blends grief. Determinants, metaphorically, paint the *portrait of loss*.

The portrait of loss is comprised of those things that influence the grief colors. Determinants include whether the death was anticipated or sudden, the cultural milieu in which the bereaved lives, and previous losses. Psychological factors, such as the survivor's personality, self-esteem, and coping skills, also influence grief. A history of mental illness and depression plays a role in how a person copes with the death of someone close to him or her. Other determinants in grieving individuals include grief patterns, relationships and attachments, social status, physical and social environments, working conditions, age and gender, historical backgrounds, religion and culture, and types of death.

Grief Patterns

Although few studies have examined gender differences beyond the first months of grief, Doka and Martin (2001) offered two patterns of grief expression – intuitive and instrumental – for understanding grieving styles. Simply stated, intuitive-style grievers express their emotions. Society acknowledges the loss by attempting to offer support. The authors indicated that the intuitive pattern of grief expression occurs when feelings are intensely experienced; expressions such as crying and lamenting mirror the inner experience, and successful adaptive strategies facilitate the experience and expression of feelings. There may be prolonged periods of confusion, inability to concentrate, disorganization, disorientation, physical exhaustion, and anxiety. Intuitive grievers are usually women, who tend to be more expressive in their grief and benefit from sharing their losses.

On the other hand, Martin and Doka (2000) maintain that an instrumental pattern of grief expression occurs when thinking is predominant over feeling as an experience, and feelings are less intense. Bereaved men are socialized to manage instrumental tasks, which can interfere with the grief process. There is general reluctance to talk about feelings; control of oneself and the environment are most important; and problem solving as a strategy enables mastery of feelings and control of the environment. Any emotional expression is done in private. Brief periods of cognitive dysfunction are common and energy levels are enhanced, but symptoms of general arousal go unnoticed. Men are often more behavioral or cognitive in their orientation. Instrumental grievers, whether male or female, do not express their emotions overtly and are therefore less supported by those around them. Because these individual do not express emotions openly, society does not offer them assistance. Being who they are, instrumental grievers would likely reject comfort anyway.

When using the metaphor palette of grief, we can see how the palette can hold colors that are either vibrant or pastel. Although instrumental grievers experience emotions similar to intuitive grievers (e.g., sadness, anxiety, loneliness), the difference is in the intensity of the feelings or the colors of the loss. "For the intuitive griever, feelings are vibrant, intense 'colors;' for the instrumental

griever, they are pastels" (Martin & Doka, 2000, p. 41). It is also possible to have a blend of style or colors "common to both instrumental and intuitive patterns, but with a greater emphasis on one or the other" (Martin & Doka, 2000, p. 51).

***

Personal Insight

Do you consider yourself an intuitive or instrumental griever? Describe why you came to that decision.

***

Gender

It is no secret that most men grieve differently then women. Numerous studies suggest that more women then men show their grief, experience psychiatric symptoms, and seek psychiatric help during the first year after bereavement (Parkes, 2001). Men and women often grieve in different ways. Stillion and Noviello (2001) noted several differences.

Therapists, regardless of gender, believed that men and women express grief differently, men and women differ in the coping mechanisms they use for dealing with grief, and friends and acquaintances respond to grieving men and women differently. Specifically, therapists described men's experience of grief as being briefer and their behavior as more stoic, more task oriented, more pragmatic, and less supported than women's experiences. (p. 254)

Grieving men may display a public image of strength and control and may want to shield their wives and children. Grieving men may avoid seeking help, which they have been conditioned to perceive as not masculine. Men need to be able to ask for and receive support, and professionals can give them permission to do so.

Profound gender differences in grief expression often occur after the sudden death of a couple's child. In a study of parents whose children died by accident, homicide, or suicide between the ages of 12 and 28, fathers' coping strategies included being restrained and cautious. Mothers reported seeking emotional and instrumental support and turning to religion. This suggests that fathers may be more resigned to the death as a fact that cannot be changed and mothers may be more likely to search for answers and have difficulty accepting the death (Murphy, Johnson, & Weber, 2002).

If bereaved men do not express their grief, they are likely to become marginalized grievers, and the pain of their loss will not be supported or validated (Zinner, 2000). After the death of their wives, grieving spouses attempt to find meaning in the death by looking at themselves as survivors with new attitudes and life choices. As men learn to adjust to a world in which their wives are missing, they may experience depression and a decline in health.

Whether or not men accept grief support, professionals should continue to offer support and understanding to male grievers. Mastrogianis and Lumley (2002) found that although social support diminishes the effects of bereavement, society assumes that men grieve silently and alone. The results of their study indicate that bereaved men prefer alternative types of aftercare services, such as golf or bowling, cooking classes, legal assistance, and health promotion classes. The authors found that those men who had a more negative mood were interested in stress management classes.

The assumption that men grieve silently and by themselves may not be true. Recommendations need to be made that best fit a man's style of grieving. Whatever their style, grieving men can find great comfort and support from nurses who recognize and respect their way of grieving.

Culture and Ethnicity

Unfortunately, cultural and ethnic variations in death and grief are not always addressed. As DeSpelder and Strickland (2005) note,

> Ethnic groups and other minorities are underrepresented in the resource materials commonly used in death education courses. Although this situation has improved somewhat over the last decade or so, many of the "lessons taught" are still based on studies of a predominantly middle-class, white population. (p. 536)

Culture and ethnicity are significant determinants of grief. Culture is a shared set of beliefs, values, and practices that structure behaviors and the way people act at the end of life. A culturally competent healthcare system recognizes and incorporates cultural diversity, the assessment of cross-cultural relations, cultural differences, the expansion of cultural knowledge, and services to meet culturally unique needs (Cort, 2004). Although some nurses may make generalizations about grief based on their own past experiences and backgrounds, it is important to look at grieving individuals as part of a cultural group. Cultural competence involves assessing, understanding, and taking responsibility for one's own beliefs and attitudes; learning about and expanding understanding and experience with diverse individuals and groups; and becoming respectful proponents of multiculturalism (Marsh, 2004).

Even though dying patients and their families are of a particular ethnicity, there are differences in customs due to their religions, economic levels, educations, and primary languages. Nurses need to be sensitive to and aware of cultural variables affecting end-of-life care, such as the patient's country of origin, age at time of immigration to the United States, length of time living in the United States, where they live, and the degree of cultural integration in their community.

Experiences of loss are melded onto a core system of cultural values, beliefs, and identity that are continuously edited by grieving individuals (Hunter, 2007-2008). As individuals assimilate into American culture, their grief, bereavement, and mourning traditions are being diluted. The American influence on these norms will gradually bring an end to traditional cultural expressions that may appear strange to those who have no understanding of their origins (Kauffman, 2008).

Knowing and respecting ethnicity and cultural backgrounds of patients and their families will help nurses understand the choices made regarding care. Nurses can reinforce the traditional beliefs and practices and recognize that certain beliefs bring comfort. They can utilize questions as opportunities to learn about the significance of the cultural beliefs. Basic questions to reflect upon when treating terminally ill patients of various cultures include:

- What are the patient's attitudes about Western medicine?

- What are the patient's beliefs about diagnosis and treatment?

- Where did the patient go for health information?

- Who are the religious leaders and what are their roles at the end of life?

Cultural variations in end-of-life practices exist in non-White racial or ethnic groups due to their lack of knowledge regarding advance directives and their less likelihood of supporting advance directives (Kwak & Haley, 2005). African Americans were consistently found to prefer the use of life support, and Asians and Hispanics are more likely to prefer family-centered decision making, than other racial or ethnic groups (Kwak & Haley, 2005). Mexican Americans, Korean Americans, and members of Canadian First Nations prefer family-based decision making at the end of life, whereas European Americans prefer patient autonomy (Thomas, Wilson, Justice, Birch, & Sheps, 2008).

Asian culture is centered on the extended family, with the entire family making all decisions regarding the patient. Older Asian Americans often look to their family members to help them make their healthcare decisions. Younger Asians may believe it is their duty to assume the decision-making roles. Asian Americans represent a diverse group of cultures, including Japanese, Korean, Vietnamese, Chinese, and more. Their culture stresses family

obligation and burying the dead. Although women perform rites, men are responsible for the more elaborate rites as well as rituals of the dead. Rituals usually take place on the 21st, 35th, and 49th days after the funeral. Friends visit the mourners in their homes, where a plate with wrapped candy is placed on the table. Visitors take the candy, eat it, and throw away the wrappers before they reach home, as the candy wards off bad luck for those who came into proximity of death.

Chinese culture is greatly influenced by the philosophies and religions of Confucianism, Taoism, and Buddhism. Social sharing of bereavement is not highly valued by the Chinese after the death, as their culture is influenced by Confucian philosophy, which focuses on maintaining harmony in social relationships (Chow, Chan, & Ho, 2007). If they outwardly express their grief with others it will contradict the harmony of those relationships. Therefore, the goal of many bereaved Chinese is to follow the flow and to peacefully accept fate (Chow et al., 2007).

Religion

Many individuals find comfort from faith based upon a belief in and reverence for a higher power and a creator of the universe. Most Americans are fairly religious. According to a CBS News Poll conducted in April, 2006, 82% of Americans believe in God; 9% believe in some sort of universal spirit or higher power; and 85% consider religion at least somewhat important in their daily lives (PollingReport.com, 2006). Based on one's religion, individuals maintain a set of principles, beliefs, values, and practices. Although over one third of Americans are not members of a religious congregation, the vast majority of them mark deaths through communal rituals performed by religious professionals (Garces-Foley, 2002-2003). These communal rituals and ceremonies can be based on religious or philosophical systems.

Individuals express their faith through both public experiences and private activities. A public experience includes attending a house of worship. A private experience includes praying or watching a religious program on television. A 74-year-old widow illustrated the significance of prayer in stating, "When the doctor told me there was nothing more to do, I remember smiling and saying I can always pray" (Martin & Doka, 2000, p. 142).

Although clergy and chaplains are trained to perform grief ceremonies and rituals, all healthcare professionals should be aware of the importance of these death-related healing experiences. By appreciating the significance of such ceremonies, nurses are better able to understand what was and continues to be significant to the patient and family. The teachings of spiritual leaders and religious practices may sustain the bereaved, although Murphy, Johnson, Lohan, and Tapper (2002) found that personal and family prayer and church attendance did not improve outcomes over time for parents bereaved by a child's violent death.

A crisis of faith occurs when one's normal, established relationship with their higher power is violated and apparently leaves them helpless in making sense of their loyalty to God and acceptance of principles of their religion (Webb, 2001). A grieving individual may feel abandoned by God, have difficulty praying, see no purpose in life, and have no sense of joy or hope (Webb, 2004).

Every religion has among its doctrines a point of view regarding death. These views can range from seeing death as a punishment to viewing it as a transition to a better existence. Lester et al. (2001-2002) examined university undergraduates' beliefs about the afterlife. Questions asked regarding feelings about life after death were:

- "Do you believe that there is life after death?"

- "Do you believe that the afterlife is in a specific place?"

- "Is there a Heaven?"

- "Is the afterlife the same for everyone?"

- "Is the afterlife affected by the timing of one's death?"

- "Is there a Hell?" (p.125)

Lester's study found that 89% of the subjects believed in life after death. Ninety percent reported that there is a Heaven and 95% reported the belief that they would be reunited with family and friends in the afterlife. A significant number of students (93%) reported that belief in the afterlife is comforting.

A significant body of research indicates that people use religion and spirituality in situations of bereavement (Brown, Nesse, House, & Utz, 2004; Wortmann & Park, 2008). Whether supporting bereaved Jews, Catholics, Buddhists, Muslims, Hindus, or those of other faiths, nurses must be sensitive to various belief systems; make appropriate referrals to religious community resources; avoid insincere expressions of condolences; and recognize that everyone grieves in their own ways. Therefore, the following sections illuminate some beliefs and practices of various religious bodies of faith.

> **Personal Insight**
> *Do you believe there is a life after death?*
> *Does that belief bring you comfort?*

Jewish Beliefs and Practices

Jewish customs depend upon whether the individual practices Orthodox, Conservative, or Reform Judism. Most Jewish patients want to be told when they are near death. They want to be treated with dignity and respect during the time of their dying and immediately after death. After death, bodies must be watched over by persons for 24 hours until burial. Autopsies are usually forbidden unless there was a criminal action that caused the death. Within the Jewish culture, the bodies of deceased Jews are ritually cleansed by a Jewish individual. The deceased is then dressed in a white linen shroud and placed in a simple wooden casket, which is closed. There is no viewing of the body.

The spouse takes full responsibility for making arrangements for the funeral, which usually takes place the day following the death. Years ago, the rabbi would tear a small piece of the mourner's clothing, usually their shirt, to symbolize mourning. Today, most Jewish mourners wear a torn black ribbon to symbolize being inwardly torn by their grief. The service takes place at the funeral home or at the cemetery and is officiated by a rabbi. Though cremation is contrary to Jewish law, the practice is permitted by Reform Jews.

At the cemetery, Jewish mourners will say the kaddish, a prayer that praises God. Jews may find comfort reading from their prayer book, the siddur. No headstone is placed at the gravesite until 6 months to a year later. This ritual of placing the headstone on the grave is called an unveiling. It is customary for family members to attend the funeral.

After the funeral, friends and family return to the mourner's home, which signifies the beginning of the shivah period, which lasts for 7 days. If nurses wanted to express their condolences they could visit the mourners during the shivah period. It is customary for anyone who attended the funeral to ritually wash their hands before entering the home. A small pitcher and towels are usually left at the entrance to the front door for the mourners entering the home. Food is brought to the home from neighbors. Hard-boiled eggs, in particular, symbolize the continuation of life. As signs of mourning, family members sit on low wooden stools and all the mirrors are covered in the home. It is not customary to send flowers to Jewish mourners. In lieu of flowers, a donation to a hospital, hospice, or other medical foundation is appreciated.

Christian Beliefs and Practices

The branches of Christianity include Protestantism, Eastern and Oriental Orthodoxy, and Catholicism. After a Christian death, the body is usually embalmed and placed in a casket, which may be plain or ornate. Cremation is also accepted by Christians. For approximately 2 days after the death, mourners, friends, and family pay their respects at a vigil. This sharing of time at the funeral home is called a wake, and the casket may be open or closed.

Christians believe that after death they go to Heaven, where one day all Christians will be reunited. The vast majority of Christians believe in some kind of Heaven and a slightly lesser majority of Christians believe in the existence of Hell, where unbelievers or sinners are punished (Religion Facts, 2009). Exline (2003) studied the belief in Heaven and Hell among Christians in the United States and found only 8% of Christian participants in the study believed Hell definitely existed and 62% of Christian participants believed that Heaven definitely existed.

Symbols unique to Christians are images of Jesus Christ crucified and resurrected. These symbols help the bereaved identify that even though they are suffering, their Lord also suffered. Christians are comforted by Psalm 23, which speaks of the deceased walking through the valley of death without fear because God is with them on their journey. Flowers are sent to the funeral home. The casket, covered in flowers, is brought to the cemetery in a hearse with the procession of mourners following behind. After the funeral and burial, friends or fellow church members may provide a meal for the family and friends.

There are certain practices unique to Catholics. Common symbols are the use of holy water or consecrated oil to bless the deceased. Dying Catholics are given last rites, a ritual of anointing. The funeral is incorporated into the Mass, officiated by a priest, and consists of prayers, Bible readings, and celebration of the Eucharist. Mass cards are left indicating that prayers are being said for the deceased.

Being that there is a rapid growth of the Hispanic population in the United States, learning about the practices of Hispanic Christians is also of importance. Hispanics include several subcultures, such as Mexican Americans, Cubans, Central and

South Americans, and Puerto Ricans. The Hispanic culture is male dominated. Family and extended family are very important. Husbands generally make the decisions at the end of life. Hispanics are very spiritual, and with deep sorrow, they sob for what is lost. Some Hispanics appoint a pastor to commend the body with a prayer. The wake, a social celebration, usually lasts one whole day with the view of the body. Diaz-Cabello (2004) notes that Hispanic mourners will grieve openly, drink hot chocolate, play dominos or cards, and talk about and remember the deceased. Every member of the family is included in the rituals. A significant day for Hispanics is the Day of the Dead as a time to remember those who have died.

Approximately 70% of adult Hispanics are Catholic, and 20% are Protestant or another Christian faith (Perl, Greely, & Gray, 2004). The followers of Catholicism may request the sacrament of the sick. Priests anoint dying persons with oil that has been blessed by a bishop. It is then massaged into the person's forehead. For nine days after the death, the mourners gather at the house of the deceased to pray the Rosary. On the last day, the cross is raised. For one year, the family can request a Mass once a month, and then once annually.

Buddhist Beliefs and Practices

Buddhists look at death and dying in a unique way. According to Buddhism, there are eight stages in the dying process. For many centuries, Buddhists have believed that as individuals go through each stage, changes occur bringing them closer to death. Through the stages, the eyesight fades, the body becomes weak, the hearing dissolves, the body becomes numb, and the need to eat diminishes, until the person finally enters an unconscious state. Although there are eight stages in the dying process, Buddhists do not look at the last stage, death, as the end of a person's existence. In the eighth stage, the person journeys into a new spiritual dimension. Death is considered an awakening, and dying is viewed as being reborn.

The dying person's state of mind is of great importance. Friends, family, and monks who recite Buddhist scriptures and mantras usually surround dying Buddhists. This death-related ritual helps the dying person achieve a peaceful state of mind. After a death, Buddhists say prayers, meditate, and do a good deed such as making a donation to a charity. They can also donate some of the deceased's money to a worthy cause, which allows the deceased to have a good rebirth and attain enlightenment. The funeral is simple and dignified.

Though cremation is the preferred funeral rite of Buddhists, contemporary Buddhist practice includes both burial and cremation. Many Buddhists who cremate their loved ones find comfort in watching the cremation, as in the case of a Buddhist couple whose infant died while they were living in the United States. The parents insisted on watching as their infant's body was cremated. This scenario speaks to the concerns of individuals who have different belief systems from professional helpers.

> Funeral directors explained that igniting the fires with the changer doors open was against crematorium procedures in that state – it would endanger anybody present. After days of negotiations, a remote facility was located where the director found no problem in granting the request. Crematorium operators, however, were appalled to see the parents leaning forward to watch the tiny body being placed inside the furnace. (Moody & Arcangel, 2001, p. 61)

Muslim Beliefs and Practices

Islamic faith defines death as an obligatory transitional experience connecting "life before death" and "life after death" (Hossain & Siddique, 2008). In the religion of Islam, Muslim mourners acknowledge Allah as God. A Muslim may say, "It is the will of Allah" to the deceased person's family, as death is a transition from a temporary life to immortal life. Although no one knows the exact time of his or her death, devoted Muslims believe that God has determined the exact time of death for every individual (Al-Sabwah & Abdel-Khalek, 2006).

Dying Muslims may choose to face toward Mecca surrounded by their family members who recite Muslim scripture from the Koran. This encourages the terminally ill person to be patient with his or her suffering. After the death, the body is washed and covered completely with a white scented shroud; feet should be directed toward Mecca, their holy city. Burial is performed as soon as possible. Hossain and Siddique (2008) found that the more religious Muslims are, the better their adjustment to death. Women may shout and wail at the time of announcement of the death, whereas men may remain silent, quietly weeping (Yasien-Esmael & Rubin, 2005). Muslims may weep as long as the crying is without shouting. Cremation is not common among Muslims.

Hindu Beliefs and Practices

Nurses working with Hindus should expect family and friends to chant and recite religious prayers. Fathers or elder males are the primary spokespersons regarding patients' healthcare decisions. The followers of Hinduism fast on a regular basis, and a family member may fast on behalf of a dying relative. They do this hoping to please a god who can bestow health. Hindus look at death as a passage from one life to another.

Traditionally, Hindus die in their own homes. Holy water or butter is placed on their lips while family members sing devotional prayers and mantras. Some Hindus place the person on the floor as they die. Hindus believe that when a person dies, a rebirth takes place. Males younger than 11 years of age and females 7 years of age and younger are buried, rather than cremated. For all others, Hindus believe that the physical body must be cremated in order for the soul to carry on into another incarnation on its karmic journey.

Prior to the cremation, the body is washed. Wearing a shroud, the body is surrounded by flowers and carried to the funeral pyre. The closest relative (usually male) lights the funeral pyre. Mourners usually wear white. The cremains are then collected and immersed in a holy river. After the funeral, mourners take a purifying bath, and after several days, mourners eat a ceremonial meal and give to charity. Only males can perform the death rites, which are believed to help the deceased on his or her journey.

> ### Personal Insight
> *What rituals of your faith will most likely sustain you when your loved one is dying or when your loved one has died?*

Historical Background

The past history and background of loss is another determinant of grief. How bereaved individuals handled previous losses and whether those losses were resolved impacts their current grief experiences. The number of losses, the age at which those losses occurred, the suddenness or anticipation of those losses, and the types of deaths experienced are all factors that affect how individuals respond to their current losses.

Bereaved Older Adults

The usual indicator for old age is chronological age. Although humans' maximum potential life span is about 115 years, most Americans live about 76 years. Aging is a natural and gradual process. With more and more older people living into their 70s, it is estimated that by the year 2030, the number of older Americans will have more than doubled to 71 million (CDC, NCHS, 2008).

As our population ages, we will encounter an increasing number of older persons who will need our assistance in coping with the cumulative impact of the unintentional and intentional losses encountered through their lifetimes. Sadly, many of them will live their last years widowed. Gamino, Hogan, and Sewell (2002) found that bereaved elderly persons experience inner voids, a loss of part of themselves, and a sense of finality and permanence; they lack companionship, interdependence, and an anticipated future (p. 809). Elderly bereaved persons placed the death of their friends in the context of their life course and history of losses, with a profound sense of survivorship due to their outliving the significant people in their lives (de Vries, Blieszner, & Blando, 2002, p. 235). In 2007, an estimated 74,632 Americans died of Alzheimer's disease and the preliminary age-adjusted death rate from Alzheimer's disease did not change significantly between 2006 and 2007 (CDC, 2010a). Many older people lose long-time friends due to Alzheimer's disease, which passed diabetes to become the sixth leading cause of death in the United States in 2007 (CDC, 2010a).

Often, family members ignore their elderly loved one's loss of friends to death and do not acknowledge the bond that they shared. One woman commented that she missed "not being necessary to anyone." One man, describing the circumstances following the death of his friend, said: "His family didn't seem to care much about him in his life. After his accident, they all came out to the coast, formed a sort of human shield around him denying us access to him or even knowledge about his condition. They swept through the house taking his belongings and left us with nothing – not even a chance to speak at the funeral" (de Vries et al., 2002, p. 235).

Grandparents experience a double grief when a grandchild dies. They grieve the personal loss of their grandchild, and they grieve for their own children's pain of loss. As they see their children grieving, they may attempt to be strong in order to provide support. Nursing interventions could include encouraging grieving grandparents to express their grief openly in front of their children and grandchildren. Sharing their grief with their children will give the entire family an opportunity to talk with and listen to each other during this time. Bereaved grandparents should support and

comfort those they love without losing sight of their own needs.

Research has shown that older individuals experience the same grief reactions as younger individuals (deVries et al., 2002). As with other grieving individuals, the older person's grief response could include appetite changes, sleep disturbances, crying, anger, sadness, guilt, and helplessness. Boelen and Van Den Bout (2002-2003) found the course of traumatic grief symptoms appears to be relatively independent of the age of the bereaved and the nature of the death.

WHAT DO NURSES NEED TO KNOW ABOUT GRIEF?

As nurses provide comfort to those who mourn, they need to recognize that grief is a normal process. Although grief can be distasteful, painful, and excruciating to watch, nurses cannot walk away from the experience of loss. Nurses are responsible for understanding the grief process, recognizing that each person's grief is a unique experience, and respecting all faiths' and cultural expressions of loss.

Balk (2004) notes that positive grief outcomes are frequently accompanied by better problem-solving skills, personal growth, and maturity among the bereaved. The Project on Death in America commissioned the Center for the Advancement of Health to assess the state of research on grief in order to make recommendations that guide high-quality, appropriate grief and bereavement care (Genevro, Marshall, & Miller, 2004). It is important for nurses to understand that the field has become theoretically diversified, and multiple models and theories are applicable when providing support to the bereaved.

Genevro et al. (2004) report that although loss may be universal, responses are widely variable. Grief is not an exclusively medical problem, but an individual and societal event with potential medical implications. Advances have been made in identifying, measuring, and understanding the biological effects of bereavement, especially in terms of neuroendocrine, immunologic, and sleep responses. The Genevro report also noted that studies are being done to identify risk factors for normal and complicated grief and the significance of maintaining continuing bonds with the deceased. Two additional findings from their research are: (a) Some grieving individuals experience positive emotions and don't experience distress or grief; and (b) Counseling may not be helpful for many people experiencing normal grief and may even have negative effects. Although the sorrow one feels over the loss of a loved one can last a lifetime, most people cope with their grief and integrate the loss into their lives without professional help. However, individuals who experience disenfranchised or complicated grief may benefit from supportive interventions.

Disenfranchised Grief

Typically, when individuals experience losses, social support is received from their communities, but society may not appreciate or acknowledge certain losses and therefore social support for the grieving person is denied. Disenfranchised grief is the name given to an experience of a loss that is not or cannot be openly acknowledged, publicly mourned, or socially supported (Doka, 2002).

During the early years of the AIDS epidemic, the causes and transmission of the disease were poorly understood. Individuals with AIDs were often ostracized. When persons died of AIDS, bereaved individuals often became disenfranchised grievers as other individuals disconnected behaviorally and emotionally from them. Those in the gay community lost many of their friends to AIDS. These grieving individuals experienced anxiety, anger, and depression due to the multiple deaths, and the cumulative impact of these deaths affected the survivors' abilities to mourn. The loss of their support systems were other losses felt by those who

had loved ones die of AIDS (Ingram, Jones, & Smith, 2001). Therefore, this type of disenfranchised grief was likely experienced by thousands in the United States.

Disenfranchised grief can occur after a miscarriage, abortion, or early infant death. Gerber-Epstein, Leichtentritt, and Benyamini (2009) studied women who had experienced a miscarriage and found that physicians can cause women to feel disenfranchised in their grief. A mother reported her feelings in response to her doctor's remarks during an examination:

We came for a routine check-up…"Yes, I see a pregnancy sac, but I don't, I don't see an embryo, there is no embryo." What does it mean, no embryo?! After the examination I try to ask questions, what does it mean, I'm sort of frightened, what – no embryo?…"No, look, you've got nothing to worry about, you'll have a bleed in a few days." And…that's it. Something like this, tossed into the air, and we're trying to ask, to understand. I'm not a stupid person [laughs]. What do you mean, no embryo! What do you mean, a bleed, no bleed! And – nothing. He simply brushed us off. I started to cry, but right away put my hand on my mouth, because I felt awkward…I sat in the doctor's waiting room, crying and trembling. (p. 11)

Another grieving mother offered the following advice to other grieving women, doctors, and those around them,

Emphasize this aspect, that it's all right to mourn, know how to say it to people – perhaps it's different for each one, one may need more time and another less…The professionals also must emphasize to these mothers, these women, that they're not alone or that they're not freaks. (Gerber-Epstein, Leichtentritt, & Benyamini, 2009, p. 21)

These mothers clearly felt disenfranchised in their grief. Disenfranchised grief can also be experienced after abortions, when women may still grieve the loss of their fetuses and the loss of their innocence. Although any infant death may cause grief, many individuals don't openly acknowledge their losses or publicly mourn. Though painful, the grief may be disenfranchised because society did not acknowledge the loss (Gajdos, 2002).

Disenfranchised grief can occur in those who have developmental disabilities and reside in residential communities. Hoover, Markell, and Wagner (2004-2005) found that after a loved one's death, only a small percentage of individuals with disabilities attend funerals and memorial meals, a slightly lower percentage take part in rituals at burial or cremation, and less than half of them participate in other rites, rituals, and death activities. The authors indicated that only 7% help plan the funeral and 3% receive counseling or support.

Disenfranchised grief can also occur in children, employees, suicide survivors, ex-spouses, and nursing home residents. Children are often unrecognized grievers. If a child has a friend or peer die, the loss is rarely openly acknowledged as adults attempt to shield the child from the pain of loss. Unrecognized grievers include employees who are not given time off to attend funerals of close friends. Another death that is not socially sanctioned is suicide, especially if the suicide was caused by autoerotica asphyxia. People may be uncomfortable expressing grief to the mourners due to the type of death. There are special problems for ex-spouses who become disenfranchised in coping with their ex-spouse's terminal illness and dying. Another group of grievers often unrecognized and disenfranchised are older men and women who reside in nursing homes; often the death of a fellow resident is handled quietly without opportunity for social support and direct expression of grief by the other residents.

Healthcare professionals, including nurses, frequently experience loss and grief related to patient deaths. This is especially true for those working in long-term care facilities, hospices, and oncology units. Nurses need to recognize their own grief responses when patients die and seek out support.

Personal Insight

If you have ever cried after a patient died, how did your coworkers respond to you as you grieved the patient's death?

If you have not experienced the death of a patient, how do you think your coworkers would respond to you if you cried?

PROLONGED GRIEF DISORDER (COMPLICATED GRIEF)

In 1997, Horowitz and his associates created the diagnostic criteria for complicated grief disordcr. In 2001, Prigerson and Jacobs modified Horowitz's complicated grief criteria. Further testing and empirical work is necessary to evaluate the reliability, validity, sensitivity, specificity, and diagnostic efficiency of the criteria proposed for complicated grief (Hogan, Worden, & Schmidt, 2005-2006; Prigerson & Maciejewski, 2005-2006). There is debate regarding whether "complicated" grief should be officially recognized as a mental disorder and included in the fifth edition of the *Diagnostic and Statistical Manual of Mental Disorders* (American Psychiatric Association [APA], 2000).

Horowitz (2005-2006) maintains complicated grief should be included with posttraumatic stress disorder in a new category of stress response syndromes. Prigerson and Vanderwerker (2005-2006) report that complicated grief should be included in a new category of attachment disorders. Parkes (2005-2006) maintains that complicated grief could be included with personality disorders, whereas Goodkin et al. (2005-2006) indicate that complicated grief should be included in the *DSM-V,* but only within Appendix B as a disorder proposed for further study.

Hogan et al. (2005-2006) noted that complicated grief disorder was formerly called traumatic grief and Goldsmith, Morrison, Vanderwerker, and Prigerson (2008) refer to complicated grief as prolonged grief disorder. Other terms used to describe complicated grief include chronic, conflicted, continued, dysfunctional, impaired, prolonged, unfinished, and unresolved. To resolve the differences between the consensus diagnostic criteria for traumatic grief and complicated grief disorder, the criteria for both disorders have been integrated to become the criteria for prolonged grief disorder, the diagnostic standard proposed for inclusion in *DSM-V* (Prigerson et al., 2009).

Prolonged grief disorder occurs when the momentous event of death devastates a mourner to a point of suffering intense grief that involves at least one of two symptoms of separation distress (i.e., yearning, intense pangs of separation distress); and the mourner has had significant functional impairment for at least 6 months from experiencing daily (or to a disabling degree) a minimum of five of the following:

1. feeling emotionally numb
2. feeling stunned or shocked
3. feeling that life is meaningless
4. confusion about one's role in life
5. diminished sense of self
6. mistrust of others
7. difficulty accepting the loss
8. avoidance of the reality of the loss
9. bitterness over the loss, and difficulty moving on with life.

(Schaal, Elbert, & Neuner, 2009)

Symptoms

Complicated grief symptoms appear to be relatively independent of the age of the bereaved and type of death (Boelen & Van den Bout, 2002-2003). Symptoms include: intense grief with longing; yearning; pining that exists for at least 6 months; feelings of bitterness; anger; preoccupation with and/or avoiding memories; inability to accept the death; and estrangement from others (Monk, Houck, & Shear, 2006). Complicated grief has also been found to be related to a heightened risk of suicidal thoughts and actions among young adult friends of adolescents who completed suicide (Prigerson et al., 1999). Complicated grief has been shown to predict decreased social function, mental health, and energy level in contrast to those bereaved individuals who do not have symptoms of complicated grief (Silverman et al., 2000).

Prigerson et al. (2002) point out that complicated grief symptoms have been assessed in those whose family members died in violent ways. Such symptoms included longing, yearning, anger, and bitterness. Although complicated grief is often provoked by violent deaths, the symptoms have also been observed in those whose family members died from health problems or surgery. The bereaved experienced pain in the same parts of their bodies as their loved ones had during their illnesses and deaths. Other symptoms included being envious of those who were not bereaved. They could not imagine being fulfilled and felt a lost sense of security and trust. Prigerson and Vanderwerker (2005-2006) maintain that most complicated grievers feel somewhat paralyzed by grief. They don't want to be socially isolated and very much want help. Wilsey and Shear (2007) found that the absence, rudeness, or aggression of others caused distress to and angered individuals experiencing complicated grief. The authors found people with complicated grief are especially sensitive of those who are not around, and those who are present but outwardly insensitive to their losses.

Several participants in the study noted noticeably harsh behaviors on the part of family, friends, or professionals that initiate emotions in the grieving individual that were beyond the limits of effective coping. Laurie and Neimeyer (2008) found that overall, African Americans reported higher levels of complicated grief symptoms than Caucasians, particularly when they did not take a lot of time sharing their losses with others. Monke et al. (2006) examined 64 patients participating in an ongoing complicated grief treatment study and found certain elements of their routine were added or missed due to their loved ones' deaths. Participants reported adding an afternoon nap and an evening snack or drink significantly more frequently. The authors found that individuals suffering from complicated grief were significantly more likely to miss personal contacts, breakfast, lunch, dinner, work, exercise, and going outside compared with 64 participants in a non- complicated grief comparison group.

Treatment for Complicated Grief

Individuals with severe grief symptoms may tend to have positive attitudes about a diagnosis of complicated grief, and this may not differ if they met the proposed criteria for this disorder (Johnson et al., 2009). A majority of bereaved in a recent study reported that if they met criteria for a grief disorder, they would be relieved to know they had a recognizable problem; they would find it helpful to know their grief symptoms were due to a bereavement-related distress syndrome (Johnson et al., 2009).

Although some have found bereavement interventions for complicated grief to be ineffective (Holland, Neimeyer, Currier, & Berman, 2007), Shear, Frank, Houck, and Reynolds (2005) reported encouraging findings related to the efficacy of a complicated grief treatment program. This treatment program included interpersonal psychotherapy focused on restoring a satisfying life. The intervention also focused on identifying trauma-like symptoms and retelling the traumatic story.

There is also a difference of opinions regarding when professionals should assess and intervene. Ott and Lueger (2002) found that professionals should assess individuals for complicated grief at 6 months and also at 9, 12, 15, and 18 months or later. Actual interventions should take place when the bereaved want help for their impaired social and occupational functions. Among ways to support these grieving individuals is to review how they have reacted to the losses and the factors that influence their reactions. Some of the factors include the circumstances of the events, the nature of the relationships, the interactions between the survivors and society, and the physical condition of the bodies.

Botella, Osma, Palacios, Guillén, and Baños (2008) treated complicated grief using virtual reality called EMMA's World. This innovative treatment program used an adaptive display consisting of computers and projectors. Patients experiencing complicated grief were shown virtual environments (e.g., a desert, an island, a threatening forest, a town covered in snow, and meadows) that reflected emotions. The display was adapted to various landscapes (e.g., from day to night; from sunlight to cloudy) which helped the complicated grievers confront and manage their own emotions. Virtual reality treatment helped individuals in this study to process the death by:

- engaging in mindfulness strategies.
- finding meaningful sense to the loss.
- working with narratives, meanings, and symbols in therapy.
- addressing the trauma-like symptoms by confronting the avoided memories.
- educating themselves on the bereavement process.
- slow breathing training to deal with physiological symptoms.
- exposure.

- cognitive restructuring.

More research is needed to support the treatment efficacy of interventions for those experiencing complicated grief.

CASE STUDY

*B*arbara, a 30-year-old Caucasian, is 33 weeks pregnant with triplets. She is brought into the emergency room in labor and is given medication to stop the contractions. The patient is given a private room on the maternity ward in a section of high-risk mothers. Due to the high-risk level of her pregnancy, she is admitted to the hospital where she remains until the babies are born 3 weeks later. She gives birth by cesarean delivery to triplets weighing 5 lbs; 5 lb, 11 oz; and 6 lb.

Later that day, the babies are brought into their mother's room for their first feeding. Yet unnamed, they are Triplet #1, Triplet #2, and Triplet #3. As the nurse wheels in one of the infants to Barbara, she notices a patient, a young woman, in the room directly across from her in bed facing the door. That woman watches as Triplet #1 is brought to his mother. With tears streaming down her face, she stares at Barbara who is excited to see her triplets. Barbara notices her crying but is not aware that she had, that same morning, given birth to a disabled infant who died during childbirth.

The nurse places the first of the three babies by Barbara's bedside and leaves to retrieve the second of the triplets. In a moment, the nurse returns with the second baby, cheerfully exclaiming in the doorway, "Here's Triplet #2. Barbara looks up to watch as her triplet is brought in for his feeding and notices the patient across the hall gasp and loudly cry out, "Two babies? Why does she have two babies and my baby died?" Although the nurse also heard what the patient said, she does not enter the young woman's room, acknowledge her grief, nor does she close Barbara's door. As the nurse leaves the room to retrieve Triplet #3, Barbara is left alone with her two sons for the first time. Because she has

had a cesarean delivery she cannot get up to close the door. Although she attempts to focus on her two sons, she cannot help but see the young woman staring at her and her babies through her tears.

Barbara realizes that Triplet #3 is about to be brought in. She knows the nurse will be cheerful and excited about bringing the third baby into her room for the first time. The mother is torn between the pleasure of being with her sons and bearing witness to another woman's painful experience of grief caused by the death of her infant. As Triplet #3 is wheeled in, Barbara is wracked with guilt as she hears the young mother scream, "Three babies? She has three babies? That's not fair. Why did God give her three babies and take my baby?"

Without saying a word, the nurse immediately leaves the room, walks into the young woman's room across the hall and closes her door. She does not speak of the incident when she later checks on Barbara.

Questions

1. What is important for nurses to understand about loss, the bereavement field, and theories of grief?

2. What could the nurse have said to the mother of triplets before going into the other patient's room?

3. What would you have said to the grieving patient?

4. Should the patient who experienced the perinatal death have been moved to another room after her loss?

5. What should the nurse have said to the mother of triplets after she left the other patient's room?

6. How do you think the mother of triplets was affected by the experience?

Discussion

One of the biggest challenges of nursing is balancing joyous moments with devastating ones, from saving lives to watching patients die. The nurse in this case study had to balance joy and grief at the same time. She could have been more effective doing both. The nurse was uncaring to the grieving patient. The babies should have been brought into their mother's room without any exclamations in the doorway in consideration of the close proximity of the grieving patient. It is obvious the nurse is excited about bringing in the babies and not considering the grief of the patient across the hall.

Nursing interventions include providing for basic emotional needs. If the nurse was aware that the patient experienced a perinatal death that morning, she could have had the patient moved to another room. She could have called pastoral care to offer support to the bereaved mother whose emotional needs were clearly neglected. Upon realizing the situation, the nurse could have stayed with the bereaved patient and asked another nurse to bring in Triplet #2 and Triplet #3 to their mother. At the very least, she could have shut the door so the bereaved mother would not have to observe a scene so devastating to her.

After the third baby was brought into the mother's room, the nurse could have talked to the mother of the triplets about the incident and helped her deal with the patient's outbursts. The nurse could assess the triplet mother's psychological needs, noting such clues as the stress of a cesarean delivery, having three babies to feed at one time, and the incident of the grieving mother. Being with her triplets for the first time was an exciting experience for the mother that was made painful by awareness of the other mother's loss. The nurse could encourage the mother of triplets to discuss the incident later that day when she went to check on her or see if she needed to talk to pastoral care. Being that the mother was in a high-risk section of the maternity floor, the nurse could advise her that she may meet mothers who experienced the death of their children. Ideally, bereaved mothers should not be placed in close proximity to mothers with surviving newborns.

Note: This scenario actually happened to the author of this book on the day she gave birth to triplets.

SUMMARY

This chapter highlighted grief's origins and defined grief as a process that includes the blending of physical, emotional, cognitive, and behavioral reactions due to loss. Nurses can educate themselves about grief to be more effective in providing support to bereaved patients and families. As individuals describe their journey of grief, nurses should realize that metaphors are often part of the language of loss. It does not matter what phrases grieving individuals use to describe their losses, what matters is that they are allowed to express themselves openly with nurses who are comfortable sharing those experiences with them.

WEB RESOURCES

AARP
    http://www.aarp.org

A Program of National Grief Support Services
    http://www.griefsupportservices.org

The Dougy Center
    http://www.dougy.org

Hospice Foundation of America
    http://www.hospicefoundation.org

Tragedy Assistance Program for Survivors (TAPS)
    http://www.taps.org

EXAM QUESTIONS

CHAPTER 6
Questions 45-51

Note: Choose the one option that BEST answers each question.

45. Physical, emotional, behavioral, and cognitive reactions after a final separation or loss are referred to as

   a. grief.
   b. hysteria.
   c. major depressive disorder.
   d. culture.

46. Determinants of grief are

   a. defined stages in the mourning process.
   b. factors, such as religion, culture, and gender, that impact the loss experience.
   c. phases of bereavement.
   d. the same for each person who grieves.

47. Which of the following best describes the intuitive griever?

   a. Thinking dominates feeling as an experience.
   b. Feelings are less intense.
   c. Has a general reluctance to talk about feelings.
   d. Feelings are intensely and overtly experienced.

48. Individuals who express their grief through an instrumental pattern

   a. are reluctant to talk about feelings.
   b. express emotions publicly.
   c. have feelings that are more intense.
   d. receive great support from those around them.

49. The type of grief that occurs when a loss is not or cannot be openly acknowledged, publicly mourned, or socially supported is known as

   a. insincere.
   b. disenfranchised.
   c. complicated.
   d. traumatic.

50. Complicated grief is

   a. officially recognized as a mental disorder.
   b. also known as prolonged grief.
   c. experienced by a majority of bereaved individuals.
   d. never responsive to professional interventions.

51. Symptoms of complicated grief are

   a. initial denial of a death.
   b. a short-term change in sleep patterns following a death.
   c. ongoing, intense grief and decreased social functioning.
   d. weight loss during the first months after a death of a loved one.

CHAPTER 7

PUBLIC TRAGEDY AND MASS TRAUMA

CHAPTER OBJECTIVE

After completing this chapter, the reader will recognize the impact of public tragedies and methods for assisting survivors during and after such tragedies.

LEARNING OBJECTIVES

After studying this chapter, the reader will be able to

1. describe what factors cause an event to be viewed as a public tragedy.
2. describe the effects of terrorist acts.
3. identify components of psychological first aid.
4. discuss the phases of a disaster.
5. name common factors that increase the risk of lasting problems for individuals following a disaster.
6. describe the importance of rituals after a disaster.

INTRODUCTION

This chapter can guide nurses in understanding the community's response after a tragedy. Although most deaths are personal, community-wide tragedies can impact hundreds, if not thousands, of individuals. We live in a time when traumatic events are becoming all too common and often, we too, are touched by the tragedy. Public tragedies include disasters, terrorist acts, and the deaths of public figures.

In the wake of Princess Diana's death, thousands mourned. Who was not touched by the plight of misplaced families due to Hurricane Katrina? Thousands watched on television and felt helpless, wondering how they could provide support in some small way. And who did not weep on September 11, 2001? Whether watching what transpired on television or functioning in the heart of the situation, nurses are very much aware of the personal impact of public tragedies.

Although most nurses impacted by disasters will be those working in hospitals or public health, other nurses affected include visiting nurses, nursing home nurses, and school nurses. Visiting nurses will have to check on victims and visit them in their homes. Victims may need to go into nursing homes and nurses in those settings will assume responsibility for their care. School nurses will also be affected as they care for students injured or otherwise affected by the trauma. This chapter explores four examples of traumatic events: deaths of public figures, homicides, terrorist acts, and natural disasters. These types of deaths are distinguished from other modes by their sudden nature and the violence often involved (Currier, Holland, & Neimeyer, 2006).

PUBLIC TRAGEDY

Doka (2003) notes, "The greater the consequences resulting from a tragic event, the more likely that event will be perceived, even retrospectively, as a public tragedy" (p. 7). The author maintains that there are certain characteristics that influence the public's perceptions, including the scope of the tragedy, the extent to which individuals identify with those involved, the social value of the victims, the consequences of the death, and the duration of the event. Individuals also struggle with issues related to the cause of the tragedy.

In a natural disaster, individuals may be angry at God. In a human-caused tragedy, the anger may be directed toward the person that caused the death. Another characteristic that influences perceptions is the degree of intentionality: If it was a random act, the public may perceive the event as one that could have happened to them; if the public perceives the tragedy as intentional, they will assign blame. Although assigning blame will not make the public any safer, it will give them an illusion of safety. Expectedness, preventability, and the degree of suffering inflicted also influence public perception of a tragedy.

When a Public Figure Dies

Deaths of public figures produce an outpouring of sympathy. The sudden death of Michael Jackson was met with hysteria by millions of mourners across the United States and other parts of the world. The death of John Kennedy, Jr., in an airplane crash was also met with public shock, disbelief, and sadness. The death of Princess Diana, caused by an intoxicated driver and paparazzi, was a public tragedy that affected millions. Thousands of individuals, like Diana, are killed each year in motor vehicle crashes, leaving behind family members and friends who mourn the losses in their social network. Mourning is an important process of interaction between the bereaved and society (Kastenbaum, 2004.), and media is very much a part of that society.

The media provides viewers an opportunity to witness the effects of a death and observe others coping in its wake. In the cases of Kennedy and Princess Diana, most television stations interrupted regular programming to broadcast the aftermath of the deaths. Scenes were replayed multiple times. Newscasters described and analyzed the losses for their respective countries and broadcast to the world. People watched on their televisions at home and in public places and talked with friends and strangers about the incidents. Rituals marking the deaths of these public figures were also viewed through the media. Through television, radio, and print, individuals were able to recognize the significance of the individual, community, and worldwide loss.

Though many individuals do not seek out assistance after public figures die, some people need help in coping with their perceived losses. Bull et al. (2002-2003) found that those seeking assistance after Diana's death wanted to talk at length about her death, had resurfacing grief issues, and were expressing sorrow.

Personal Insight
Describe a public tragedy that happened in your lifetime. What emotions did you experience during and afterwards?

Did the media coverage affect your response to the tragedy?

MASS TRAUMA

Although many are traumatized by the deaths of public figures, those deaths do not constitute mass trauma. Mass trauma refers to events that are extremely frightening, possibly life threatening, and experienced by a large number of people at the same time. There are five components used to classify events causing mass trauma (Boyd Webb, 2004, p. 6):

1. Single versus recurring traumatic event:

- *Type I:* Acute, one single event, as in the case of the shootings at Columbine High School.

- *Type II:* Chronic or ongoing trauma, as in the case of the events of September 11th, when several planes attempted to fly into buildings in several states.

2. Proximity (emotional or geographic) to the traumatic event:

   - On site, on the periphery, or through the media.

3. Extent of exposure to violence/injury/pain:

   - Witnessed and/or experienced.

4. Nature of losses/deaths/destruction:

   - Personal, community, and/or symbolic loss.

   - Danger, loss, and/or responsibility traumas.

   - Loved one "missing"/no physical evidence.

   - Death determined by retrieval of body or fragment(s).

   - Loss of status/employment/family income.

   - Loss of a predictable future.

5. Attribution of causality:

   - Random/"act of God" or deliberate/human-made.

Mass trauma events include homicides, terrorist acts, and disasters.

HOMICIDE

In 2006, there were 573 deaths by homicide in the United States (Heron et al., 2009). Generally, homicide refers to death from criminal actions that are intentional. All too often the public is not aware of the number of homicides that occur in their own communities. It is when the media brings those deaths into the homes of television viewers that one can understand the depth of the pain homicide victims feel.

Whether we know the victims or learn about their deaths through the media, intentional criminal acts that end lives can be devastating to watch. This was true in the case of two teenagers at Columbine High School who brought guns to school, killed 13 classmates and teachers, and then took their own lives. Many individuals did not know the students or teachers who were killed or the teens who took their own lives. However, viewers were affected by this mass trauma as they watched these traumatized children and communities respond.

Homicide is the fourth leading cause of death for children 1 to 14 years of age, the second for teens 15 to 24, the third for 25 to 34 years of age, and the sixth for 35 to 44 years of age (CDC: NCIPC, 1999-2006). Firearms were used in 64.5% of homicide deaths, followed by sharp instruments (12.2%) and blunt instruments (5.3%) (Karch et al., 2009). In 2005, males were almost 10 times more likely than females to commit murder (Fox & Zawitz, 2010) and most homicides were committed by individuals who knew their victims. Many homicides are committed by current intimate partners, previous boyfriends, or ex-spouses (Table 7-1). Approximately one in three female homicide deaths are committed by an intimate partner, but only 5% of male victims are killed by intimate partners (Paulozzi, Saltzman, Thompson, & Holmgreen, 2001). The gender distribution of homicide victims and offenders differs by the manner of homicide (see Table 7-2).

In 2005, homicide victimization rates for Blacks were six times higher than the rates for Whites and offending rates for Blacks were more than seven times higher than the rates for Whites. From 1976 to 2005, 86% of White homicide victims were killed by Whites and 94% of Black victims were killed by Blacks. The race distribution of homicide victims and offenders differs by whether the homicide was due to felony murder; sex, drug, or gang activities; an argument; or a workplace occurrence (Fox & Zawitz, 2010).

TABLE 7-1: VICTIM–OFFENDER RELATIONSHIP BY VICTIM GENDER, 1976-2005		
	Percent of homicide victims by gender	
Victim/Offender relationship	*Male*	*Female*
Total	100.0%	100.0%
Intimate	5.0%	30.0%
Spouse	3.0	18.3
Ex-spouse	0.2	1.4
Boyfriend/Girlfriend	1.8	10.4
Other family	6.8%	11.8%
Parent	1.3	2.8
Child	2.1	5.4
Sibling	1.2	0.9
Other family	2.2	2.8
Acquaintance/Known	35.3%	21.8%
Neighbor	1.1	1.3
Employee/Employer	0.1	0.1
Friend/Acquaintance	29.4	17.0
Other Known	4.6	3.4
Stranger	15.5%	8.7%
Undetermined	37.4%	27.6%

Note. From "Homicide Trends in the U.S." by Office of Justice Programs, Bureau of Justice Statistics. Available at http://www.ojp.usdoj.gov/content/homicide/gender.cfm

Laurie and Neimeyer (2008) examined the African American experience of grief, focusing on identity change, interpersonal loss dimensions, and continuing attachments with the deceased. Although African Americans don't usually seek professional support, they report more frequent losses due to homicide, maintenance of a stronger continuing bond with the deceased, greater grief due to extended-kin death beyond the immediate family, and a sense of community support in their grief.

Research on families after the violent death of a child or young adult by accident, homicide, or suicide indicates that the grief experienced by both parents may disrupt the cohesion and function of the family, leading to mental distress (Lohan &

Murphy, 2002). According to Wickie and Marwit (2000-2001), parents of murdered children report more negative views of the benevolence of the world; these negative views are often a result of the special circumstances surrounding homicide, such as the act of murder itself, the additional trauma of investigations, prolonged judiciary proceedings, increased isolation, and intense anger at perpetrators (p. 110).

Parents whose children die suddenly tend to isolate themselves from society. Their tendency to withdraw may be linked to factors common in parents whose child died in sudden traumatic ways, including feelings of guilt and self-blame about their child's death (Dyregrov, Nordanger, & Dyregrov, 2003). However, Hatton (2003) found that less than one fifth of homicide survivors identified guilt or self-blame as a major difficulty. This finding may be due to victims' rights advocates who have been helping homicide survivors cope with their losses. Respondents in Hatton's study reported severe emotional pain as the greatest difficulty. They also reported constantly searching for reasons for the murder and experiencing related rage and anger.

Although violent death is a major public problem in the United States, there is no gold standard for bereavement services offered to family survivors to help them adjust (Murphy, 2000). Gamino et al. (2000) found,

> When focusing on personal growth as a positive outcome following bereavement, four factors emerged as correlates of better adjustment: ability to see some good resulting from the death, having a chance to say good-bye to the loved one, intrinsic spirituality, and spontaneous positive memories of the decedent. (p. 638)

In a hospital setting, immediate support should be provided to bereaved victims after a homicide by giving them the opportunity to be with their dead loved one and providing a private area to share the experience while validating their loss.

TABLE 7-2: HOMICIDE TYPE BY GENDER, 1976-2005

Homicide Type by Gender, 1976-2005				
	Victims		Offenders	
	Male	*Female*	*Male*	*Female*
All homicides	76.5%	23.5%	88.8%	11.2%
Victim/offender relationship				
Intimate	35.2%	64.8%	65.5%	34.5%
Family	51.5%	48.5%	70.8%	29.2%
Infanticide	54.6%	45.4%	61.8%	38.2%
Eldercide	58.1%	41.9%	85.2%	14.8%
Circumstances				
Felony murder	78.4%	21.6%	93.2%	6.8%
Sex related	18.8%	81.2%	93.6%	6.4%
Drug related	90.2%	9.8%	95.5%	4.5%
Gang related	94.7%	5.3%	98.3%	1.7%
Argument	77.8%	22.2%	85.6%	14.4%
Workplace	79.1%	20.9%	91.3%	8.7%
Weapon				
Gun homicide	82.7%	17.3%	91.3%	8.7%
Arson	56.4%	43.6%	79.1%	20.9%
Poison	55.3%	44.7%	63.5%	36.5%
Multiple victims or offenders				
Multiple victims	63.3%	36.7%	93.5%	6.5%
Multiple offenders	85.6%	14.4%	91.6%	8.4%

For the years 1976-2005 combined, among all homicide victims, females were particularly at risk for intimate killings and sex-related homicides.

Note. From "Homicide Trends in the U.S." by J.A. Fox & M.W. Zawitz (2010). Retrieved February 4, 2010 from http://bjs.ojp.usdoj.gov/content/pub/pdf/htius/pdf

The National Organization for Victim Assistance (2008) notes,

> Experts in the field of victim assistance have learned over the years that crime victims who are treated with dignity, compassion and respect will learn to cope more effectively with the pain of being a crime victim. They will also be more willing in the future to report crimes, trusting that they will be believed and treated well. (para #3)

Although nurses may not choose to work in the victim assistance field, they may encounter victims of violent crimes at some point in their careers. When a patient dies in the Emergency Department due to a stab wound, gun shot, or other fatal injury, family members are considered victims of crime. When family members first learn of the homicide, they are preoccupied with the nature of the injuries inflicted on the victim, the brutality of the killing, the weapon used, the victim's suffering, and the identity of the murderer (Miller, 2008). These crime victims rely on compassionate nurses to help them cope with their pain. Prigerson and Jacobs

(2001) indicated that after a patient's death, medical staff should consider:

- offering a direct expression of sympathy.

- acknowledging that the clinician does not know exactly what the bereaved person is going through.

- talking about the deceased, including saying his or her name.

- eliciting questions about the circumstances of the death.

- asking questions about feelings and about how the death has affected the person.

Terrorist Acts

Terrorism is a form of psychological warfare. Goals of terrorism are to coerce, instill fear, punish, blame victims, and induce psychological toxicity by targeting a large number of people (Everly, 2003). A terrorist's goal is to induce fear and intimidation (Martino, 2002). Forms of terrorism include hijacked airlines and cruise ships, building sieges, airport attacks, and bombings. Bombings are designed to cause death, destruction, fear, and confusion. In comparison to natural disasters, intentional mass casualty events are associated with higher rates of long-term psychological symptoms (CDC, 2008a). Nurses may treat those injured in the blast or those whose family members have been injured or died. Being separated from loved ones or witnessing the devastation causes psychological symptoms including:

- *Physical reactions:* fatigue/exhaustion, gastrointestinal distress, tightness in throat/chest/stomach, headache, worsening of chronic conditions, somatic complaints, or racing heartbeat.

- *Emotional reactions:* depression/sadness, irritability/anger/resentment, anxiety/fear, despair/hopelessness, guilt/self-doubt, unpredictable mood swings, emotional numbness, or inappropriately flat affect.

- *Cognitive reactions:* confusion/disorganization, recurring dreams or nightmares, preoccupation

with the disaster, trouble concentrating/remembering things, difficulty making decisions, questioning spiritual beliefs, disorientation, indecisiveness, worry, shortened attention span, memory loss, unwanted memories, or self-blame.

- *Behavioral reactions:* sleep problems, crying easily, excessive activity, increased conflicts with others, hypervigilance/startle reactions, isolation/social withdrawal, distrust, irritability, feelings of rejection or abandonment, emotional distancing, judgmental or over-controlling thoughts and behaviors, abuse of substances and/or alcohol.

(CDC, 2008a)

On September 11, 2001, approximately 3,000 people were killed in a series of hijacked airplane crashes. Following the September 11th terrorist attacks, the U.S. Department of Health and Human Services offered grief and emotional response advice for children and adults. Resources for grief counseling and mental health services after a disaster were included. Brief crisis intervention to New York City employees of the World Trade Center was also provided. These interventions were clinically effective and beneficial up to 2 years after treatment (Boscarino, Adams, & Figley, 2004). The authors found a positive effect on the mental status of employees, which included a reduced risk for binge drinking, alcohol dependence, posttraumatic stress disorder (PTSD) symptoms, major depression, somatization, anxiety, and global impairment, compared with similar New York City employees who did not receive brief crisis intervention counseling.

Trauma after a terrorist attack is not limited to direct survivors. Nurses are at personal risk during and after the attack. There are clinical challenges after a terrorist act. Nurses may fear contamination by biological, chemical, or nuclear agents and also worry about the safety of their own families (DiGiovanni, Reynolds, Harwell, Stonecipher, & Burkle, 2003). These agents can produce changes in a person's mental state, impaired concentration, psychomotor changes, slowed speech, anxiety, and irritability (Shalev, 1996). Nurses who treat victims initially do so not knowing if the symptoms are the result of a psychiatric disorder or the terrorist act.

Professionals deployed to the scene are also vulnerable to increased risk of personal emotional trauma, but most do not seek out professional mental health support. A recent study examined treatment utilization by responders at the World Trade Center during or after September 11, 2001. Among 174 workers who accepted psychotherapy referrals following psychiatric screening for World Trade Center-related symptoms, 74 (42.5%) attended at least one session, whereas 100 (57.5%) did not (Jayasinghe et al., 2005).

Although some nurses are also mental health professionals, those who are not often work side by side with mental health professionals offering psychological first aid to traumatized individuals during the first 48 hours after an event. Ritchie (2003) described six components of psychological first aid:

1. Protect survivors from further harm.
2. Reduce physiological arousal.
3. Mobilize support for those who are most distressed.
4. Keep families together and facilitate reunions with loved ones.
5. Provide information; foster communication and education.
6. Use effective risk communication techniques. (p. 45)

In 2003, the Institute of Medicine formed a committee to review the critical issues in responding to psychological needs of individuals after a terrorist act. The first recommendation of the committee was to "develop evidence-based techniques, training, and education in psychological first aid to address all hazards and all members of society during the pre-event, event, and immediate post-event phases of a terrorism event in order to limit the psychological consequences of terrorism" (Stith Butler, Panzer, & Goldfrank, 2003, p. 137).

Tsui and Cheung (2003) suggested the following actions that professionals could take to restore the community's strength after a terrorist attack: (a) offer counseling for those in fear or depression; (b) provide material and emotional assistance for those injured or bereaved; (c) facilitate communication among ethnic and religious groups; (d) promote programs that encourage young people to respect differences and diversity; and (e) protect and advocate for marginalized and vulnerable people in the community.

> *__Personal Insight__*
> *Have you experienced multiple traumatic losses in your life? If so, have you experienced emotionally painful thoughts?*
>
> *What were the thoughts and how did you cope with them?*

DISASTERS

Disasters, such as earthquakes, tornadoes, and explosions, can impact many people at one time, whether due to natural or human causes. In 2005, an estimated 162 million people worldwide were impacted by disasters causing over 105,000 deaths and $176 million in damages (Hall & Hamaoka, 2005). Those affected include the dead, survivors, witnesses, first responders, bereaved relatives and friends, other responders, and local citizens. A disaster can happen at any moment and can cause major loss of health, life, and property.

Disasters can be due to natural or accidental causes. Geophysical disasters include earthquakes, volcano eruptions, and tsunamis. Other natural disasters can be caused by hurricanes, tornadoes, ice storms, droughts, and floods. Human-generated accidental disasters include industrial accidents, hazardous material exposures, chemical and nuclear explosions, and transportation disasters such as a bridge collapse (FEMA, 2010).

The Role of the Hospital Nurse After a Disaster

Hospital nurses may assist in the aftermath of disasters, such as large-scale bus or auto accidents, collapse of buildings, or disease outbreaks. Numerous victims with multiple injuries can result.

When unexpected injury-causing events produce large numbers of casualties, a representative of emergency management will contact the hospital detailing the type of disaster, anticipated/estimated number of victims, and estimated time of arrival in order to warn the emergency department (ED) of the anticipated influx of multiple victims.

The role of the ED charge nurse on duty or care director/manager is to notify the hospital's chief nursing officer and the medical director of emergency services of the disaster. The charge nurse implements the disaster plan and is advised of the degree of mobilization, assigns RNs to triage and treatment rooms, and advises noncritical ED patients and families that the disaster plan has been implemented and that treatment may be delayed. The ED nurse responds to assignments delegated by the patient care manager and charge RN.

Nurses working in an ED (triage center) during a disaster report to the incident triage nurse who will be assigned by the ED manager/charge nurse/Assistant Director of Nursing. The victims arrive with disaster tags from the field medics. At the time of triage, a mass casualty packet is generated for each victim. Critical patients are triaged as *priority* and the incident triage nurse will assess the victims, place color tape that corresponds with a patient's condition around the victim's wrist, and write the time of triage on the tape. A corresponding small piece of that color tape will be placed in the front pouches of triage belts. This will enable nurses to maintain a total patient count. For deceased patients, the time of triage becomes time

of death and is written on their foreheads with a grease pen found in the disaster kit. Depending upon the conditions of the victims, some may be sent to the operating room. Burn and trauma victims will be stabilized and transferred as ordered by the ED physician. Nurses deal with chemical/ biological exposures and refer them according to their institution's policy. Victims requiring decontamination are decontaminated prior to entering the healthcare facility.

In the United States, priority treatment in EDs is given to those individuals with the most severe injuries, but this may not be the case during disasters. If resources are scarce, not all injured will received aggressive care. Treatment may be intentionally withheld from seriously injured persons who are likely to die because of their injuries. Kipnis (2007) notes, "What would be a serious wound in a hospital with an untapped surge capacity can become a fatal injury in a hospital coping with disaster" (p. 89). Treatment preference may be given to those who are less wounded, rather than the more severely wounded or hopeless. This reverse or military triage has ethical, moral, and religious implications and controversies. Who lives? Who dies? Who decides who lives and who dies? Are nurses protected from litigation when making those life-saving decisions?

On August 29, 2005, Hurricane Katrina struck the coastal areas of Alabama, Florida, Mississippi, and Louisiana. The hurricane caused floods and significant numbers of deaths and infrastructure damage. Hundreds of individuals were stranded in hospitals waiting for help. Three days after the hurricane, those in the hospital were told they would be on their own and no help was forthcoming (Deichmann, 2007, p. 110). Medical resources were in short supply. Clinicians were working in the heat, darkness, and stench. Kipnis (2007) asks, "Are there conditions that, had they been present in New Orleans (or anywhere else), would have excused ending the lives of patients, conditions under which both law and professional ethics should withhold condemnation?" (p. 82).

In the aftermath of Katrina, former Louisiana Attorney General Foti accused Dr. Pou, a cancer surgeon, and two nurses, Cheri Landry and Lori Budo, of killing four hospital patients, 62 to 90 years of age, after the August 29, 2005 hurricane. The district attorney eventually dropped the charges against the two nurses and a grand jury refused to indict Dr. Pou. Many doctors and nurses who stayed to serve during Hurricane Katrina faced civil lawsuits for patient deaths that occurred while waiting for evacuations (Foster, 2008).

On June 8, 2008, Louisiana Governor Bobby Jindal signed into law the last of a three-piece legislation effort designed to protect medical personnel during declared disasters in the state of Louisiana (Committee for Disaster Medicine Reform, 2008). The new Louisiana law limits civil lawsuits against medical professionals during a declared disaster and allows prosecutors to use a medical panel to review evidence when a doctor or nurse is suspected of euthanasia or other criminal medical actions during a disaster (Foster, 2008). The law also protects medical workers when "reverse" triage protocols are used because those protocols make patients who are not expected to survive the last to be evacuated. Hopefully, other states will follow suit to protect their nurses from litigation in future disasters. Had September 11th resulted in more casualties instead of deaths, this issue may have been addressed in New York City prior to Louisiana.

> **_Personal Insight_**
> _If your life would be in danger if you stayed to care for your patients, would you stay?_

Phases of a Disaster

Nurses may be called upon to provide psychological support to their communities during and after disasters. During the pre-disaster period, warning systems, preparedness plans, and recruitment and training of mental health liaisons and responders are put into place (McCabe, Everly, Siegel, Heitt, & Kaminsky, 2004). This is the time when communities initiate safety mechanisms that will reduce the effects of the disaster (DeWolfe, 2000).

Although many years have passed since the American Red Cross identified the four phases of a disaster, these phases are still used to describe the relationship between patients and activities of disaster recovery. After the impact, these phases are characterized as:

1. heroic
2. honeymoon
3. disillusionment
4. reconstruction.

During the *heroic* phase, immediately post-disaster when there is disruption of services, people watch out for one another and individuals risk their own safety to save strangers. Survivors take inventory and the focus is on rescue, food, warmth, and safety (Raphael & Newman, 2000). The time immediately after the disaster is when first responders attempt to save lives and property (Raphael & Newman, 2000). After doing all that they can do, they then leave the disaster area.

One week to 6 months later, individuals enter into the *honeymoon* phase. People help each other and collaborate; they are hopeful about recovery. The next phase, *disillusionment,* often begins about 2 months after the disaster and lasts from 1 to 2 years. Resources are seen as "too little, too late." People work through their grief, come to terms with their losses, and may be frustrated with the slowness of recovery. The last phase is *reconstruction,* when recovery and rebuilding are realized.

The implications of a disaster may last for some time, perhaps a lifetime. The impact of a disaster on an individual's functioning will depend on many factors. Studies show that middle-aged adults are at the most risk for complicated grief as they have greater stress and burden, even before the impact of the disaster, and assume even more obligations afterward (Norris, Byrne, Diaz, & Kaniasty, 2001). Assumptions and Principles about Psychosocial Aspects of Disasters (International Work Group on Death, Dying and Bereavement, 2002) lists common factors that increase the risk of complicated grief:

a. prior vulnerability to stress and loss

b. deaths that are unexpected and untimely

c. experience or witness of horrific or terrifying events

d. deaths attributable to human agency

e. multiple losses and concurrent crises

f. losses by children whose parent(s) dies in the disaster

g. losses by parents whose child dies in the disaster

h. absence of or undue delay in the recovery of intact bodies of those killed in the disaster.

(p. 458)

Psychological reactions to a disaster include depression, generalized anxiety disorder, panic disorder, increased substance use (alcohol, drug, and tobacco), and PTSD (Hall & Hamaoka, 2005). After a disaster, psychiatric nurses may come in contact with individuals who are experiencing stress reactions, major depression, personality disorders, rage reactions, or either lost or depleted medications (Federation of Texas Psychiatry, 2005). Nurses would benefit from developing disaster counseling skills in order to be better equipped to provide support to a disaster victim with lasting problems (Table 7-3). The primary focus after obtaining medical attention for any physical injuries is establishing shelter and safety.

Kolski, Avriette, and Jongsma (2001) maintain that nurses should inform patients of common reactions to disasters that include irritability, fatigue, decreased appetite and sleep, nightmares, sadness, headaches, hyperactivity, decreased concentration, and increased alcohol or drug consumption. The

---

TABLE 7-3: PATIENT COUNSELING TIPS

How Do You Interact with Patients after a Traumatic Event?

The clinician should be alert to the various needs of the traumatized person.

- Listen and encourage patients to talk about their reactions when they feel ready.
- Validate the emotional reactions of the person. Intense, painful reactions are common responses to a traumatic event.
- De-emphasize clinical, diagnostic, and pathological language.
- Communicate person to person rather than "expert" to "victim," using straightforward terms.

What Can You Do to Help Patients Cope with a Traumatic Event?

Explain that their symptoms may be normal, especially right after the traumatic event, and then encourage patients to:

- Identify concrete needs and attempt to help. Traumatized persons are often preoccupied with concrete needs (e.g., How do I know if my friends made it to the hospital?).
- Keep to their usual routine.
- Identify ways to relax.
- Face situations, people, and places that remind them of the traumatic event – not to shy away.
- Take the time to resolve day-to-day conflicts so they do not build up and add to their stress.
- Identify sources of support, including family and friends. Encourage talking about their experiences and feelings with friends, family, or other support networks (e.g., clergy and community centers).

Note. From "Coping with a Traumatic Event," by Centers for Disease Control and Prevention, 2005. Retrieved August 23, 2010, from http://emergency.cdc.gov/masscasualties/copingpro.asp

authors recommend the following ways that nurses can provide emotional support to patients following a disaster:

- Assist in locating a disaster shelter established by the American Red Cross.

- Encourage patients to eat well-balanced, hot meals offered through community resources.

- Utilize the American Red Cross communication hotline to provide assistance in locating significant persons.

- Reinforce the importance of asking for help from volunteers.

- Gently ask patients to recall actions taken before, during, and immediately following the disaster being careful not to press them into being overwhelmed.

- Express the appropriateness of grieving material losses (possessions) as well as the loss of future hopes and plans.

- Educate patients about resources that can assist with providing financial and material support. (p. 57)

Collaborating with Relief Agencies

Nurses can become better informed by reaching out to other organizations and developing protocols for working together in times of disasters. Government agencies, such as the Federal Emergency Management Agency (FEMA) and the Center for Mental Health Services, provide assistance in a disaster's aftermath. Nonprofit organizations, including the National Voluntary Organizations Active in Disaster (NVOAD), the National Organization for Victim Assistance (NOVA), and the American Red Cross can help nurses gain valuable information in providing support after a disaster.

PSYCHOLOGICAL TRAUMA

Research indicates that between 15% and 35% of Americans have experienced a life-threatening, traumatic event (Bromet & Havenaar, 2002). The term "trauma" derives from the Greek, meaning "wound." This section will focus on psychological wounds caused by death and traumatic loss. *The Diagnostic and Statistical Manual of Mental Disorders, 4th Edition,* Text Revision (*DSM-IV-TR*) (APA, 2000) defines trauma as:

Direct personal experience of an event that involves actual or threatened death or serious injury, or other threat to one's physical integrity; or witnessing an event that involves death, injury, or a threat to the physical integrity of another person; or learning about unexpected or violent death, serious harm or threat of death or injury experienced by a family member or other close associate (criterion A1). The person's response to the event must involve intense fear, helplessness, or horror (or in children, the response must involve disorganized or agitated behavior) (criterion A2). (p. 463)

Traumatic Loss

Reactions to traumatic loss are subjective (Currier et al., 2006). Reactions to loss can include a loss of meaning and purpose, questioning good versus evil and one's basic beliefs, and withdrawal from places of worship (McPherson, 2004). Grief will be more intense for those bereaved after a traumatic death, especially if the deceased was young and the death seemed preventable (Gamino et al., 2000). To find meaning in a traumatic loss, individuals have to identify the traumatic event and their responses or reactions to it. Once people understand that they are experiencing normal reactions to abnormal events, they can then focus on finding meaning in the tragedy (see Table 7-4).

TABLE 7-4: COMMON RESPONSES TO A TRAUMATIC EVENT			
Cognitive	**Emotional**	**Physical**	**Behavioral**
• poor concentration	• shock	• nausea	• suspicion
• confusion	• numbness	• lightheadedness	• irritability
• disorientation	• feeling overwhelmed	• dizziness	• arguments with friends and loved ones
• indecisiveness	• depression	• gastrointestinal problems	
• shortened attention span	• feeling lost	• rapid heart rate	• withdrawal
• memory loss	• fear of harm to self and/or loved ones	• tremors	• excessive silence
• unwanted memories	• feeling nothing	• headaches	• inappropriate humor
• difficulty making decisions	• feeling abandoned	• grinding of teeth	• increased/decreased eating
	• uncertainty of feelings	• fatigue	• change in sexual desire or functioning
	• volatile emotions	• poor sleep	• increased smoking
		• pain	• increased substance use or abuse
		• hyperarousal	
		• jumpiness	

Note. From "Coping with a Traumatic Event," by Centers for Disease Control and Prevention, 2005. Retrieved August 23, 2010, from http://emergency.cdc.gov/masscasualties/copingpro.asp

Deaths due to homicides, multiple deaths, shocking or grotesque deaths, and children's deaths especially shatter the lives of survivors and can lead to trauma symptoms (Green 2000; Sanders, 2001). The *DSM-IV-TR* provides a list of traumatic events such as being in combat, a disaster, a severe automobile accident, having a life-threatening illness, or witnessing death. Common responses are shattered assumptions about the world, flashbacks, fear and anger, survivor guilt, attempts to find meaning, crying, wailing, and difficulty in making sense of the violent death. These traumatic events are crisis situations and disrupt the victim's ability to cope. Problem-solving abilities are challenged as victims are physically, emotionally, cognitively, behaviorally, and spiritually overwhelmed. Such reactions may lead to PTSD, which can include distressing dreams, flashbacks, hypervigilence, and avoidance behaviors.

Posttraumatic Stress Disorder (PTSD)

Some of the traumatically bereaved family members treated by nurses will experience PTSD (Table 7-5). PTSD was first introduced as a diag-

nositc category in 1980. The *DSM-IV-TR* explains that directly experienced or witnessed traumatic events can lead to PTSD, an intense physical and emotional response to thoughts and reminders of the event that lasts for weeks or months after the traumatic event. Individuals who have experienced a past trauma and those who are living in dangerous situations where trauma may occur might be more likely to develop PTSD after being exposed to a new traumatic event (Physicians Postgraduate Press, 2001). All nurses should be aware of possible PTSD symptoms in their patients, as many persons do not correlate their death-related experiences to their present physical conditions. Characteristic types of PTSD symptoms include reliving, avoidance, and increased arousal.

TABLE 7-5: POSTTRAUMATIC STRESS DISORDER

What Is PTSD?

Posttraumatic stress disorder (PTSD) is an intense physical and emotional response to thoughts and reminders of the event that lasts for many weeks or months after the traumatic event. The symptoms of PTSD fall into three broad types: reliving, avoidance, and increased arousal.

- Symptoms of reliving include flashbacks, nightmares, and extreme emotional and physical reactions to reminders of the event. Emotional reactions can include feeling guilty, extreme fear of harm, and numbing of emotions. Physical reactions can include uncontrollable shaking, chills, or heart palpitations and tension headaches.

- Symptoms of avoidance include staying away from activities, places, thoughts, or feelings related to the trauma, or feeling detached or estranged from others.

- Symptoms of increased arousal include being overly alert or easily startled, having difficulty sleeping, experiencing irritability or outbursts of anger, and being unable to concentrate.

Other symptoms linked with PTSD include: panic attacks, depression, suicidal thoughts and feelings, drug abuse, feelings of being estranged and isolated, and not being able to complete daily tasks.

What Can You Do for Yourself?

There are many things you can do to cope with traumatic events.

- Understand that your symptoms may be normal, especially right after the trauma.
- Keep to your usual routine.
- Take the time to resolve day-to-day conflicts so they do not add to your stress.
- Do not shy away from situations, people, and places that remind you of the trauma.
- Find ways to relax and be kind to yourself.
- Turn to family, friends, and clergy for support, and talk about your experiences and feelings with them.
- Participate in leisure and recreational activities.
- Recognize that you cannot control everything.
- Recognize the need for trained help, and call a local mental health center.

What Can You Do for Your Child?

- Let your child know that it is okay to feel upset when something bad or scary happens.
- Encourage your child to express feelings and thoughts, without making judgments.
- Return to daily routines.

Note. From "Coping with a Traumatic Event," by Centers for Disease Control and Prevention, n.d.-a. Retrieved August 23, 2010, from http://cdc.gov/masstrauma/factsheets/public/coping.pdf

COPING WITH COMMUNITY-WIDE GRIEF

To meet the needs when public figures die or in any type of community-wide grief response, employers should have guidelines in place to support their staff. Hotlines can be established through national and local agencies, religious organizations can offer meetings, and media must cover the story in a sensitive manner. Bull et al. (2002-2003) recommended the following suggestions to assist in future occurrences of community-wide grief.

- Organizations should have distinct guidelines detailing appropriate strategies to deal with increased requests for assistance and support during such occurrences of grief.

- Organizations should ensure availability of adequate numbers of support workers/staff, even if this requires utilizing "reserve" volunteers.

- Support staff should have access to their own support meetings and be able to implement additional debriefing sessions.

- Literature concerning grief and relevant support services should be available at large gatherings such as memorial services.

- Literature should detail elements of grief and other relevant issues, such as resurfacing of previous losses, and community members should be reassured their reactions to such devastating circumstances are normal.

- Such literature and information should be accessible in the print media, on television, and on radio.

- Hotlines should be established to disseminate information as well as to advise people on more comprehensive paths of assistance.

- Large-scale services by religious and other groups should be offered as an option for those wishing to express their grief.

- Media should be alerted to ways of sensitively and responsibly covering tragedies, in recognition of the potential impact of media coverage on vulnerable grievers. (p. 44)

Finding Meaning in the Tragedy

The challenge of understanding the effects of disasters is to describe the nature and the meaning of the events from the individual and community perspectives (Benight & McFarlane, 2007). When significant individuals or public figures die, those grieving the loss will react to that loss and attempt to find meaning in it. Making meaning is defined "generally as finding some degree of coherence, orderliness, predictability, purpose, or value in what happened" (Gamino et al., 2002, p. 794). Meaning is found when individuals establish an understanding of the tragedy (O'Connor, 2002-2003).

Spiritual and religious meaning reduces anxiety. In a cross-campus study, Ai, Cascio, Santangelo, and Evans-Campbell (2005) found that after the September 11th terrorist attacks, a greater sense of spiritual meaning was related to lower levels of anxiety and depression in 457 undergraduate and graduate students. Murphy and Johnson (2003) found that one of the predictors of parents finding meaning 5 years after the death of a child was the use of religious coping.

Attig (1996) notes that the bereaved can relearn their relationships with the deceased. The love felt does not die, and the relationship is not dead. The bereaved can continue to hold close those who die, even though the person is no longer alive. The author maintains that letting go entirely is not necessary. The bereaved should not fear being morbid if they continue to talk about their loved one or decide to keep their child's clothes. Such behaviors can even be life affirming, as meaning is found in the sharing of stories and the act of smelling or touching the clothes worn by the deceased.

Meaning is also found as the bereaved carry on in the absence of the deceased. Life is not ended for them, although the person they cared for is dead. Life goes on, and decisions still must be made with the deceased in mind. Promises made to the deceased are kept and by so doing, the bereaved continue to maintain the connection. As stories of the deceased are shared, bereaved individuals become self-transformed and inspired (Attig, 1996). There is a spiritual connection and a reason and purpose in life as well as death. Many individuals may have difficulty finding meaning in a public tragedy and struggle with why it happened for many years. Understanding why gunmen shoot students and teachers or why children are killed in a school building by a tornado that missed countless buildings around them, can take a lifetime, and for some, meaning is never found.

Sudden Death Rituals

Rituals may be defined as ceremonial actions that have meaning and significance to the individual performing or observing the act. Death rituals are acts in response to a loss situation that bring comfort to those who mourn. After a public tragedy it is not uncommon for eulogies, a common ceremonial ritual, to be attended by hundreds of people and sometimes televised. Respect is paid as words are spoken about the deceased – the relationships shared and the meaning of the life now ended.

If grieving individuals do not have any rituals, they can invent them (Sanders, 2001). Through these inventions, something meaningful is created that sustains survivors as they reflect upon the tragedy. Pollack (2003) pointed out how frequently memorials and gravesites are constructed after a tragedy. The author notes, "From the tombs of the unknown warrior to the cemeteries in Normandy, memorials and rituals are commonly constructed in the aftermath of tragedy" (p. 125).

> ### *Personal Insight*
> *Have you ever seen a ritual or spontaneous memorialization after a public tragedy? If so, describe it.*

After 9/11, mourners created rituals that represented their grief. These rituals empowered those who were grieving. Doka (2003) maintains:

> Rituals permit meaningful action at a disorganized time; it allows people to "do something." By doing something, even engaging in ritual, we feel that we have symbolic mastery over events. Ritual allows a reorganization of community and continuity in a chaotic time. Collectively, it offers a reassurance that while we cannot control the tragedy itself, we have reasserted control in its aftermath. (p. 180)

Doka (2003) describes spontaneous rituals, planned rituals, ongoing rituals, and therapeutic rituals as four kinds of rituals in public tragedy. After the September 11th public tragedy, many Americans donated to those intimately affected by the terrorist attack. The tragic deaths of thousands of men and women brought about many spontaneous rituals. Survivors felt a need to do something positive, which helped them cope with the situation.

Spontaneous memorials are immediate expressions of grief. Roadside death memorials bring comfort to the bereaved. After a motor vehicle accident in which several members of a wedding party were killed, individuals who knew them or who heard about the tragedy on television left crosses, flowers, ribbons, notes, and other mementos at the site of the accident. These objects are reminders to all who pass the site that someone special died there. As a memorialization, roadside death memorials provide a way to express intense grief and are a means of communication with and about the deceased (Reid & Reid, 2001).

Doka (2003) maintains that planned rituals can be done in private to honor those who died, organizational rituals can honor a victim of that organization, and public rituals can bring grieving communities together. Ongoing rituals also bring comfort when performed annually on the anniversary of the event. These rituals bring communities together to remember and pay tribute to the lives that were lost. Therapeutic rituals include writing letters, planting trees, or lighting candles. To eternally recognize public tragedies, permanent memorials can also be created. These memorials are lasting impressions and acknowledgments at the site.

CASE STUDY

At 10 a.m. on a Tuesday morning, a call was received in the emergency room (ER) stating that there was an explosion at a local elementary school. The ER nurse was told that there were at least 40 victims (teachers and students). The ER physician instructed the charge nurse to inform the nursing supervisor that the triage center needed to be activated in anticipation of the casualties. The administrator on call, in coordination with the nursing supervisor, decided to activate the command center (staffed by safety officers, vice presidents, emergency management coordinators, and security).

The local police department and EMS began transporting children and teachers to the hospital. Injuries ranged from nonserious to life-threatening. The incident commander in the hospital command center implemented full-scale center activation. Individual centers activated were family waiting (staffed by pastoral care, guest relations, and behavioral health specialists), triage (staffed by ER nurses, doctors, and medical intensive care unit [MICU] specialists), physician response (a designated area where physicians sign in and document contact information should they be needed), and disaster care/discharge planning (staffed by nurses, techs, and physicians). Also activated during this mass casualty event was the manpower pool where employees reported for alternate duties as assigned. The media center was located in the front lobby and staffed by security and persons from public relations/marketing.

More children and teachers arrived. Some were on stretchers and others walking. Loud moaning and crying could be heard from everywhere. Kids were screaming and parents were storming through the doors in hysteria. Families had to be contacted. School officials worked with the local police and the office of emergency management. Criminal investigations were underway. Police and prosecutor office officials roamed the ER halls asking questions.

Some of the nurses on duty had children in that school and one of the ER doctors had a husband who taught at the school. They were anxious to receive word regarding the safety of their loved ones. Unfortunately, several of the nurses' children were seriously injured and the nurses were understandably released from duty.

All elective surgeries were cancelled and inpatients had to be discharged to make room for the victims. All surgeons and respiratory physicians were called in to handle the trauma and smoke inhalation victims. Many required immediate surgery. There were 56 victims and still more were anticipated. Other neighboring hospitals offered assistance and local MICUs accepted transfers. It was difficult to track all of the patients because many had to be transferred immediately. Severe burn victims and intense traumas had to be transported via helicopter to trauma centers and burn units. Families were frantic as they tried to locate their children.

The event lasted over 14 hours. All employees were exhausted. There were multiple deaths but the morgue only held 4 so arrangements had to be made for additional refrigeration for the black-tagged victims. Several firefighters were injured from the flames and structural damage.

By midnight, many employees had been relieved, but some insisted on remaining on duty until all had been treated or transferred.

Questions

1. Were there enough staff, especially on the off shifts, to make phone calls and manage the chaos of such a disaster?

2. How should a nurse explain to inpatients and their families that they need to be discharged to make room for the victims?

3. What about the nurses who spent 12 to 14 hours at the hospital during the disaster and couldn't get home to their own children?

4. How do nurses who usually care for adults handle the deaths and traumatic injuries of little children?

Discussion

Emergency department nurses are prepared to handle casualties in a local hospital emergency room during disasters. Other nurses in the hospital setting may not be well trained to offer proper assistance after explosions.

This disaster was a stressful event for the community and for the staff. Hospital nurses who work in other departments were not accustomed to the extreme pace of an ER. This may cause a great deal of stress. Some nurses may have never treated children and may not know how to handle the pediatric patient. While caring for these children, it is possible the nurses are worrying about the safety of their own children and loved ones.

Some nurses had their loved ones hurt in the explosion and were dismissed from duty, which left a shortage of support. Most of the nurses, though exhausted, worked for 14 hours, refusing to leave. Additionally, some of the nurses who stayed may have been approached by the media. Knowing how to respond to media requests for information is paramount. Finally, if the hospital does not have the equipment needed to handle the disaster, additional stress is placed upon staff. Nurses must be aware of the emotional support and spiritual counseling available at their hospitals for those in the community and, most importantly, for themselves.

SUMMARY

This chapter focused on the aftermath of violence, public tragedies, and mass trauma. Unfortunately, no community or person is protected from the possibility of a traumatic event. In recent years, communities across the United States have been hit hard by traumatic events. These events have not only changed the landscape, but have brought attention to the need for nurses to understand their roles and prepare for the decisions and situations they may face.

WEB RESOURCES

American Red Cross
http://www.redcross.org

Emergency Nurses Association
http://www.ena.org

FEMA: U.S. Department of Homeland Security
http://www.fema.gov/news/disasters.fema

Substance Abuse and Mental Health Services Administration (SAMHSA)
http://www.mentalhealth.samhsa.gov

National Institute of Mental Health
http://www.nimh.nih.gov/health/publications/ generalized-anxiety-disorder-listing.shtml

National Organization for Victim Assistance (NOVA)
http://www.trynova.org

National Voluntary Organizations Active in Disaster (NVOAD)
http://www.nvoad.org

National Student Nurses' Association Guidelines for Establishing and Implementing Disaster Preparedness, Recovery, and Relief Projects
http://www.nsna.org/portals/0/Skins/NSNA/pdf/ Disaster_Guidelines.pdf

EXAM QUESTIONS

CHAPTER 7
Questions 52-61

Note: Choose the one option that BEST answers each question.

52. According to Doka, the greater the consequences resulting from a tragic event, the more likely that event will be perceived as

    a. public perception.

    b. an illusion of safety.

    c. a public tragedy.

    d. a suffering tragedy.

53. Which of the following statements about homicide is true?

    a. It is seldom committed by an intimate partner.

    b. It is the second most frequent cause of death for teens 15 to 24 years of age.

    c. In most cases, individuals do not know their victims.

    d. Homicide victimization rates are higher for Whites than Blacks.

54. Inducing a state of fear, punishing and blaming victims, and instilling psychological toxicity by targeting a large number of people is the goal of

    a. a disaster.

    b. a public tragedy.

    c. disenfranchised grief.

    d. a terrorist act.

55. A component of psychological first aid is to

    a. induce physiological arousal.

    b. mobilize support for those who are less distressed.

    c. separate families and discourage reunion during trauma.

    d. protect survivors from further harm.

56. The phase of a disaster in which warning systems, preparedness plans, and recruitment and training of mental health liaisons and responders are put into place to reduce the effects of a disaster is known as

    a. pre-disaster period.

    b. heroic phase.

    c. reconstruction phase.

    d. death phase.

57. According to the American Red Cross, four phases of a disaster are

    a. reconstruction, impact, honeymoon, safety.

    b. impact, death, honeymoon, disillusionment.

    c. heroic, honeymoon, disillusionment, and reconstruction.

    d. rescue, food, warmth, safety.

continued on next page

58. The risk of complicated grief after a disaster may be increased if

    a. one has no prior vulnerability to stress or loss.

    b. bodies are recovered intact and without delay.

    c. the deaths that occur were expected.

    d. the person experiences multiple losses and concurrent crises.

59. According to Doka, rituals empower those grieving after a disaster by

    a. concealing unacceptable emotions.

    b. allowing people to "do nothing."

    c. offering symbolic mastery over events.

    d. offering reassurance that we can control the tragedy itself.

60. Three characteristic types of symptoms experienced by persons with posttraumatic stress disorder (PTSD) are

    a. gastrointestinal, respiratory, and cardiac.

    b. mental illness, psychosis, and personality disorders.

    c. reliving, avoidance, and increased arousal.

    d. amnesia, forgetfulness, and cognitive impairment.

61. Doka (2003) describes spontaneous rituals, planned rituals, ongoing rituals, and therapeutic rituals as four kinds of rituals in

    a. anticipatory grief situations.

    b. pre-disaster phases.

    c. public tragedies.

    d. inducing psychological arousal.

CHAPTER 8

SUICIDE

CHAPTER OBJECTIVE

After completing this chapter, the reader will be able to discuss the magnitude and significance of suicide as a public health concern and related implications for healthcare professionals.

LEARNING OBJECTIVES

After studying this chapter, the reader will be able to

1. differentiate between suicide, suicidal ideation, suicide threat, and suicide attempt.

2. explain how demographic, psychological, biological, and societal factors influence suicidal behaviors.

3. identify groups at risk for suicide and related prevention efforts based on these populations.

4. discuss warning signs of suicide.

5. describe nursing interventions to help bereaved survivors of suicide.

INTRODUCTION

There are 95 suicides and 2,369 attempts each day (McIntosh, 2010) making suicide the 11th ranking cause of death in the United States (CDC: NCIPC, 2010a). Risk of attempted (nonfatal) suicide is greatest among females and the young (American Association for Suicidology [AAS], 2009b). There is one sui-

cide every 15.2 minutes and an attempt every 38 seconds (McIntosh, 2010), which makes suicide a serious health problem caused by an interaction of psychological, biological, and sociological factors.

Nurses are often in key positions to identify persons at risk, intervene to prevent suicide, and support the survivors of suicide. Developing an understanding of the risk factors, causes, warning signs, and types of suicides, coupled with learning appropriate assessment and intervention skills, will equip nurses to respond effectively on professional and personal levels.

Although prevention and treatment approaches are still evolving, nurses can use the information in this chapter to gain a better understanding of patients' motivations toward suicide, actions for preventing suicide, and means to help survivors as well as themselves cope with this type of traumatic, sudden loss.

WHAT IS SUICIDE?

A death is considered a suicide when a person acts to end his or her life (CDC: NCIPS, 2008). The suicide process begins with suicide ideation. With suicide ideation, the person ruminates about the idea of suicide, possibly makes a verbal or written threat of suicide, and may end life with the completed act.

Gutierrez, Rodriguez, and Garcia (2001) define the spectrum of suicidal behaviors as follows:

> Suicide is a death by self-inflicted means where there is evidence that the intent was to cause death. Suicide attempts are nonfatal acts, with or without injury, where there is evidence that the person had some intent to cause death. Suicide threats may be spoken or unspoken and do not involve a self-harmful act, but the intention is to communicate that a specific act of self-harm may happen soon. (p. 320)

The phrase "committed suicide" has been commonly used to describe the action of taking one's own life. "Died by suicide," "died of suicide," or "died from suicide" are phrases that more accurately describe the reality of suicide, respect the needs of both the person who died and the survivors, and do not carry the stigma of criminality. This terminology is also consistent with how individuals describe other types of death such as "died of cancer," "died by accident," and "died from heart disease." The Alberta Mental Health Board notes,

> Changing the language used to describe suicide is not easy. For such change to occur the involvement of many stakeholders to help lead and support this change is essential. The outcome is well worth it – helping to reduce the stigma and barriers to supporting survivors through the tragedy of a death by suicide. (2008, p. 2)

Why Suicide?

Suicidal ideation and failed attempts symbolize intense types of personal suffering and are risk factors for eventual completed suicide (Cox, Enns, & Clara, 2004). Lack of coping skills and problem-solving ability may be factors contributing to increased depression and suicide ideation (Olvera, 2001). However, more recent research indicates that suicide is increasingly associated with depression, hopelessness, and social isolation (Anderson, Lester, & Rogers, 2008).

Why do people choose to die by suicide? Explanations are sometimes found through psychological autopsy, also called psychiatric autopsy or retrospective death assessment. A psychological autopsy attempts to reconstruct a person's psychological makeup including lifestyle, thoughts, feelings, behaviors, intentions, risk factors, motivations, psychodynamics, life circumstances, and the mode and details of the suicide (Hawton, Houston, Malmbergand, & Simkin, 2003). The autopsy is based on personal interviews, examination of records, and analysis of suicide notes and identifies the sociological, psychological, and biological aspects of the suicide.

DEMOGRAPHIC VARIABLES IMPACTING SUICIDE

Age

In 2001, an average of 1 young person killed himself or herself every 2 hours and 7 minutes. If the 184 suicides of persons younger than 15 years of age are included, 1 young person died by suicide every 2 hours and 1.6 minutes (McIntosh, 2010). Although most people believe that the highest rate of suicide is among teenagers in the United States, this is not true. An average of 1 elderly person kills himself or herself every 1 hour and 37 minutes (McIntosh, 2010). Two of the most vulnerable groups are those 45 to 54 years of age and 75 to 84 years of age (McIntosh, 2010). Elderly adults have rates of suicide close to 50% higher than that of the nation as a whole (all ages) (AAS, n.d.a). In a study of 83 elderly people in a nursing home, the residents reported high levels of depression, suicidality, and hopelessness. Such residents are often left in facilities without any visits from family or friends. Many older people have outlived their friends and family members and must cope with the changes in their social lives and family status.

Loneliness is an important variable influencing suicidal behavior in older adults, whether they reside in nursing facilities or their homes. Other risk factors for elderly persons include a sense of loss and disabilities (Ron, 2002).

Gender

Suicide is the seventh leading cause of death for males and the sixteenth leading cause for females. In 2007, 27,269 males and 7,329 females died by suicide (McIntosh, 2010). For every female suicide there are 3.6 male suicides; however, twice as many females as males attempt suicide. Research suggests that the highest rate of suicide among males is with those 75 years of age and older (a rate of 35.7 per 100,000 population). For females, the highest rate of suicide is among those 45 to 54 years of age (a rate of 8.4 per 100,000 population) (CDC, 2009b).

Ethnicity

Approximately 83% of those who die by suicide annually in the United States are Americans of European descent (Leong & Leach, 2007). Caucasians (a rate of 12.4 per 100,000 population) have higher rates of completed suicides than African Americans (a rate of 4.9 per 100,000 population) (AAS, n.d.a). In the case of African Americans, known risk factors for suicide include: psychological distress (i.e., depression, hopelessness, trauma, and psychotic symptoms); alcohol and illicit drug use; accessibility to lethal means; social isolation; family dysfunction; impaired interpersonal functioning; maladaptive coping; racial inequality; and a previous suicide attempt (Anglin, Gabriel, & Kaslow, 2005; Willis, Coombs, Drentea, & Cockerham, 2003). With the exception of racial inequality, these same risk factors are true for suicides in general. The group that has the lowest suicide rate in America is African American women. Marion and Range (2003) note that these women may possess defenses such as culture, reli-

gion, and social support, along with a negative attitude toward suicide.

As of 2008, there were approximately 4.9 million American Indian and Alaska Native people in the United States (Office of Minority Health, 2009). One of the highest suicide rates in an ethnic group is among American Indians. Suicide is the second leading cause of death among American Indians and Alaska Natives 15 to 34 years of age. Suicide rates among American Indian and Alaskan Native adolescents and young adults 15 to 34 years of age (19.7 per 100,000) are 1.8 times higher than the national average for that age group (11.1 per 100,000) (CDC, 2009b). Yoder, Whitbeck, Hoyt, and LaFromboise (2006) maintain that suicide risk factors for this group include discrimination, negative life events, depression, and substance abuse.

Regional Differences

The highest ranking suicide rate is in the western part of the United States, followed by the southern states, the Midwest, and the Northeast. The highest ranking state for suicide is Alaska, followed by Montana and New Mexico; the lowest ranking states for suicide are the District of Columbia, New Jersey, and New York (McIntosh, 2010).

Common Methods of Suicide

Of the 34,598 suicides in the United States, the most common method is by use of firearm, with the latest official final data for 2007 estimating that 17,352 men and women die annually. Estimates of other methods are 8,161 by suffocation, 6,358 by poisoning, 619 by cut/piercing, and 358 by drowning (McIntosh, 2010). Firearms is the most common method of suicide among men and poisoning is most common among women (CDC, 2009b). A recent study by Stack and Wasserman (2009) found that women were 47% less apt than men to shoot themselves in the head. The authors reported that women are less apt to use shotguns and rifles in their suicides as they are more concerned than men with facial disfigurement and have a lower desire to die than do men (Stack & Wasserman, 2009).

EXPLAINING SUICIDE

Psychological Explanations

Psychological explanations of suicide include *psychache,* tunnel vision, and high risk factors. Edwin Shneidman (1993), the father of suicidology, points out the psychache is a general psychological and emotional pain that reaches intolerable intensity. If individuals do not cope with the psychological pain caused by the frustration of psychosocial needs, they may attempt or complete suicide. One other psychological explanation includes having tunnel vision such that the suicidal person only sees one way of coping with the problem.

If a patient's psychache is identified as problematic, emotional and physical details can be assessed and risk factors explored. Ullman and Najdowski (2009) found a correlation between serious suicidal ideation and attempts for younger, minority, bisexual female adult sexual assault survivors. Another risk factor is for those living with illnesses associated with later-life depression, such as Parkinson's disease, heart disease, stroke, and Alzheimer's disease. Approximately 25% of cancer patients suffer from clinical depression, which can also lead to suicide ideation (American Foundation for Suicide Prevention [AFSP], n.d.a). As stated earlier, elderly persons (especially males) who are lonely also are more likely to contemplate or complete suicide.

Biological Explanations

Many people who die by suicide have a psychiatric disorder that is biologically based and caused by a biochemical brain imbalance. There is a relationship between low concentrations of the serotonin metabolite 5-hydroxyindoleacetic acid (5-HIAA) in cerebrospinal fluid and an increased incidence of attempted and completed suicide in

psychiatric patients (AFSP, n.d.c). This biochemical imbalance can lead to depression and suicide ideation (Table 8-1). Those at increased risk for suicide are individuals with affective disorders, bipolar disorders, alcoholism, and substance abuse diagnoses. Psychological autopsy studies reflect that more than 90% of people with completed suicides had one or more mental disorders (AAS, n.d.a).

TABLE 8-1: THE LINKS BETWEEN DEPRESSION AND SUICIDE
• Major depression is the psychiatric diagnosis most commonly associated with suicide.
• About two thirds of people who complete suicide are depressed at the time of their deaths.
• About seven out of every hundred men and one out of every hundred women who have been diagnosed with depression in their lifetime will go on to complete suicide.
• The risk of suicide in people with major depression is about 20 times that of the general population.
• People who have had multiple episodes of depression are at greater risk for suicide than those who have had one episode.
• People who have a dependence on alcohol or drugs in addition to being depressed are at greater risk for suicide.
• People who are depressed and exhibit the following symptoms are at particular risk for suicide:
1. Extreme hopelessness
2. A lack of interest in activities that were previously pleasurable
3. Heightened anxiety and/or panic attacks
4. Global insomnia
5. Talk about suicide or a prior history of attempts/acts
6. Irritability and agitation

Note. From "Some Facts about Suicide and Depression," by American Association of Suicidology, 2009b. Accessed August 7, 2009, from http://www.suicidology.org/c/document_library/get_file?folderID=232&name=DLFE-157.pdf

Sociological Explanations

In 1897, Emile Durkheim developed a comprehensive sociological model explaining suicide as the result of interaction patterns between individuals and society (Kastenbaum, 2009). Durkheim (1897a, 1897b, 1951) maintained that the social suicide rate was defined by two distinct social characteristics: the degree of the social integration of the individual and the solidarity or cohesiveness of the society or culture. Based upon the interactions between these two variables (social integration and social solidarity), Durkheim identified four types of suicide.

Altruistic Suicide: This type of suicide occurs when a person is highly integrated into a very cohesive or solidified culture and believes that it is his or her duty to die for the group.

Lester (1999) claimed the primary purpose of altruistic suicide is to make peace. Older persons may want to end their lives for peace of mind as the burden of their care is lifted from the significant others in their lives. Chronically ill, disabled, or dependent individuals may also have unselfish motives and take their own lives.

Egotistical Suicide: this type of suicide is committed by persons who are not well integrated into society. Corr, Nabe, and Corr (2003) note, "Egotistic suicide depends on an under involvement or under integration, a kind of disintegration and isolation of an individual from his or her society" (p. 470). Celebrities, intellectuals, artists, and the wealthy are also candidates for egotistical suicide as they may make their own rules and live outside of the constraints and rules of the culture (Kastenbaum, 2009).

Those ostracized by society because they are not mainstream in their beliefs and practices are also subject to egotistical suicide. Risk factors for egotistical suicide include lack of employment, financial difficulties, substance use, physical and sexual abuse, and social isolation (Cooperman & Simoni, 2005; Roy, 2003). A study by Komiti et al.

(2001) found that individuals who have HIV infection may have a higher rate of suicide ideation and attempts than those who are not infected because they are stigmatized by society. Researchers have also noted that negative attitudes about one's appearance and sexual identification within a community can be a sociological reason for suicide. Brausch and Gutierrez (2009) studied the role of body image and disordered eating as risk factors for depression and suicidal ideation in adolescents. They reported that disordered eating contributed to both suicide ideation and depressive symptoms, whereas body image only contributed to depressive symptoms (Brausch & Gutierrez, 2009).

Fatalistic Suicide: This occurs when a person feels overcontrolled by society, stifled, and suppressed. The person may feel that opportunities are blocked and there is no hope for the future in his or her society. The suicide of Sigmund Freud is an example of fatalistic suicide.

In 1923, Freud was diagnosed with cancer of the mouth and jaw. His notable problems were compounded in 1939, when he had to adjust to leaving his home in Vienna due to Nazi persecution. He died by suicide in 1939, in unbearable pain and depressed over having to leave his homeland.

Anomic Suicide: In anomic suicide, people are in a crisis situation and are confused due to major changes in their society. Social breakdown and the failure of established social institutions render people unable to cope with the rules and the changes. This is especially true during periods of financial crisis. Those forced to leave their jobs because of age or those who lose their jobs during periods of high unemployment are susceptible to anomic suicide as they feel they may no longer have a place in society. Ying and Chang (2009) studied suicide and socioeconomic factors. They found that in a low-income family in which the woman was employed but the man was not, the unemployed adult man was at high risk for suicide (Ying & Chang, 2009).

The Social Impact of Media

Research supports a strong association between media coverage of suicide and increased suicidal behavior in the community (Blood, Pirkis, & Holland, 2007; Gould, 2001; Stack 2005). Suicide coverage in print media such as newspaper has been shown to increase imitative suicide behaviors. U.S. suicide statistics were compared with the number of suicides appearing on the front page of the New York Times from 1948 through 1968. Monthly suicides significantly increased during months of high suicide media coverage. This study also found that the rate of suicide imitation increased when pictures were included in the reporting. Pirkis, Burgess, Blood and Francis (2007) maintain that no description of how the suicide occurred should be mentioned in the media. Extensive coverage and the use of the word suicide in a large headline were also found to increase the frequency of imitative behavior. This phenomenon of suicide imitation has become known as the "Werther effect" named after Goethe's literary hero (Werther) whose suicide was imitated by others (Etzersdorfer & Sonneck, 1998; Martin, 1998; Phillips, 1979). Media needs to exercise caution when reporting suicide to vulnerable groups such as young people, who are known to be susceptible to the copycat effect (Pirkis et al., 2007).

The American Foundation for Suicide Prevention (n.d.b) has made the following recommendations for language in the media:

- Whenever possible, it is preferable to avoid referring to suicide in the headline. Unless the suicide death took place in public, the cause of death should be reported in the body of the story and not in the headline.

- In deaths that will be covered nationally (as of celebrities), or those apt to be covered locally (as of persons living in small towns), consider phrasing for headlines such as: "Marilyn Monroe dead at 36," or "John Smith dead at 48." Consideration of how they died could be reported in the body of the article.

- In the body of the story, it is preferable to describe the deceased as "having died by suicide," rather than as "a suicide" or having "committed suicide." The latter two expressions reduce the person to the mode of death, or connote criminal or sinful behavior.

- Contrasting "suicide deaths" with "non-fatal attempts" is preferable to using terms such as "successful," "unsuccessful" or "failed." (Paragraph 10)

Lee, Chan, Lee, and Yip (2002) noted that a Hong Kong newspaper reported a complete account of a suicide by burning charcoal in a confined space. Within 3 years of the person's death, there was a dramatic increase in suicides using burning charcoal, with the number of suicides rising from 0% to 10% (Lee et al., 2002).

Etzersdorfer and Sonneck (1998) summarize the potential social impact of media reports on suicide as follows:

The trigger-effect will be bigger, the more details of the special methods are reported, the more suicide is reported as being inconceivable ("he had everything life can give"), the more the motives are reported to be romantic ("to be forever united"), the more simplifications are used ("suicide because of bad news"). The attention will be bigger if the report is printed on the front page, if the term "suicide" is used in the headline, if there is a photograph of the person who committed suicide, if the attitude of the person is implicitly described as being heroic and desirable ("he had to do that in this situation"). The effect will be smaller if more alternatives are shown ("where is it possible to find help in such a situation?"), if there are reports about a crisis that was overcome and did not result in suicide, if readers are provided with background information on suicide behavior and suicide in general (such as what to do when someone expresses suicidal thoughts). (p. 69)

> ***Personal Insight***
>
> *Consider a current movie or television program you saw which deals with a suicide or suicide attempt. How were you influenced by what you saw?*

Samaritans (2009) has recommended 13 tips for reporters when interviewing family members and friends after a suicide:

1. Avoid explicit or technical details of suicide in reports.

2. Avoid simplistic explanations for suicide.

3. Avoid brushing over the realities of a suicide.

4. Avoid disclosing the contents of any suicide note.

5. Discourage the use of permanent memorials.

6. Avoid labeling places as suicide "hotspots."

7. Don't overemphasise the "positive" results of a person's suicide.

8. Encourage public understanding of the complexity of suicide.

9. Expose the common myths about suicide.

10. Don't romanticise suicide or make events surrounding it sound melodramatic.

11. Include details of further sources of information and advice.

12. Remember the effect on survivors of suicide – either those who have attempted it or who have been bereaved.

13. Look after yourself.
(Paragraph 2)

SUICIDE PREVENTION

Public Health Strategies

Current suicide prevention programs and public health strategies were initiated as a result of the 1999 Surgeon General's Call To Action to Prevent Suicide (Table 8-2), which began a series of initiatives to bring attention to the problem of suicide and to recognize suicide as a public health problem (U.S. Public Health Service, 1999). In response to this initiative, the U.S. Public Health Service recommended a four-step strategy:

- *Step one:* Define the problem. Gather information about the characteristics of suicidal persons, incidents, and events that precipitate suicidal acts and effective supportive measures.

- *Step two:* Identify causes, risk factors, and groups of people at risk. Identify protective factors that can prevent suicide, such as clinical care for mental, physical, and substance abuse disorders; access to interventions; restricted access to lethal methods; support; learned skills in problem solving; and cultural and religious beliefs that discourage suicide.

- *Step three:* Develop and test the effectiveness of interventions.

- *Step four:* Implement interventions that have demonstrated effectiveness in preventing suicide and suicidal behavior.

The U.S. legislative bodies continue to fund prevention efforts. The Senate's spending bill for the fiscal year 2008 included $30 million for suicide prevention activities under the Garrett Lee Smith Memorial Act (American Psychological Association, 2007). Introduced by former Senator Gordon Smith in memory of his son who had died by suicide, the goal of this legislation is to amend the Public Health Service Act to support the planning, implementation, and evaluation of organized activities directed toward preventing suicide in young people (One

TABLE 8-2: SURGEON GENERAL'S CALL TO ACTION TO PREVENT SUICIDE

Awareness: Appropriately broaden the public's awareness of suicide and its risk factors

1. Promote public awareness that suicide is a public health problem and, as such, many suicides are preventable. Use information technology appropriately to make facts about suicide and its risk factors and prevention approaches available to the public and to healthcare providers.

2. Expand awareness of and enhance resources in communities for suicide prevention programs, and mental and substance abuse disorder assessment and treatment.

3. Develop and implement strategies to reduce the stigma associated with mental illness, substance abuse, and suicidal behavior and with seeking help for such problems.

Intervention: Enhance services and programs, both population-based and clinical care

4. Extend collaboration with and among public and private sectors to complete a national strategy for suicide prevention.

5. Improve the ability of primary care providers to recognize and treat depression, substance abuse, and other major mental illnesses associated with suicide risk. Increase the referral to specialty care when appropriate.

6. Eliminate barriers in public and private insurance programs for provision of quality mental and substance abuse disorder treatments, and create incentives to treat patients with coexisting mental and substance abuse disorders.

7. Institute training for all health, mental health, substance abuse and human service professionals (including clergy, teachers, correctional workers, and social workers) concerning suicide risk assessment and recognition, treatment, management, and aftercare interventions.

8. Develop and implement effective training programs for family members of those at risk and for natural community helpers on how to recognize, respond to, and refer people showing signs of suicide risk and associated mental and substance abuse disorders. Natural community helpers are people such as educators, coaches, hairdressers, and faith leaders, among others.

9. Develop and implement safe and effective programs in educational settings for youth that address adolescent distress, provide crisis intervention, and incorporate peer support for seeking help.

10. Enhance community care resources by increasing the use of schools and workplaces as access and referral points for mental and physical health services and substance abuse treatment programs, and provide support for persons who survive the suicide of someone close to them.

11. Promote a public/private collaboration with the media to assure that entertainment and news coverage represent balanced and informed portrayals of suicide and its associated risk factors, including mental illness and substance abuse disorders and approaches to prevention and treatment.

Methodology: Advance the science of suicide prevention

12. Enhance research to understand risk and protective factors related to suicide, their interactions, and their effects on suicide and suicidal behaviors. Additionally, increase research on effective suicide prevention programs, clinical treatments for suicidal individuals, and culture-specific interventions.

13. Develop additional scientific strategies for evaluating suicide prevention interventions and ensure that evaluation components are included in all suicide prevention programs.

14. Establish mechanisms for federal, regional, and state interagency public health collaboration toward improving monitoring systems for suicide and suicidal behaviors, and develop and promote standard terminology in these systems.

15. Encourage the development and evaluation of new prevention technologies, including firearm safety measures, to reduce easy access to lethal means of suicide.

Note. From "The Surgeon General's Call To Action To Prevent Suicide" by U.S. Public Health Service, 1999, Washington, DC. Retrieved August 7, 2009, from http://www.surgeongeneral.gov/library/calltoaction/calltoaction.htm

Hundred Eight Congress of the United States of America at the Second Session, 2004).

POPULATION-BASED PREVENTION

Nurses often have contact with individuals at risk for suicide. Examining population-based prevention strategies that focus on at-risk groups may enable nurses to take effective action to prevent suicides. These at-risk include students; lesbian, gay, transgender, and bisexual youth; individuals with mental illness; alcoholics; older adults; individuals with guns in their homes; police officers; and those in the military. Prevention efforts include depression screenings, public information campaigns that encourage a healthy lifestyle and help-seeking behaviors, and efforts to educate physicians and other healthcare providers on signs of depression and suicide risk factors (Fiske & Abore, 2000-2001).

Population-based prevention should also focus on those who have previously attempted suicide. In 2007, data indicated there were 864,950 suicide attempts or one attempt every 38 seconds in the U.S. (McIntosh, 2010). For every death by suicide there were 25 attempts, with three female attempts for each male attempt (McIntosh, 2010).

Adolescent, High School, and College Age Students

Among young adults, 15 to 24 years old, there is 1 completed suicide for every 100 to 200 attempts (Goldsmith, Pellmar, Kleinman, & Bunney 2002). The CDC (2008c) reported that in 2007:

- 14.5% of students, grades 9 to 12, had seriously considered suicide in the previous 12 months (18.7% of females and 10.3% of males).

- 6.9% of students reported having made at least one suicide attempt in the previous 12 months (9.3% of females and 4.6% of males).

- 2.0% of students reported having made at least one suicide attempt in the previous 12 months

that required medical attention (2.4% of females and 1.5% of males).

Research has shown that adolescents and young adults who most strongly believe that it is acceptable to end one's life are more than 14 times more likely to make a plan to kill themselves as those who do not hold those beliefs (Joe, Romer, & Jamieson, 2007). Nurses who ask the right questions to children can help identify those at highest risk. Such a question might be: "What are your beliefs about suicide?"

One group with substantial risk is Hispanic students. Hispanic female high school students in grades 9 to 12 reported a higher percentage of suicide attempts (14.0%) than their White, non-Hispanic (7.7%) or Black, non-Hispanic (9.9%) counterparts (CDC, 2008c).

It is estimated that 1,100 college students die by suicide annually in the United States (Joffe, 2008). A recent study examined factors that contributed to a college student's suicide attempt. The most frequent reasons given, in order of importance, were depression, trouble with relationships, stress, hopelessness, family problems, anxiety, and social isolation (Westefeld et al., 2005). The authors found that 24% of 1,865 college students had thoughts about attempting suicide and 5% had attempted.

Nurses should also assess whether a student has been arrested. Male and female students with a history of being arrested were more likely to have been diagnosed with depression and to have engaged in suicide ideation in the past, suggesting complex links between depression, delinquency, and suicidal behavior in college students (Langhinrichsen-Rohling, Arata, Bowers, O'Brien, & Morgan, 2004).

Student Barriers to Seeking Help

A strategy for prevention must also address the barriers that keep adolescent students from seeking help for themselves or their friends. Cigularov, Chen, Thurber, and Stallones (2008) studied factors preventing adolescents from seeking help after a suicide education program. Identified barriers to seeking help for oneself were:

- problems with adults
- lack of self-confidence
- fear of hospitalization
- lack of closeness to school adults.

Barriers to seeking help for troubled friends were:

- friendship concerns
- inapproachability of school adults
- fear of friend's hospitalization
- underestimation of friend's problems.

Nurses should be aware of such barriers and should work closely with counselors and social workers to eliminate factors that prevent students from seeking help.

As part of a comprehensive school-based suicide prevention program, Stuart, Waalen, and Haelstromm (2003) studied the efficacy of training peer helpers in suicide risk assessment. The authors found that peers needed basic training in empathy and active listening as well as training in suicide risk assessment and encouragement to seek out the angry and isolated peers in their schools. With training, peer helpers can develop relationships with these peers, even when such relationships might be resisted or difficult (p. 331).

Lesbian, Gay, Transgender, and Bisexual Youth

Population-based prevention should also focus on lesbian, gay, bisexual, and transgender youth. Among adolescents, sexual minority status is a key risk indicator for suicidal behaviors (Russell, 2003). When D'Augelli, Hershberger, and Pilkington

(2001) studied the suicidality patterns and sexual orientations of 350 lesbian, gay, and bisexual youths 14 to 21 years of age, they found that suicide attempts often occurred after the subjects became aware of their sexual feelings and before they told their parents or any one else of their sexual orientation. The authors concluded that over a quarter of the adolescents sampled reported a suicide attempt within their families. The findings show that nurses can prevent suicide in this population by being sensitive to their unique needs, fostering family and social supports, and encouraging professional counseling.

The term *transgender* refers to an individual's self-identity or gender expression that is different from his or her sex at birth; transgendered individuals include transsexuals, cross-dressers, and gender benders (Grossman & D'Augelli, 2007; Sears, 2005). Grossman, D'Augelli, Howell, and Hubbard (2005) studied transgender youth and their parents' reactions to their gender nonconformity and identity. All of the youth reported feeling different from others in early childhood. Increased gender nonconformity was associated with increased verbal and physical abuse by both parents. Grossman and D'Augelli (2007) found that half of transgender youth thought seriously of taking their lives, half of those related their thoughts to their transgender identity, and one quarter reported a suicide attempt.

Mental Illness

Another population-based strategy includes recognizing the risk of suicide among those with mental illnesses, such as schizophrenia, borderline personality disorder, and bipolar disorder. Schizophrenics have an increased risk of suicidal behavior (Fenton, 2000; Roy, 2001). Donatelle (2003) noted that schizophrenia is characterized by "alterations of the senses (including auditory and visual hallucinations); the inability to sort out incoming stimuli and make appropriate responses; an altered sense of self; and radical changes in emotions, movements, and behaviors" (p. 45). In the United States, case management or individual psychotherapy with medication is probably the most common treatment for schizophrenia (Fenton, 2000). Also, cognitive behavior therapy has been shown to reduce symptoms in schizophrenics (Bateman, Hansen, Turkington, & Kingdon, 2007).

Individuals at a high risk for suicidal behavior include those with borderline personality disorder, which may be accompanied by multiple lethal suicide attempts set off by apparently minor incidents and, less commonly, by high lethality attempts attributed to impulsiveness or comorbid major depression (Brodsky, Groves, Oquendo, Mann, & Stanley, 2006). Major depressive, panic, and bipolar disorders are also major illnesses that can lead to suicide. Mood stabilizers such as lithium may help control bipolar disorder. Newer medications such as lamotrigine (Lamictal), gabapentin (Neurontin), and topiramate (Topamax) are being studied to determine their effectiveness on bipolar individuals (National Institute of Mental Health [NIMH], 2008).

Alcohol and Drugs

Use of alcohol compounds depression, impairs judgment, and increases the risk of impulsive behavior. A history of alcohol abuse is often linked with a history of mood disturbance and other impulsive and violent behavior (Miller, 2004). Drinking within 3 hours of a suicide attempt has been shown to be associated with nearly lethal attempts. Alcohol-dependent men and women have been found to be more than twice as likely to attempt suicide as nondrinkers (Preuss et al., 2003) The National Violent Death Reporting System examined toxicology tests of those who died by suicide in 16 states: 33.3% tested positive for alcohol, 19.1% for opiates, 10.3% for cocaine, 8.1% for marijuana, and 4% for amphetamines (Karch et al., 2009).

Prevention strategies must focus on both younger persons and older adults. Pfaff, Almeida, Witte, Waesche, and Joiner (2007) emphasized the relationship between binge drinking and suicide among older persons. The authors found that older adults who use alcohol less frequently but in greater quantities are more likely to have a history of suicide attempts. Roy (2001) notes strategies to treat alcoholism include Alcoholics Anonymous meetings, prescribing naltrexone and acamprosate as aids in prolonging abstinence from alcohol, and treating comorbid depression.

Elderly Persons

Although suicide is the second leading cause of death among 25 to 34 year olds and the third leading cause of death among 15 to 24 year olds, the highest rates of suicide are found among those older than 75 years of age. The rate of suicide for adults 75 years of age and older was 15.9 per 100,000. Among adults aged 75 and older, there is 1 completed suicide for every 4 suicide attempts (CDC, 2009b).

White elderly males are most at risk. In 2006, 5,299 elderly people killed themselves in the United States, which means there were about 14.5 elderly person suicides each day. One elderly person completes suicide every 99.2 minutes. Among males, adults 85 years of age and older have the highest rate of suicide (a rate of 48.4 per 100,000 population) (AAS, 2009a).

Geriatric suicide is differentiated by fewer warning signs, more lethal means of ending life, and greater incidences of depression and physical illness than suicide in children and adults. Segal, Mincic, Coolidge, and O'Riley (2004) conducted a study to examine attitudes of older persons about suicide. Older persons reported that an attempter can't be dissuaded by a concerned listener, suicidal behaviors are normal in some situations, and suicide attempts are not a cry for help.

Nurses should pay careful attention to elderly patients who are physically ill and who exhibit any of the following warning signs of suicide (Holkup, 2003):

- stockpiling medications

- buying a gun

- giving away money or cherished personal possessions

- taking a sudden interest, or losing their interest, in religion

- failing to care for themselves in terms of their routine activities of daily living

- withdrawing from relationships

- experiencing a failure to thrive, even after appropriate medical treatment

- scheduling a medical appointment for vague symptoms.

Interventions in primary care settings and community outreach to isolated and at-risk elderly individuals are two recommended approaches in preventing geriatric suicide (Conwell, 2001). Suicidal older adults rarely seek out mental health services, but Préville, Boyer, Hébert, Bravo, and Seguin (2005) found that 53.5% of suicidal elderly adults consulted general practitioners or specialists during the 2-week periods prior to their suicides. Hopelessness, depression, physical illness, and access to a gun can lead to geriatric suicide. Religious beliefs and having children are a stronger reason for older adults not to complete suicide. It may be difficult to identify older clients who are at risk because they are less inclined to reveal their suicidal intentions than younger age groups (Miller, Segal, & Coolidge, 2001). Older patients often meet with their nurses to discuss their physical complaints prior to seeing the doctors, and it is during this time that nurses can use their knowledge related to suicide risk factors to assess the patient and determine the potential for suicidal behavior.

The Center for Elderly Suicide Prevention (CESP) seeks to prevent suicide in the elderly by identifying and addressing possible risk factors (e.g., social isolation, bereavement, depression).

CESP provides a 24-hour friendship line, individual counseling, friendly home visits, and psychotherapy home visits for seniors 60 years of age and older.

Individuals with Guns in the Home

Regions with higher rates of gun ownership have higher rates of suicide (Ilgen, Zivin, McCammon, & Valenstein, 2008).

All patients at risk for suicide must be asked if guns are available or easily accessible or if they intend to buy a gun (Simon, 2007). Dahlberg, Ikeda, and Kresnow (2004) maintain that there is a higher risk of dying by firearm suicide than by suicide from another means when there are guns in the home.

Police Officers

More police officers die by suicide than are killed in the line of duty. The stressors in police work include work overload, shift work, exposure to violent and life-threatening situations, the pressures of the criminal justice system, and problematic relationships with the community (Loo, 2003). Increased exposure to traumatic events places police officers at high risk for developing posttraumatic stress disorder and related symptoms (Violanti & Gehrke, 2004). If such distress and symptoms are not addressed, the risk of suicide is higher. Alcohol use has been identified as a problem among police officers (Davey, Obst, & Sheehan, 2000). Suicide prevention for police should involve psychological screening of new officers, periodic reassessments, a referral system, and in-service programs or outside continuing education that reduces stigma of depression, police stress, and suicide (Miller, 2005).

United States Military

Population-based prevention must also include the military. The suicide rate in the Army is at a 26-year high and male veterans are twice as likely to die by suicide as male non-veterans (Suicide Prevention Action Network [SPAN], 2010). Many who serve in the armed forces experience catastrophic events, which can include life-altering injuries, such as amputations, spinal cord injuries with paralysis, and traumatic brain injuries (TBI). A TBI is caused by a blow or jolt to the head or a penetrating head injury that disrupts the normal function of the brain. Injuries can range from "mild," causing a brief change in mental status or consciousness, to "severe," resulting in an extended period of unconsciousness or amnesia after the injury (CDC, 2008a). The leading causes of TBI are bullets, fragments, blasts, falls, motor vehicle-traffic crashes, and assaults. TBI can result in the disturbance of behavioral or emotional functioning, which can put the individual at risk for suicide. Those who served in the military may be at a higher risk for suicide if they experienced a TBI.

Simpson and Tate (2007) conducted a systematic search of the literature addressing suicidality after TBI. The authors reported that results from population-based studies concluded that people with TBI have an increased risk of death by suicide (three to four times greater than for the general population) and significantly higher levels of suicide attempts and suicide ideation. Clinical studies have also reported high levels of suicide attempts (18%) and clinically significant suicide ideation (21% to 22%) in TBI samples (Simpson & Tate, 2007).

Many soldiers have experienced TBI in recent wars. Although victims often show no outward sign of injury, contact with a bomb blast can affect vital brain functions, such as short-term memory, problem solving, and sleep. TBI can cause extensive functional changes that affect thinking, sensation, language, and/or emotions. Corrigan, Whiteneck, and Mellick (2004) found about 40% of those hospitalized with TBIs had at least one unmet need for services one year after their injuries. Unmet needs could contribute to suicidal thoughts and/or actions. The most frequent unmet needs were for services to help with:

- improving memory and problem solving.
- managing stress and emotional upsets.

- controlling one's temper.
- improving one's job skills.

The U.S. Army confirmed that 115 active-duty soldiers died by suicide in 2007, making the overall rate nearly 19 per 100,000 soldiers. Twenty-six percent of the soldiers who died by suicide in 2007 had never been deployed to Iraq or Afghanistan (Voice of America, 2008). Although officials say personal issues, such as relationship problems, trouble at work, and legal or financial difficulty are among the main causes of suicide in the military (Voice of America, 2008), suicide is a complex problem, not one issue that causes persons to end their lives. The U.S. military is predominantly young adults (85% male) from many races and ethnic backgrounds. About one half of the troops are between 17 and 26 years of age, a group already at high risk for suicide (Eaton, Messer, Garvey, Wilson, & Hoge, 2006).

It is possible that some suicides in the military are not being reported. Carr, Hoge, Gardner, and Potter (2004) used sources other than official records and found 17% more suicides than were reported by the military. The authors also found an additional 4% of deaths that were suspect, which suggested errors were made in reporting. Proper classification could possibly account for 21% additional suicides in the military.

The majority of military members who died by suicide did not have a known history of a mental disorder; 6% of suicides and 8% of suicide attempts were reportedly by persons who had a prior diagnosis of PTSD, and 50% of soldiers who completed suicide had a recent failed intimate relationship (U.S. Army Behavioral Health Technology Office, 2007). Nurses supporting veterans can save lives by understanding the significance of TBI, depression, PTSD, and combat stress as warning signs for suicide among those who are serving or who have served in the military. In 2007, the Veterans Suicide Prevention Act was signed into law. The bill directs the Secretary of Veterans Affairs to develop and implement a comprehensive program designed to reduce the incidence of suicide among veterans. The benefits of the bill include 24-hour mental health care for veterans found to be at risk for suicide, and development of an outreach and education program to enable veterans and their families to recognize readjustment problems and promote mental health.

ASSESSING SUICIDAL BEHAVIORS

The focus of this chapter thus far has been on describing and defining suicide and its prevalence in society, and exploring population-based prevention efforts for those at risk for suicide. With this basic understanding of suicide established, the focus will now shift to the role of the nurse in assessing suicidal behaviors in healthcare settings.

Primary Care

Beaudin, Vigil, and Weber (2004) found that 50% of practitioners underdetected suicide ideation in patients. The failure to detect this risk is one of the most prevalent and preventable clinical errors in behavioral health.

In order to form a clinical judgment of a patient's risk for suicide, nurses need to identify the factors that contribute to suicidal behaviors, the level of risk, and protective factors. Jacobs and Brewer (2004) maintain the following areas need to be evaluated during the assessment:

- patient's current and past psychiatric diagnoses, with attention to any comorbidity

- family and personal history of suicide attempts and mental illness

- individual strengths and vulnerabilities

- acute and chronic life stressors

- possible protective factors (things that reduce the likelihood of suicide)

- current complaints, symptoms, and mental state; in particular,

  - the presence or absence of any hopelessness, anxiety, and/or substance abuse

  - current suicidal thoughts, plans, and behaviors

  - input from collateral sources, if the patient is not forthcoming. (p. 374)

Warning Signs

Rudd et al. (2006) offered a definition of a warning sign as:

the earliest detectable sign that indicates heightened risk for suicide in the near-term (i.e., within minutes, hours, or days). A warning sign refers to some feature of the developing outcome of interest (suicide) rather than to a distinct construct (e.g., risk factor) that predicts or may be casually related to suicide. (p. 258)

Van Orden et al. (2006) maintain that "warning signs for suicide are the behavioral manifestations of precipitating conditions in a particular individual; they are directly observable, reflect the current state of the individual, and indicate the presence of a suicidal crisis." (p. 273)

In 2003, a working group convened by the American Association of Suicidology reached a consensus on a set of warning signs for suicide (see Table 8-3). Mandrusiak et al. (2006) sampled 50 websites and found that the warning signs for suicide most frequently mentioned by persons posting on the Internet are: giving away prized possessions, isolation or withdrawal, use or increased use of alcohol or drugs, changes in sleeping patterns, and indirect verbal statements (talking about dying or not being around).

The Impact of the Nurse's Attitudes

The attitudes nurses have toward suicide, their own history of suicidality, and death acceptance are all factors contributing to suicide intervention competencies (Neimeyer, Fortner, & Melby, 2001).

TABLE 8-3: HOW DO YOU REMEMBER THE WARNING SIGNS OF SUICIDE?

Here's an Easy-to-Remember Mnemonic:

IS PATH WARM?

Ideation

Substance Abuse

Purposelessness

Anxiety

Trapped

Hopelessness

Withdrawal

Anger

Recklessness

Mood Change

These warning signs were compiled by a task force of expert clinical-researchers and "translated" for the general public.

Note. From "Fact Sheet: Suicide in the U.S.A." by American Association for Suicidology, n.d.a. Retrieved August 7, 2009. from http://www.suicidology.org/c/document_library/get_file?folderID= 232&name=DLFE-159.pdf

Nurses' personal histories and discomfort in discussing suicide can affect their ability to develop therapeutic communication with suicidal patients (Neimeyer et al., 2001).

A good strategy for improving prevention of suicide in a hospital is improved training of healthcare personnel. Botega et al. (2007) studied 317 nurses working at a general hospital. Nurses attended a 6-hour program on suicide prevention that focused on stigma, common mental disorders associated with suicide in a hospital, the concept of psychache, interviewing skills, assessment, and management of the suicidal patient. The authors found that positive changes in nurse's attitudes were significantly maintained at a 6-month follow-up evaluation.

Emergency Room Assessment

Many who have attempted suicide pass through local emergency rooms (ERs) and more than 325,000 to 425,000 people with self-inflicted injuries are treated in ERs each year (CDC, 2007).

Nurses must be confident in evaluating suicidal patients and ensuring that social workers and mental health professionals, who include psychiatric advanced practice nurses (APRNs) and/or psychiatrists, see at-risk patients for intensive evaluation. Training and experience in identifying depression and suicide ideation is therefore essential for the ER nurse.

Suicide assessments should never be postponed in patients suspected to be at risk. It is critical that the patient is not left alone and remains visible to staff at all times. Rather than having the mental health professional see the patient at the end of the medical workup, the patient should be seen periodically throughout his or her time in the ER to identify any changes in behavior.

Depression and Suicide Assessment

Education in identifying depression in patients is key to reducing suicide rates. Experts from 15 countries completed an extensive review of the literature from 1966 to June 2005 and found that education in depression recognition and treatment, as well as restricting access to lethal means, such as a gun, reduces the suicide rate (Mann et al., 2005).

It is currently impossible to distinguish between patients with depression who will make a suicide attempt and those who will not. Prevention, therefore, must be based on the assumption that any patient with more than mild symptoms of depression is at risk for suicide and can only be effective if it is applicable to all patients with moderate to severe depression (Matakas & Rohrbach, 2007, p. 507).

The National Institute of Mental Health has made recommendations regarding diagnostic evaluation for depression. The professional should take a comprehensive history of any symptoms of depression: how severe they are, when they began, and how long they have lasted. The history takes account of the patient's past symptoms and treatment. Questions asked should address alcohol and drug use, suicide ideation, family history of depression, and past treatment and its effectiveness. The physician can also perform a mental status examination to establish if speech, cognition, or memory has been affected (NIMH, 2009).

Mental health professionals can assess signs of depression by using specific risk assessment instruments. These assessments include: the Reasons for Living Inventory (Linehan, Goodstein, Nielsen, & Chiles, 1983); the Scale of Suicide Ideation with outpatients (Beck, Brown, & Steer, 1997); and the Beck Depression Inventory, the Beck Anxiety Inventory, and the Beck Hopelessness Scale (Rudd et al., 2006). To assess signs of mental pain, clinicians can use the Mental Pain Scale (Orbach, Mikulincer, Sirota, & Gilboa-Schechtman, 2003) or the Psychological Pain Assessment Scale (Shneidman, 1999). A recent study by Pompili, Lester, Leenaars, Tatarelli, & Girardi (2008) noted that when a psychiatrist used the Psychological Pain Assessment Scale during a structured clinical interview, it was found that current and worst-ever psychache were significantly higher in patients considered to be at risk of suicide.

Initial Assessment

As a nurse cultivates a therapeutic alliance with a suicidal patient, an assessment is made by identifying risk factors for suicide (Table 8-4). It is essential to get a detailed history of suicidal behaviors as 20% to 70% of people who die by suicide have made at least one suicide attempt before and 3% to 10% of individuals who attempt will eventually complete suicide (Tremeau et al., 2005).

The presence of risk factors is a signal for the provider that the patient needs help. Hirschfeld and Russell (1997) list clinical risk factors as hopelessness, clinical depression or schizophrenia, substance abuse, history of suicide ideation, panic attacks, and severe anhedonia. Another risk factor is spousal bereavement. Johnson, Zhang, and Prigerson (2008) found that widowed adults with

TABLE 8-4: RISK FACTORS FOR SUICIDE

- Previous suicide attempt
- Mental disorders – particularly mood disorders such as depression and bipolar disorder
- Co-occurring mental and alcohol and substance abuse disorders
- Family history of suicide
- Hopelessness
- Impulsive and/or aggressive tendencies
- Barriers to accessing mental health treatment
- Relational, social, work, or financial loss
- Physical illness
- Easy access to lethal methods of suicide, especially guns
- Unwillingness to seek help because of stigma attached to mental and substance abuse disorders and/or suicidal thoughts
- Influence of significant people – family members, celebrities, peers who have died by suicide – both through direct personal contact or inappropriate media representations
- Cultural and religious beliefs – for instance, the belief that suicide is a noble resolution of a personal dilemma
- Local epidemics of suicide that have a contagious influence
- Isolation, a feeling of being cut off from other people

Note. From "The Surgeon General's Call To Action To Prevent Suicide 1999," by U.S. Public Health Service, Health and Human Services. Retrieved January 11, 2010, from http://www.surgeongeneral.gov/library/calltoaction/calltoaction.htm

low self-esteem and dependency on their spouses have elevated risk for depressive symptoms and suicidality.

When assessing suicide ideation, the initial assessment involves looking at imminent risk. Depending upon the acute risk, hospitalization may be necessary. Phrases, such as "I wish I were dead" or "I'm going to end it all" are verbal clues that an individual may be suicidal. Phrases, such as "What's the point of going on?" or "You would be better off without me," and "I can't go on anymore" are phrases that are not as direct, but still provide clues to nurses that their patients may have suicide ideation.

During the initial assessment, a suicide intent checklist can be used. This checklist is designed to measure the likelihood to engage in self-harm and includes questions on suicide ideation and formulated plan; access to a means; desire to die or fear of dying; use of alcohol or drugs; family history of suicide; prior attempts; support systems; future orientation; disorganized thoughts or hallucinations; recent personal losses; recent diagnosis of physical illness; guilt, blame, or shame for personal behaviors; and preparations for death (Lee & Bartlett, 2005).

Nurses need to become comfortable with asking questions about suicide.

• Start by telling the person you are concerned and give examples.

• If depression is indicated, don't be afraid to ask whether the person is considering suicide or has a particular plan or method in mind.

• Ask if the person has a therapist and is taking medication.

• Do not attempt to argue someone out of suicide. Rather, let the person know you care, that he or she is not alone, that suicidal feelings are temporary, and that depression can be treated. Avoid the temptation to say, "You have so much to live for," or "Your suicide will hurt your family" (AFSP, n.d.d, Paragraph 9).

To evaluate the lethality of the plan, nurses assess the intent, behaviors, and predictable consequences of that behavior. Predictive behaviors can include purchasing a gun, giving away possessions, or putting personal and business affairs in order. Additionally, individuals who have suffered from depression and suddenly exhibit opposite behaviors of elation are considered high risk. This time fol-

lowing a depression can be considered a vulnerable one, for it is at this time that many individuals complete suicide. Therefore, someone considered at risk should be monitored by their primary care physician or psychiatric care provider for months following a depression.

When managing a suicidal patient, the nurse should continuously monitor the lethality of the plan, consult with a peer (e.g., psychiatrist, social worker, physician, nursing supervisor), hospitalize the patient if necessary, show personal concern, involve significant others in the patient's life, and carefully qualify the issue of confidentiality to convey that statements regarding suicide will not be treated as a secret between patient and professional (Shneidman, 1993).

NURSING INTERVENTIONS

When a patient has attempted suicide, is having suicidal ideations, or is assessed to be at risk for suicidal behaviors, it is essential that the nurse intervene by facilitating appropriate referrals to mental health professionals or specialized services.

Referral to a Mental Health Professional

The American Association of Suicidology recommends some ways nurses can be helpful to individuals threatening suicide (Table 8-5). Nurses who are not trained mental health professionals can refer patients at risk for suicide to mental health professionals including psychiatrists, psychologists, clinical social workers, and psychiatric clinical nurse specialists or psychiatric nurse practitioners. Often these professionals are licensed by the state in an effort to maintain quality and protect the public from unqualified practitioners.

Psychiatrists are medical doctors specializing in mental disorders. They look at emotional problems as illnesses, can prescribe related medications, and may have admitting privileges at local hospitals.

TABLE 8-5: PREVENTING SUICIDE

The American Association of Suicidology recommends these interventions for someone who is threatening suicide:

1. Be aware. Learn the warning signs.
2. Get involved. Become available. Show interest and support.
3. Ask if he or she is thinking about suicide.
4. Be direct. Talk openly and freely about suicide.
5. Be willing to listen. Allow for expression of feelings. Accept the feelings.
6. Be non-judgmental. Don't debate whether suicide is right or wrong or feelings are good or bad. Don't lecture on the value of life.
7. Don't dare him or her to do it.
8. Don't give advice by making decisions for someone else to tell them to behave differently.
9. Don't ask 'why.' This encourages defensiveness.
10. Offer empathy, not sympathy.
11. Don't act shocked. This creates distance.
12. Don't be sworn to secrecy. Seek support.
13. Offer hope that alternatives are available, do not offer glib reassurance; it only proves you don't understand.
14. Take action! Remove means! Get help from individuals or agencies specializing in crisis intervention and suicide prevention.

Note. From "Understanding and Helping the Suicidal Individual" by American Association of Suicidology, n.d.b. Retrieved August 7, 2009, from http://www.suicidology.org/c/document_library/get_file?folderID=232&name=DLFE-30.pdf

Psychiatric clinical nurse specialists and psychiatric mental health nurse practitioners are nurses who have education and training in psychiatric illness and treatment at the graduate school level. They also can prescribe certain medications and may have admitting privileges at local hospitals.

Mental health counselors have extensive education and clinical training treating mental health problems via individual and group therapy.

Psychologists treat individuals using psychological techniques and are usually skilled in testing for psychological problems. Clinical social workers have at least a master's degree in social work and 2 years of experience in a clinical setting. Social workers counsel those with emotional problems and also arrange for needed social services. Psychoanalysts are psychiatrists or psychologists with special training in psychoanalysis, an approach involving intense exploration of the patient's unconscious mind in order for patients to remember early traumas that have been blocked.

Regardless of which profession intervenes, it is crucial that the environment will enable the individual to feel most comfortable and will support a rapport leading to an effective evaluation of the severity of suicide ideation and a plan for effective intervention.

No-Suicide Contracts

Mental health professionals frequently use no-suicide or no-harm contracts enlisting the patient's agreement to seek ways to reduce emotional stress, not kill oneself and, if suicidal, to call for help. The contract is signed with copies going to the person at risk and the clinician. The no-harm contract is not recommended for use with new patients, in emergency room settings, or with psychotic or impulsive patients (Jacobs & Brewer, 2004). The existing research does not support the use of these no-harm contracts to prevent suicide, nor to protect clinicians from malpractice litigation if the patient dies by suicide (Goin, 2003; McConnell & Lewis, 2007).

> *Personal Insight*
> *Suppose a coworker or friend was suicidal. What would you do?*

Suicide Hotlines

Crisis hotlines are 24-hour, toll-free suicide prevention telephone services available to anyone in suicidal crisis. The National Suicide Prevention Hotline (1-800-273-TALK) can route the suicidal caller to the nearest crisis center where immediate assistance and referral can be provided. Kalafat, Gould, Munfakh, and Kleinman (2007) studied the effectiveness of telephone crisis services and hotlines. They found significant decreases in crisis states and hopelessness of the callers during the telephone session, with decreases in crisis states and hopelessness in the weeks following the call. However, the authors maintain that, "despite strong theoretical and practical justification as a suicide prevention strategy, hotlines' empirical effectiveness has yet to be demonstrated unequivocally" (p. 339).

POSTVENTION

Shneidman (1993) coined the term *postvention,* meaning "those things done after the dire event has occurred that serve to mollify the after-effects of the event in a person who has attempted suicide, or to deal with the adverse effects for the survivor-victims of a person who has committed suicide."

Individuals Bereaved by Suicide

It is estimated that for every suicide there are at least six individuals bereaved by that suicide. It is estimated that 4.6 million Americans became survivors of suicide between 1990 and 2006, with an estimated 207,588 survivors of suicide added in 2007 (McIntosh, 2010). Grief after a suicide encompasses emotional, mental, social, spiritual, and intellectual dimensions and there is considerable evidence that the bereaved may have elevated risk for developing complicated mourning (Jordan & McMenamy, 2004).

In the first systematic review of individuals bereaved by suicide compared with survivors of other deaths, no significant differences between those bereaved after a suicide and other bereaved groups were found regarding general mental health, depression, PTSD, anxiety, and suicidal behavior (Sveen & Walby, 2008). However, the authors found that suicide survivors report higher levels of rejection, shame, stigma, need for concealing the cause of death, and blaming than survivors of other deaths. Bereaved parents by suicide have an increased likelihood of guilt, remorse, and self-blame in the mourning process if their child had a psychiatric illness, they had a troubled relationship with their child, and if their child had made previous attempts (Feigelman, Gorman, & Jordan, 2008-2009).

Because of the historical stigma associated with suicide, survivors often perceive stigma when, in fact, there is none. It is helpful if nurses give survivors the option of being open, rather than reinforcing (and thus perpetuating) the "stigma of suicide." Nurses do need to be aware that the suicide may actually be a relief for survivors if the person's mental illness caused them emotional turmoil, but they may also feel guilt for that initial sense of relief.

While providing help to suicide survivors, nurses may be called upon to answer some difficult questions. Why did their loved one take his or her own life? When responding to the question, one must realize that there may never be an answer. It is most important to simply be able to explore the questions openly and honestly and help survivors understand that suicide is rarely just the result of one thing. Suicidal deaths are often sudden, and survivors have little, if any, chance to say goodbye. Most survivors are surprised by the news and then must adjust to a loss that was unnatural in many ways.

McMenamy, Jordan, and Mitchell (2008) note that individuals bereaved by suicide report high levels of distress, depression, guilt, anxiety, and trauma and may find it difficult talking with others about the suicide. The pain of loss can last for many years. Although in time survivors work through their grief and integrate the loss into their lives, it is not uncommon for survivors to reflect on those professionals who supported them in the immediate aftermath of the suicide. Survivors may need support to be direct and honest about the suicide with friends, family, faith community, and workplace associates. Improved societal understanding about depression, mental illness, and suicide itself has contributed to increased compassion and understanding for survivors.

A suicide survivor's sudden loss experience may elevate his or her own suicidal risk due to the disruption in attachment, any substance abuse involved, or genetic predispositions, such as depression and bipolar disorder. Best predictors of reduced general health and posttraumatic distress for suicide survivors are isolation, low level of education, short time period since the loss, and female gender. Variables predicting complicated grief reactions for survivors are self-isolation, female gender, and absence of other children if a parent (Dyregrov, Nordanger, & Dyregrov, 2003). A critical aspect of standard aftercare procedures for nurses should include the provision of verbal and written information to family members that stresses grief as a normal but individualized process affecting each member of the family and the family system (Dyregrov, 2002).

Support Groups for Individuals Bereaved After a Suicide

Support groups have proven to be beneficial for bereaved survivors. Murphy and Johnson (2003) studied 138 grieving parents after the violent death of a child. The authors found that parents who went to bereavement support groups were four times more likely to find meaning in their child's death than parents who did not attend such a group. Geron, Ginzburg, and Solomon (2003) reported that members join support groups to develop relationships with others in similar situations, gain coping skills, and make contact with experts in the field of bereavement. McMenamy et al. (2008) found that individuals bereaved by suicide viewed professional help as beneficial and valued one-to-one contact with others who were bereaved by suicide.

Common statements made by group members can include "No one mentions his name," and "I

haven't told anyone the truth about how he died." Guilt is a common feeling among suicide survivors who often believe they could have done something to prevent the suicide. Survivors may need to find someone to blame for the suicide (i.e., the doctor, therapist, family members, friends, themselves, as well as the victim). The suicide survivor group gives them the opportunity to ask questions and focus on their most pressing issues and concerns. Suicide survivors may feel as though no one understands what they are going through, and they may find it difficult to talk about suicide with survivors of other types of losses. Studies show that homogeneous groups are a valuable tool to facilitate an identification with and a connection to group members (Davies, 2004; Dean, McClement, Bond, Daeninck, & Nelson, 2005; Jordan & Neimeyer, 2003) because survivors feel as though fellow group members understand their experiences.

During the group experience, grieving individuals can be empathetic toward one another, feel accepted and safe, learn new coping mechanisms, help others in the group, focus on their strengths, and view themselves as resources and experts (Anderson-Butcher, Khairallah, & Race-Bigelow, 2004). The group becomes a place where grieving individuals can share their grief and come to realize that what they are feeling is normal. High-risk mourners benefit from support groups (Dunne, 2004).

Suicide Survivors' Perceptions of Clinicians

Approximately 12 clinicians lose one of their patients to suicide each week in the United States. Because suicide survivors are upset, grieving, possibly feeling guilty, and frequently looking for compensation through a claim of negligence, the number of lawsuits keeps on rising (Lee & Bartlett, 2005). Peterson, Luoma, and Dunne (2002) examined what behaviors of clinicians, who were caring for the patient prior to suicide, were most and least helpful to the bereaved after the suicide. Behaviors reported as being most helpful included initiating contact after the death, offering condolences, and sharing their own experiences and senses of loss. It was found that 23% felt that the clinicians made a mistake regarding medication decisions and 27% reported their attitudes and beliefs toward mental health care had changed, resulting in a lack of faith in clinicians. The study found that clinicians should contact families of their patients who die by suicide by phone or in face-to-face meetings because survivors want to connect, accept condolensces, invite them to the funeral, and discuss their loved one's illness and treatment (Peterson et al., 2002). Initiating such contact may prevent feelings of anger and distrust in survivors, as well as lawsuits.

Many clinicians experience a considerable personal loss and emotional turmoil after losing a patient to suicide and, for some clinicians, the impact reaches clinical levels of emotional problems that disrupt normal functioning (Ruskin, Sakinofsky, Bagby, Dickens, & Sousa, 2004). In addition to family, friends, coworkers, and classmates, clinicians are intimately affected by a suicide and may need support as they grieve.

Personal Insight

Have you ever known anyone who died by suicide?

If so, did you experience a considerable personal loss and emotional turmoil?

CASE STUDY

Mr. Sung, an elderly Asian patient, 65 years old and recently widowed, arrived at his physician's office for his appointment. Through the years, he had always greeted the nurse with a warm smile and cheery hello. Today he walked slowly with his head down, avoiding eye contact. Usually alert and talkative, today he seemed lost in his own thoughts and didn't offer any verbal greeting.

The nurse asked him how he was feeling and he replied in a whisper "I'm fine." She noted that

he did not seem very happy. He told her that he was lonely since his wife's death and that all his friends were gone. She noted how difficult that must be for him.

Mr. Sung said, "I am all alone now. Nobody needs me. I don't know why I keep waking up every morning."

The nurse asked, "Do you think about ending your life?"

He replied, "Yes, it has been on my mind lately, and I can't seem to get the idea out of my head."

Dr. Alexander walked into the exam room and asked Mr. Sung how he was doing. The patient replied, "I am just fine, doc."

Questions

1. What are the signs that this patient may be at risk for suicide?

2. What factors precipitated his feelings?

3. What should the nurse do next?

Discussion

Signs that Mr. Sung may be at risk for suicide include the change in his affect, his avoidance of eye contact and conversation, his feelings of hopelessness and lack of meaning in his life, his age, and his gender. He also expresses suicidal ideations. The fact that he recently lost his wife, has lost other friends, and is now living alone are precipitating factors. The nurse showed compassion and asked appropriate questions to facilitate her assessment of his risk. She now needs to make the physician aware of her findings, especially because Mr. Sung is not being candid with the physician about his feelings. The nurse must intervene to assure that the patient's feelings and needs are made known and that he receives further assessment and intervention.

SUMMARY

This chapter explored the prevalence of suicide and psychological, biological, and sociological explanations for suicidal behaviors. Terminology relevant to suicide and related processes was defined. Population-based assessment and prevention activities were described. Nursing assessment, preventive intervention, and postvention procedures and resources were delineated.

WEB RESOURCES

American Association of Suicidology (AAS)
   http://www.suicidology.org

American Foundation for Suicide Prevention
   http://www.afsp.org

Barbara Rubel
   http://www.griefworkcenter.com

National Center for Suicide Prevention Training
   http://www.ncspt.org

National Institute of Mental Health
   http://www.nimh.nih.gov

Suicide Prevention Action Network USA
   http://www.spanusa.org

Suicide Prevention Resource Center
   http://www.sprc.org

Surgeon General's Call to Action to Prevent Suicide
   http://www.surgeongeneral.gov/library/callto
   action/default.htm

EXAM QUESTIONS

CHAPTER 8
Questions 62-72

Note: Choose the one option that BEST answers each question.

62. Rumination about taking one's own life is

    a. suicide ideation.
    b. suicide threat.
    c. suicide.
    d. suicide attempt.

63. According to Gutierrez, Rodriguez, and Garcia (2001), suicide is defined as

    a. death by self-inflicted means where there is evidence that the intent was to cause death.
    b. death by self-inflicted means where there is no evidence that the intent was to cause death.
    c. spoken or unspoken thoughts with the intention to communicate that a specific act of self-harm may happen soon.
    d. nonfatal acts, with or without injury, where there is evidence that the person had some intent to cause death.

64. To explain the act of suicide, professionals should use which of the following phrases?

    a. Committed suicide
    b. Ended it all
    c. Psychological suicide
    d. Died of suicide

65. The group at highest risk for suicide is

    a. teenagers.
    b. middle-aged adults.
    c. postmenopausal females.
    d. elderly males.

66. Which of the following groups has less risk for suicide?

    a. Police officers
    b. Members of the military
    c. American Indians
    d. African American women

67. The most common method of suicide among women is

    a. suffocation.
    b. poisoning.
    c. use of firearms.
    d. hanging.

68. Psychache is best described as

    a. a negative attitude toward life.
    b. an intense desire to end one's life.
    c. intense psychological and emotional pain.
    d. physical pain brought on by grief.

69. According to Durkheim's model, the two variables interacting to cause suicide are

    a. ego and altruism.
    b. social integration and social solidarity.
    c. fatalism and anomie.
    d. social isolation and depression.

153

70. Media coverage has been shown to increase the rate of suicide imitation when

    a. it is reported that the suicide was prevented.

    b. the cause of death is reported in the text.

    c. suicide headlines and pictures are used.

    d. alternatives to suicide are described.

71. A warning sign of increased suicide risk that is frequently mentioned by people posting on the internet is

    a. taking antidepressant medications as prescribed.

    b. increased socialization and networking.

    c. giving away prized personal possessions.

    d. making a psychotherapy appointment.

72. A nurse can best help a person bereaved due to a suicide by

    a. not using the term suicide when talking about how the person died.

    b. allowing the bereaved to openly discuss the death.

    c. offering an explanation for the suicide.

    d. distracting the person from thinking about the death.

CHAPTER 9

HELPING BEREAVED ADULTS COPE WITH MOURNING

CHAPTER OBJECTIVE

After completing this chapter, the reader will be able to explain how bereaved individuals cope with mourning.

LEARNING OBJECTIVES

After studying this chapter, the reader will be able to

1. describe the experience of bereavement.

2. list effective nursing interventions for a parent whose child has died.

3. describe theoretical models related to the process of mourning.

4. describe various bereavement interventions.

INTRODUCTION

This chapter will focus on issues related to bereavement and the loss experience. Adults grieve from all types of losses and this section will focus on the death of spouses, parents, and children. The mourning process is described to explain how people adapt and adjust after significant deaths. This chapter answers questions concerning ways to support the bereaved. The significance of social support is stressed and the issue of whether bereavement intervention is needed is identified.

BEREAVEMENT

The time period following a death in which the survivor grieves and mourns the loss is referred to as the bereavement period. Individuals experience many losses in their lifetimes. The focus of bereavement moves from the deceased to one's own mortality, fears of losing the known world, losing oneself, and being lost to others (Young, 2007-2008).

Death of a Spouse

The death of one's spouse is often a loss of great significance, especially for the older adult. As Lund and Caserta (2002) point out,

Loneliness and problems associated with managing the tasks of daily living are two of the most common and difficult adjustments for older adults. These problems are even more difficult for the older spousally bereaved because the daily lives of spouses are so closely connected. In later life, especially, spouses frequently become dependent on each other for conversation, love, and sharing of tasks. Loneliness is problematic because it involves missing, sadness, and a void that does not go away simply by being with or among other people. (p. 211)

Widows experience a lower sense of coherence, less instrumental and emotional support, poorer mental health, and perceive life events and hassles as significantly intense experiences compared with married women (Ungar & Florian, 2004).

After a spouse dies, a widow may maintain an emotional and spiritual attachment to the deceased husband. The bond between a husband and wife remains, even if the surviving spouse falls in love with someone new. Many older individuals experience the death of their spouses after a lifetime of losses. They may experience personal death worries as they see their friends and loved ones dying around them. These older individuals may need to learn new skills as they adjust their roles. Although it is not uncommon to relocate, doing so should be well planned and not rushed.

A strong social network can alleviate some of the stress caused by the death of a spouse. According to Hogan and Schmidt (2002), social support during bereavement consists of having someone listen nonjudgmentally to the bereaved as they express thoughts and feelings about the grief. The bereaved should be allowed to speak about their dead partners, share stories, ask others what they recall, and create rituals and celebrations for holidays and anniversaries (Hedtke, 2002). While providing emotional support, nurses can also address practical matters and offer advice and referrals.

Death of a Child

The relationships and attachments between parents and their children are unlike any other bonds and the death of a child causes the most intense and overwhelming of all grief responses (Davies, 2004). The death of a child initiates the grief process and a multitude of responses that follow separation and loss. A bereaved mother often wants to know why her child died and whether she caused the death to happen. Whether bereaved parents are describing the brief memories of their child or blaming themselves, nurses can reassure and comfort them. As the nurse attempts to respond to unanswerable questions, it helps to focus on the need of bereaved parents to ask questions, not on the need to have answers for the questions. Sometimes, there are no answers.

Parents grieve the loss of their child whether it occurs before or after the birth. Friends, family, the community, and medical staff may misjudge the impact of pregnancy loss on bereaved parents, according them little grief for their unborn child (Rubin & Malkinson, 2001). Effective grief support and communication occurs when there is an exchange of views, an understanding of the particular language of bereaved parents, and compassionate nurses who want to help the bereaved through the tragedy of their child's death. For those grieving parents who did not have an opportunity to say goodbye to their child, saying farewell in a symbolic way in the weeks or months after the death can have a healing effect (Wijngaards-de Meij, Stroebe, Stroebe, Schut, & Van Den Bout, 2008).

Annually, approximately 4,500 infants die suddenly of no immediately obvious cause, and nearly half of these sudden unexplained infant deaths (SUIDS) are attributed to sudden infant death syndrome (SIDS) (CDC, 2009a). Causes of SUID can include suffocation, poisoning, and accidents.

SIDS is the most common cause of death in infants one month to one year of age and is the third leading cause of infant mortality (after congenital anomalies and short gestation/low birth weight) in the United States (Table 9-1). Bereaved parents have a difficult time adjusting in bereavement due to not understanding why their infant died. Factors that increase an infant's risk for SIDS include:

- tummy (prone) or side sleeping
- soft sleep surfaces
- loose bedding
- overheating
- mothers who smoked during pregnancy
- bed sharing
- preterm and low-birth-weight infants (CDC, 2009a).

TABLE 9-1: THE 10 LEADING CAUSES OF INFANT DEATH IN THE UNITED STATES

1. Congenital malformations, deformations, and chromosomal abnormalities (congenital malformations)

2. Disorders relating to short gestation and low birth weight, not elsewhere classified (low birth weight)

3. Sudden infant death syndrome (SIDS)

4. Newborn affected by maternal complications of pregnancy (maternal complications)

5. Accidents (unintentional injuries)

6. Newborn affected by complications of placenta, cord, and membranes (cord and placental complications)

7. Respiratory distress of newborn

8. Bacterial sepsis of newborn

9. Neonatal hemorrhage

10. Diseases of the circulatory system

Note. From Deaths: Final data for 2006, by Heron et al., 2009. *National vital statistics reports,* 57(14). Hyattsville, MD: National Center for Health Statistics.

Barr and Cacciatore (2008) studied problematic social emotions of 441 bereaved mothers following miscarriage, stillbirth, neonatal death, or infant/child death and found envy, jealousy, and guilt were positively correlated with maternal grief. Although it may be distressing, communicating concerns (e.g., unfairness) will help parents to cope with their loss. Some studies have shown that women who have undergone a pregnancy loss experience high levels of guilt (Barr, 2004), self-blame (St John, Cooke, & Goopy, 2006), and a sense of responsibility (Hale, 2007). However, Price (2008) found that mothers who experienced pregnancy loss are resilient. They recover from their pregnancy losses with hardly any harmful effects to their long-term mental health and future parenting.

Gerber-Epstein et al. (2009) studied the experience of miscarriage in a first pregnancy and found three central issues in the experience of an early miscarriage in a first pregnancy:

1. Internal search to find meaning in the loss of "someone" or "something" that did not exist, of an unseen embryo, which concerns the complexities of the loss

2. Interpersonal aspect and focuses on the presence of the partner in the situation

3. Treats the miscarriage as a social–cultural phenomenon and examines the woman's experience through this prism (p. 22).

Perinatal loss includes deaths in the first week of life and stillbirths. The preliminary infant mortality rate for 2006 was 6.7 infant deaths per 1,000 live births, a 2.3 percent decline from the 2005 rate of 6.9 (CDC: NCHS, 2008). After a perinatal loss, mothers continue to feel connected and close to their babies, and this continued relationship is not related to the time elapsed since the death (Uren & Wastell, 2002). Despite the passage of time, one 85-year-old mother acknowledged that she still felt guilty that her infant child had died (Riches & Dawson, 2002). Nurses can identify those things that bring comfort to the bereaved, including the belief that they will see their loved ones again. A 31-year-old bereaved father of a premature son said,

"I look forward to someday seeing his sweet little face in heaven" (Gamino et al., 2002, p. 807).

Ultrasounds are now routine prenatal care. Usually, they allow parents to see their infant moving or give them a glimpse of its beating heart. Ultrasounds can also show that an infant has died, leaving bereaved parents to experience a range of emotions and behaviors, including self-blame, denial, not eating, and suicidal ideations (McCreight, 2008). Katherine, a woman who experienced one stillbirth and two miscarriages reported:

When they showed me there was no heartbeat I was gutted. It was like someone had ripped out my heart, my heart broke and it's never gone back right. I couldn't go out of the house. I just couldn't cope with it all and I didn't eat for weeks, I just wanted to die, badly (McCreight, 2008, p. 7).

Mothers who conceive again after such a loss, may fear another ultrasound. Usually mothers are told of their child's death immediately after an ultrasound, so the procedure may remind her of the child who died in utero. Nursing interventions before such an ultrasound exam can help mothers cope with the exams. Nurses should be mindful that the last ultrasound might have been the last time the parents saw the previous baby's heart not beating. Interventions include first allowing the parents to hear the infant's heartbeat, explaining what will occur during the ultrasound, and constantly reassuring parents that flashbacks and memories of the baby in subsequent pregnancies is normal (O'Leary, 2005).

Protocols for Bereaved Parents

Bereavement protocols should offer parents the opportunity to decide if they want to spend time with their dead infant (Reilly-Smorawski, Armstrong, & Catlin, 2002), but nurses should never force parents to hold their child. Reynolds (2003-2004) reported,

These parents should be given an option to hold and see their dead infant. However, a helping professional's too rigid, overzealous adherence to perinatal bereavement protocols can deprive the patient of individualized intervention and care plan that is assessment driven. Indeed, perhaps the most serious deficit in the psychosocial management of stillbirth is the lack of a thorough psychosocial/psychiatric assessment prior to the introduction of postnatal care options for the stillborn. (p. 87)

Neonatal intensive care unit nurses can offer bereavement packets that include photos, footprints, and a memory certificate. These packets become significant mementos to grieving parents.

Reilly-Smorawski et al. (2002) created a contact sheet to guide nurses when making follow-up calls to bereaved parents. To facilitate communication, the primary nurse should contact the grieving parents about 1 to 3 weeks after the death to see how they are coping with their loss. This compassionate telephone call shows the parents that their nurse is still thinking of them during their difficult time. Reily-Smorawski et al. note that themes could include asking if there was a memorial service, if they are getting enough sleep, how their friends have been supportive, if they have other children, how they are doing, and if there are any unresolved issues they would like to discuss. In acknowledging the baby's life and death, whether by allowing the parents to hold the child, offering a bereavement packet, or making a follow-up call, parents are helped to accept the reality of their child's death.

When creating bereavement protocols in a pediatric intensive care unit (PICU), nurses also need to focus on what parents need prior to their child dying. They are connected to their child and may need pastoral care assistance as well as a compassionate nurse who communicates honestly with them during the experience of their child's life nearing its end. When creating bereavement protocols, nurses should focus on creating positive memories by creating a sacred private atmosphere where parents are allowed to say good-bye to their child.

Briller, Meert, Myer Schim, Thurston, and Kabel (2008) used qualitative methods to study factors influencing parents' grief responses after losing a baby in the PICU of an urban children's hospital. The following themes emerged from their stories, revealing important components of their experiences:

- Connection with Child: *You're in a state of shock and you're never gonna leave your child at that time.*

- Religious Practice: *Sometimes there's certain scriptures that maybe a pastor would pull that might, you know; soothe your hurt at the time.*

- Professional Support: *And I didn't know the chaplain. But I felt like I knew him by the end. I'm sure he spent several hours with me that day.*

- Compassion: *The receptionist at that front desk …She, you know, every morning greet us and would know my whole extended family, would know when we had a procedure…there was hugs, I mean for my entire family, not just for me. It was so nice.*

- Trust: *We had a good friend that's an emergency room nurse…She kind of helped us because she deals with this stuff every day. And since we trusted her, not that we didn't trust the other people, but it's another opinion and somebody that's kind of reinforcing what you're hearing and seeing.*

- Honest Communication: *I think it's hard for people to tell you that your child's gonna die. So it's – sometimes it's done in a circuitous way – instead of in a straightforward way.*

- Privacy: *But here you are in a room in PICU where it's all glass. And you're in there saying your goodbye and if you happen to turn your head, you see all these people staring in at you, watching.*

- Sacred Atmosphere: *I had a very peaceful spiritual experience when my son passed. I felt that something entered the room and I had this calm and I wasn't crying…it was a peace that came over me.*

- Enough Time: *And that was valuable to us. The fact that nobody really rushed us to make a decision. I think they gave us time*

(Briller et al., 2008, p. 255).

Meert, Briller, Myers Schim, Thurston, and Kabel (2009) found four categories of bereaved parental need in the PICU. These needs emerged from accounts of people, places, events, and interactions and reflections on the meanings and significance of the parent's loss:

1. Who Am I: Parent-child connections before, during, and after the death as well as cultural, religious, and family traditions.

2. While My Child Was Dying: Parental needs for personal and professional support and key attributes related to that support, such as compassion, trust, honest communication, and recognizing the child as a person.

3. My Child's Death Context: Environmental factors, including privacy, sacred atmosphere, enough time, and facility support that contribute to parents' perceptions of the milieu surrounding the death.

4. My Bereavement Journey: The process of coping with loss and integrating the experience into their lives through bereavement support, being given permission to grieve, and finding a sense of meaning.

MOURNING

Customs

Mourning is the explicit expression of grief and the customary response to bereavement. The term "mourning" refers to the period of time when grief goes public.

Customs of mourning vary depending upon culture. Cultural influence may play a role in the choice of clothing individuals wear during their bereavement and when to return to wearing clothing worn prior to the death. Mourning clothes have changed through the years for men and women. During the time of mourning in the late 18th century and throughout the 19th century, men in England and France wore dark clothing and women wore heavy, concealing, black garments, crepe veils, caps, and bonnets up to 4 years after their losses (Bedikian, 2008). Rules have gradually become more relaxed, and it is now acceptable in many cultures not to wear mourning clothing.

However, some individuals still dress in dark colors for up to a year after their loss.

COPING WITH MOURNING

When is mourning finished, and is it ever really over? The answer is simple. Mourning is finished when the individual says it is, or better said, when the individual feels it is. Yet, models or theories can help in evaluating the patterns of grieving people.

> *Personal Insight*
>
> *When do you think an individual should be finished mourning?*
>
> *What brings you to this conclusion?*

Over the past 20 years, researchers and grief experts have developed theories of mourning, including: Four Phases of Mourning Theory, Six "R" Process Theory, Dual Process Model, Continuing Bonds Theory, Four Task Model, Meaning Reconstruction, OTHERS(S) Model, Posttraumatic Growth Model, and Resilience Model. Brief descriptions of each of these models follow.

Four Phases of Mourning

One of the earliest mourning theories was Parkes' Four Phases in Mourning. Parkes (1970) proposed that mourning be divided into four phases based on Bowlby's attachment theory. The hypothesized four phases are as follows: (1) *shock and numbness,* during which individuals have difficulty processing the fact that their loved one has died; it is during this phase when they feel the most numb; (2) *yearning and searching,* wherein individuals experience intense separation anxiety and denial; they yearn and search for the person who died; (3) *disorganization and despair,* characterized by the inability to concentrate; and (4) *reorganization,* during which individuals realize that life will not be exactly the same as when their loved ones were

alive and they rebuild their lives accordingly. As Freud wrote:

> We find a place for what we lost. Although we know that after such a loss the acute stage of mourning will subside, we also know that we shall remain inconsolable and will never find a substitute. No matter what may fill the gap, even if it be filled completely, it nevertheless remains something else (Freud, 1961, p. 386).

Six "R" Processes of Mourning Model

Another well-known mourning theory is one that focuses on actions taken to move individuals through their unique grief processes. Therese Rando created a process-based theory and many counselors have acknowledged its significance. Rando (1993) maintains that six processes are required for healthy accommodation of loss. Complicated grief takes place when there is a compromise, distortion, or failure in completing one or more of the six "R" processes of mourning. The processes, as outlined by Rando, are: 1) *recognizing* the loss, wherein a grieving individual acknowledges and understands that the death took place and experiences the pain of that loss; (2) *reacting* to the separation, during which the individual feels the loss, expresses it, and mourns any secondary losses; (3) *recollecting and reexperiencing* the deceased and the relationship, including reviewing and remembering times shared with the loved one and reexperiencing the feelings associated with those thoughts; (4) *relinquishing* the old attachments to the deceased and the old assumptive world; (5) *readjusting,* to move adaptively into the new world, without forgetting the old; and (6) *reinvesting,* during which the individual forms new relationships and accepts the changes that have occurred in life due to the loss.

Dual Process Model

Stroebe and Schut (1999, 2001) proposed the Dual Process Model as a model of coping with grief. Mourning is viewed in the context of coping with two types of stressors – loss and restoration. If one type of coping is used disproportionately from the other, mourners are likely to experience higher levels of distress. Mourners cope via a process of oscillation between the loss-oriented (LO) approach and the restoration-oriented (RO) approach. The LO approach is concerned with coping with loss. LO behaviors include grief work, intrusion of grief, breaking bonds or ties to the deceased, relocation, denial, and avoidance of restorative changes.

The RO approach is concerned with behaviors oriented toward restoration and coping with stressors secondary to the loss (e.g., financial problems, tasks of daily living). RO processes might include attending to life changes, doing new things, finding distractions from grief, denying or avoiding grief, taking on new roles and identities, creating new relationships, dealing with secondary losses, addressing sources of stress, and adapting to loss while taking respites from grieving when needed. What differentiates this model from the six "R" Process model is the oscillation between two processes, RO and LO, throughout bereavement; conversely, the six "R" processes are hypothesized to occur in a linear fashion. By alternating between LO and RO, grieving persons can either confront their grief or avoid it. It is unclear how balanced this oscillation should be at different times during mourning. Grieving persons can manage the dosage of grieving. They can also take a respite from dealing with LO or RO, as part of their adaptive coping with death.

Caserta and Lund (2007) examined 163 recently bereaved widows 45 to 94 years of age, and found that widows who focused more on LO approach coping were found to be more depressed and lonely and experienced greater feelings of grief. Widows who focused on RO coping reported higher levels of self-care and daily living skills and personal growth (Caserta & Lund, 2007). RO

challenges include mastering new tasks, making decisions, taking on new roles, and greater self-care.

Continuing Bonds Model

For years the traditional thanatological approach focused on breaking bonds with those who died. In 1996, Klass, Silverman, and Nickman hypothesized that bereaved individuals did not have to sever the bonds, but could maintain inner representations of the deceased and hold them in their memories. Believing that the bond they shared will never be broken brings comfort and support to those who mourn. The concept of continuing bonds "challenges the traditional thanatological approach that views 'breaking the bonds' with the deceased as the major task of the bereaved, and the persistent occupation with the loss as an indicator of complicated reaction" (Ginzburg, Geron, & Solomon, 2002, p. 129).

The essential purpose of continuing the spiritual bonds is to enable grievers to develop new and meaningful relationships with the deceased. Parkes (2003) notes in regard to continuing the bonds,

> My own view is that there is a literal truth in the statement, "He or she lives on in my memory," but it is important for bereaved people to discover which habits of thought and behavior are now obsolete and must be let go and which can be retained. (p. 39)

Barrera et al. (2009) examined early parental bereavement after a childhood cancer death. Ninety percent of the parents in their study reported the ability to maintain relationships and continued spiritual bonds with their deceased children. Thoughts and behaviors that bring comfort change as time passes. However, the connection remains. Survivors sense their loved one's presence through memories and feelings, and this continues the spiritual connection with the deceased (Gamino et al., 2002). Grieving individuals have reported they felt the deceased were "watching over them" and there were still "inner connections" to their loved ones

(Gamino et al., 2002). These inner connections are particularly felt when grieving individuals create death rituals.

Four Tasks of Mourning Model

William Worden suggests that individuals accomplish tasks in mourning through a cognitive behavioral approach, rather than an emotional approach, as in Kübler-Ross's Five Stages Model for dying individuals. According to Worden (2002), abnormal grief reactions occur when people are unable to complete these four tasks of mourning. These tasks are goal oriented and are helpful to people who desire structure or steps to guide them though their grief. Healthcare providers can identify the task or tasks of mourning that are not completed and help the bereaved to resolve each task.

First, grieving persons must *accept the reality* of the loss. In accepting the reality, the bereaved understand their loved ones are truly dead. If death is unexpected, they may experience denial and find it difficult to accept that the persons are really dead and will not return. For actualization of the death to take place, mourners can view the bodies before the funeral, attend the service or funeral, or view photographs and personal belongings of the deceased.

Worden's second task of mourning is *working through the pain of grief.* The bereaved experience physical and emotional pain and may attempt to numb their pain with illegal drugs and alcohol. Others may work long hours to avoid the deep pain of loss. For some, the pain is so great that they attempt to avoid it by not visiting places their loved ones may have been.

The third task of mourning is *adjusting to an environment in which deceased individuals are missing.* If the individuals don't adjust, they may withdraw from life. Bereaved individuals have new responsibilities and must take on roles previously performed by their loved ones. If a grieving widower relied on his wife to shop and cook, he will need to find alternative ways to provide for meals. If a husband prepared the yearly taxes, a widow must learn how to do tax preparation or find another person to fulfill this role.

The fourth and final task of mourning is to *emotionally relocate the deceased and move on with life.* As bereaved people develop healthy new relationships with others, they may feel disloyal to their deceased loved ones. Their task is to create new relationships, while not forgetting their loved ones. Widowers may seek out new wives. Women may decide to get pregnant after the death of their babies. It may be difficult to emotionally relocate the deceased. Although bereaved individuals need to invest in new relationships, they may not be ready or able to do so. Establishing new relationships exposes people to vulnerability and the possibility that new relationships may also end, but Worden maintains that individuals must move on with life as part of the grieving process.

Meaning Reconstruction

Neimeyer (2000) describes mourning as a set of challenges to mourners to acknowledge the reality of the loss and to open themselves up to the pain. Neimeyer maintains that mourners must revise their basic assumptions about their worlds and reconstruct their relationships to that which has been lost. Once this is accomplished, bereaved individuals can reinvent themselves. This meaning reconstruction in response to loss is viewed as the central process of grieving (Neimeyer, 2001). Rather than breaking ties with the deceased, a continuing experience of relationship is encouraged and the bereaved develops a new sense of self without the loved one.

An example of such meaning reconstruction comes from the work of Cadell and Marshall (2007), who studied individuals' self-construals after the loss of a partner from HIV/AIDS for whom they were the caregivers. Self-construals are one's own version and explanation of the loss experience. The authors found that caregiving became a part of the self. The caregiving role gave significance and purpose to their lives. After partners die, the loss can become a crisis of meaning due to the loss of the persons and the relationships. The authors maintain that regaining meaning involves making sense of both the relationships and the caregiving roles. As they mourn, bereaved individuals attempt to reconstruct their relationships with the deceased (Neimeyer, 2006a). The individuals in the study were reconstructing their relationships with the deceased and attempted to reestablish "their self-construals in relation to the deceased partner by acknowledging the influence of the partner in their lives" (p. 545).

> **_Personal Insight_**
> *If you experienced the death of a patient, how did you acknowledge the reality of the loss?*
>
> *What made it real for you?*

OTHERS(S) Model

The OTHERS(S) model is strength based and focuses on practical skills, empowerment, education, relationships, and growth during bereavement (Fazio & Fazio, 2005). When individuals are able to look at the positive, self-question, have a sense of humor, connect with what they are feeling, remain stable and bounce back, feel connected to someone, and develop confidence in their abilities to handle loss, their symptoms will be reduced. They will return to normal levels of functioning, and they will grow from the loss (Fazio & Fazio, 2005). The OTHERS(S) Model stands for the following coping behaviors:

O – *Optimism/Hope:* belief that one can survive, learn and grow from the experience.

T – *True Meaning:* value can be found in the life lost.

H – *Humor:* one can still laugh and enjoy life.

E – *Emotional Intelligence:* ability to understand the feelings of self and others.

R – *Resilience:* ability to bounce back.

S – *Self-Confidence:* belief in one's own ability to cope.

S – *Spirituality:* belief in something outside oneself, a higher power.

Posttraumatic Growth Model

The posttraumatic growth model is defined by Tedeschi and Calhoun (2008) as "positive psychological change experienced as a result of the struggle with highly challenging life circumstances" (p. 1). A loss disrupts the individual's assumptive world or sense of self. Personal growth can result if the person subsequently views himself or herself and others differently, reevaluates priorities, and appreciates life in a new way. Optimism is positively associated with posttraumatic growth after a loss (Gillies & Neimeyer, 2006; Milam, 2006). Studies show that two groups in particular experience posttraumatic growth – individuals who accepted that their loved ones were dying and grieving parents.

Metzger and Gray (2008) found the ability to accept imminent loss was positively associated with greater gains and growth following the loss. As their loved ones were dying, these people had pre-loss acceptance and recognized the significance of existing relationships. After their loved ones died, they may have tried to maintain and improve their relationships with other survivors.

Grieving mothers reported personal growth after 3 years and felt as though they had more compassion, more tolerance, and more forgiveness as a result of their grief (Hogan, Greenfield, & Schmidt, 2001). A sense of personal growth may be perceived by some bereaved parents after the death of their child (Riley, LaMontagne, Hepworth, & Murphy, 2007), especially when they planned and problem solved when faced with life stressors. Personal growth can be achieved by creating memorial funds or becoming involved as a volunteer helping others, creating rituals prior to and after the death, and leaning on faith and belief systems that help remember the good times shared with their loved one. The experience of loss became one of positive growth after 31 months for one grieving mother who reported,

> Her death has changed my life profoundly and I feel like a completely different person. It's like a part of me died and a stronger part took its place (Uren & Wastell 2002, p. 301).

The Resilience Model

What do you do when your life is shattered? What do you do when the bright future you expected for yourself feels like it is collapsing into ruins? People who have bounced back from devastating setbacks are inspiring, real-life examples of resiliency (Siebert, 2005, p. 20).

Resilience is the ability to adapt to adversity and use effective coping strategies to "bounce back" after loss. The contextual resilience model emphasizes the central role that person-environment transactions play in bereavement (Sandler, Wolchik, Tein, & Ayers, 2008). The resilience model focuses on coping to adapt behaviorally and cognitively to the changes that occur after death and loss. The bereaved adapt to loss and find meaning through a process that is a part of their cultural belief systems, rituals, roles within their family, and community. Bonanno, Galea, Bucciarelli, and Vlahov, (2006) found that married individuals were more resilient than those unmarried, divorced, or separated, and males showed more resilience than females. Bonanno, Moskowitz, Papa, and Folkman (2005) reported that 52% of bereaved individuals in their study were considered resilient at 4 months and 18 months after the death of their spouses. Bonanno, Wortman, and Neese (2004) maintain that resilient spousally bereaved persons cope by talking and thinking about the deceased, have fewer regrets about behavior related to the deceased, and have less need to question or search for meaning in the death. Resilience has recently been recognized as a common coping response for individuals experienc-

ing disasters (Almedom & Glandon, 2007). The main objective of resiliency is to establish an experience that allows the bereaved to introspect intensely and identify, discover, nurture, and develop internal and external sources of energy for daily living and coping (Richardson, & Waite, 2002).

SUPPORTING THE BEREAVED

Social Support

Social support is defined as the amount of emotional or instrumental assistance a person receives (Goldsmith, 2007). Emotional assistance refers to thoughtfulness, care, and attention. Instrumental assistance refers to tangible support. Such social support is often found in bereavement support groups.

Rack, Burleson, Bodic, Holmstrom, and Servaty-Seib (2008) studied 105 bereaved adults' evaluations of grief management support strategies. Nurses can learn much from this study as it clearly shows the significance of the gift of presence and listening. The participants in the study reported the highest-rated helpful support strategy was offering presence (being there) followed by expressing the willingness to listen, expressing care and concern, complimenting the deceased and the bereaved, discussing being reunited, highlighting the positive, discussing memories of the deceased, and providing tangible support and a religious perspective. The lowest-ranking helpful support strategies reported was advice giving, followed by minimizing feelings and forced cheerfulness. Although the bereaved may experience relationship difficulties, significant positive changes can occur, including a greater sense of compassion, connectedness, and intimacy (Tedeschi & Calhoun, 2008).

Dyregrov (2003-2004) investigated social support for traumatically bereaved parents who lost a child or young adult due to suicide, accident, or

SIDS. Survivors reported that their social networks (i.e., family, friends, acquaintances, work colleagues, and neighbors) positively responded to them by contacting them, bringing them food, helping with housework, going for walks together, and sending letters, poems, or books. However, some individuals were socially inept and unable to help. The bereaved anticipated the support of certain people who failed to appear, did not communicate, withdrew from them, or offered unhelpful advice.

To cope with social ineptitude in others, 81% of the survivors stressed the importance of their own "openness" in being able to inform others of their loved one's death, tell their story, and clarify their needs (Dyregrov, 2003-2004). When the bereaved are able to openly share their losses, they can create rituals with caring friends and family members. After the death of loved ones, the bereaved begin self-reflective processes that help them cope, and they may create related rituals. For example, when the bereaved continually visit the gravesite, a pattern of remembrance confirms their ongoing love and promise never to forget. This ritual, marked by time, creates a sense of personal endurance that is self-stabilizing and challenges the despair associated with emptiness (Armour, 2003). It becomes a meaningful ritual, as the bereaved attempts to create some type of order to keep his or her world cohesive and predictable.

BEREAVEMENT INTERVENTIONS

The aim of bereavement intervention in healthcare and community settings is to decrease symptoms of distress, avert problems, and encourage positive coping (Shapiro, 2008).

Although much research from the 1970s to 1990s focused on issues of pathology and bereavement risk assessment, it is now generally accepted that most people will recover over time, without any professional bereavement interventions or with low-level interventions only (Bonanno et al., 2004).

Reid, Field, Payne, and Relf (2006) found that the bereaved accessed support from voluntary bereavement organizations, general medical practitioners, and churches; those who declined support had support from other sources or preferred to cope on their own. Studies find relatively small or non-existent effects of bereavement interventions for adults experiencing normal bereavement and, in a high proportion of cases, bereaved individuals would have been better off without intervention (Jordan & Neimeyer, 2003).

Somhlaba and Wait (2008) found that spousal death triggers feelings of sadness, dejection, diminished self-esteem, heightened anxiety, high stress levels, and mild depression. They point to the necessity for bereavement intervention programs and support from social networks that are aimed at mitigating feelings of social isolation. Bereavement interventions were found to be beneficial for younger, female adults with higher levels of problems who entered into the program later in their bereavement, but bereaved children have reported weak program effects (Brown, Sandler, Tein, Liu, & Haine, 2007). Clinical bereavement interventions are most beneficial when they are of a high quality, delivered by trained professionals, and targeted at the 5% to 20% of specific groups who may experience complicated grief (Nucleus Group, 2004; Brown et al., 2006).

Being that bereavement counseling may not be essential to the bereaved who are not high-risk mourners, intervention should be provided for the bereaved suffering from complicated grief without social support, especially when the death occurred under traumatic circumstances (Neimeyer, 2000). Bereavement intervention can include group therapy, individual and family treatments targeted at high-risk mourners, such as children who have lost parents, and survivors of suicide and homicide. Genevro, Marshall, and Miller (2004) recommend that, "at a minimum, however, physicians and other healthcare providers should be capable of responding compassionately to bereaved persons" (p. 557).

"Companioning" the Mourner

Alan Wolfelt (2009) has developed a philosophy of caregiving to be applied in working with grieving people. Rather than treating grief as if it is a pathological condition, Wolfelt encourages the helper to be totally present with the bereaved and "companion" them through the grief experience. He espouses 11 tenets for "companioning" as follows:

1. Be present to the person's pain; do not try to take it away.

2. Be willing to go to the wilderness of the soul with another.

3. Honor the spirit, rather than focusing on the intellect.

4. Listen with the heart, rather than analyzing with the head.

5. Bear witness to the struggles of others; don't judge or try to direct.

6. Walk alongside the bereaved; don't take the lead.

7. Allow for silence; don't fill every moment with words.

8. Be still with the bereaved.

9. Respect disorder and confusion; don't force logic and order.

10. Learn from the bereaved, rather than teaching them.

11. Be curious rather than the expert.
(p. 11)

Wolfelt's model could be practiced by any nurse who is working with bereaved persons. It is based upon a philosophy of compassion and understanding that all can apply in their work.

Bereavement Support Groups

A bereavement self-help group is a support group that offers mutual aid. Members are allowed to be honest about their feelings, identify with other grieving individuals, extend sympathy and compassion, and feel understood (Hartley, 2004). Bereavement support groups become support systems for the bereaved. Facilitators are most often individuals who have experienced deaths of someone close to them. Women, in particular, are given a forum to exchange emotions in a nonjudgmental setting (McCreight, 2008).

Bereavement support groups are not for everyone. Such groups are best suited to intuitive type grievers who want to express their losses with similarly bereaved persons (Dennis, 2009). Bereavement self-help/support groups might be appropriate where cultural barriers have prevented immigrant minority groups from accessing traditional bereavement support (Nucleus Group, 2004). Although participation in a support group makes some difference, mutual support was not found to aid in the reduction of mental illness and PTSD among bereaved parents after the violent deaths of their children (Murphy, Johnson, & Weber, 2002).

Bereavement treatment interventions might include establishing spousally bereaved support groups to offer social and emotional support (Somhlaba & Wait, 2008). A widow of 15 months stated, "I have pretty much gotten over the acute pain of my husband's death but still feel that I need to go back to my support group from time to time so I can still talk about him" (Ott & Lueger, 2002, p. 404). This widow's grief was normalized by the group process.

Grief is facilitated in support groups in a variety of ways, such as:

- discussing the changes in one's life since the death.

- remembering and sharing the memories with those who have experienced similar losses.

- normalizing feelings.

- telling and retelling one's story.

- sharing pictures and objects that once belonged to the deceased.

- providing information to the bereaved on the grief process.

- exploring spiritual activities that bring comfort.

- encouraging forgiveness.

Some mourners seek out others who want to socialize with another bereaved individual. Often, after a support group ends, several of the members will exchange telephone numbers or plan to meet for coffee. They continue to talk about the relationships they shared with those who have died, their histories of loss, and practical problems, such as medical insurance issues, work problems, isolation, managing household finances, and difficulty performing activities of daily living. Such groups work especially well for lonely bereaved spouses. Members might meet for bus trips, group walks on the boardwalk, meals at restaurants, and theatre performances. The aim of attending this type of support group is to be with other grievers and meet people.

Support groups can also be informational. Those who attend this type of group want to learn ways to live their lives in a more constructive way. After a spouse dies, making meals or filling out a tax return may be difficult tasks. Having guest speakers and experts at the group meeting to present on various topics related to the unique needs of those who mourn can assist the bereaved in making life adjustments (e.g., filling out a tax return, preparing living wills, cooking for one).

Those bereaved after suicide may choose peer-run suicide survivor support groups due to unsupportive friends and distrust of practitioners. It is common for the suicidially bereaved to experience insensitive remarks from others. They often report that close associates do not make references to their deceased loved ones, thereby invalidating their existence (Feigelman, Gorman, & Jordan, 2007). Because they are angry with and skeptical of practitioners who did not successfully treat their

lost loved ones, suicide survivors prefer being helped by their peers in a group setting, as compared to obtaining professional assistance (Feigelman, Gorman, Beal, & Jordan, 2008).

Internet Bereavement Support

Fox (2005) notes that, annually, approximately 95 million people search for health information online and 23% of those users search for information about mental health, depression, anxiety, and stress. The Internet is becoming a common source of information for bereavement support and an increasingly common tool for mental health interventions (Ybarra & Eaton, 2005). Although little research has been done on online behaviors of bereaved individuals, Vanderwerker and Prigerson (2004) found that 60% of bereaved persons use the Internet and 50% communicate by e-mail in order to receive social support.

Online bereavement support groups and networks are open to individuals around the world. The bereaved are finding self-help through mailing lists, listservs, and web sites that offer support 24 hours a day. Wagner, Knaevelsrud, and Maercker (2005) found that Internet-based intervention may be especially helpful to those persons experiencing the death of a significant person under traumatic circumstances. Suicide survivors have also reported the value of Internet support groups as a place to cope, feel safe, and share (Feigelman et al., 2008).

Social withdrawal and the stigma associated with requesting help, particularly by males, may deter the bereaved from getting professional assistance (Clark et al., 2004). Those who cannot drive to a support group or who are not comfortable sharing their grief in a group can find comfort and support in the privacy of their homes. Table 9-2 displays factors that suicide survivors online support groups' participants value in their groups. Support groups and chat rooms also exist for patients living with a life-threatening illness. Caregivers can benefit from this online support, which helps them with

TABLE 9-2: WHAT INTERNET SUPPORT GROUP MEMBERS VALUE ABOUT ONLINE PARTICIPATION

1. Offering help to cope with the pain and sadness of loss (85%);

2. Having a safe place to discuss tabooed topics (84%);

3. Sharing information and experiences (84%);

4. Having the power and opportunities to discuss grief-related subjects of importance (76%);

5. Having a help source available whenever survivor problems emerge (74%);

6. Memorializing one's lost loved one (73%);

7. Helping advance goals of suicide prevention and better mental health resources availability (64%);

8. Helping to get through the holidays and other difficult times for survivors (64%);

9. Being able to help others struggling with suicide loss issues (63%);

10. Learning how to talk about suicide openly and publicly when necessary (62%).

Note. Fom "Internet support groups for suicide survivors: A new mode for gaining bereavement assistance," by Feigelman et al., 2008. *Omega 57*(3), 217-243. Reprinted with permission.

feelings of isolation and alienation. Online support is also found in creating a personal website where an individual can tell one's story, reach out to others who share similar experiences, and share his or her approach to healing.

Psycho-educational Workshops

Psycho-educational workshops offer the bereaved an opportunity to learn about death, dying, and bereavement. An overriding goal of psycho-educational workshops is to empower the participants by offering information that guides them in understanding the topic and how it relates to their experiences. The presenter's goal in facilitating the workshop is to address the concerns and issues facing the group.

Psycho-educational workshops offer information, opportunities for understanding, and support. One such situation involves those who are affected by a death in the line of military duty. Each Memorial Day weekend, friends and families come together at the Annual National Military Survivor Seminar, TAPS, held in Washington, DC. For 3 days, leading experts in the field of trauma and grief offer workshops. These workshops are not limited to family and friends. Chaplains, ombudsmen, commanders, family support personnel, and others also attend to learn valuable information. Workshop topics can include helping families cope with loss, financial planning, and other topics related to death in the line of military duty.

Another psycho-educational workshop takes place each May during National Police Week in Washington, DC. Concerns of Police Survivors, Inc. hosts the National Police Survivors' Conference for law enforcement survivors, co-workers, family, and friends. Some of the workshops are specific to drunken driving incidents, heart attacks, natural causes, and suicides. These workshops educate and empower the survivors as they share their grief with others who have experienced similar types of losses.

CASE STUDY

Carol's routine ultrasound that morning showed the infant was in distress. She had an emergency cesarean delivery and delivered a stillborn son. Carol is overwhelmed with grief after the death of her stillborn who died from a congenital malformation. Carol repeatedly asks why her infant has died and states, "I know I caused this. I should have taken better care of myself." Her husband and Mary Lou, the nurse assigned to her care, attempt to reassure and comfort her. Mary Lou spends time with Carol and her husband, John, allowing them both to ask questions and share their grief.

Mary Lou asks Carol if she wants to hold her infant son. At first, Carol does not want to hold the infant. She is hysterical, asking why God would take her baby. Mary Lou contacts pastoral care to request a visit to the patient's room. When the chaplain appears, Mary Lou excuses herself to allow for a private interaction.

After the chaplain leaves, Mary Lou returns to the room. As Carol holds onto John's hand, Mary Lou gently asks again if she wants to hold her baby. The nurse calmly explains that it is Carol's choice and does not force the issue.

Carol eventually decides to hold her child. She and John spend some time alone with the baby. Later the nurse gives her a bereavement packet, including a photo of the baby, his footprints, and a memory certificate. The nurse's sensitivity and compassion helps Carol and John accept the reality of their child's death.

Carol is taken back to her room while her husband speaks with her doctors and pastoral care. Carol is left alone in her room with the door open when she notices that across the hall an infant is brought to its mother. Her grief is intense. She wants to close her door but after her cesarean delivery, she can't move. A moment later the nurse takes a second baby into the room. Carol screams out, "two babies? Why does she have two babies and my baby died?" Carol cries hysterically. When she looks up, she notices yet another baby being wheeled into the room.

Carol wails, "three babies? She has three babies? That's not fair. Why did God give her three babies and take my baby?" A few moments later the nurse crosses the hall and enters Carol's room. She closes her door and offers her bereavement support. She allows Carol to ask her unanswerable questions and assures the grieving mother it was not her fault. The nurse remains with Carol until her husband comes into the room a few minutes later.

Mary Lou calls Carol one week after she leaves the hospital. She speaks slowly and clearly and introduces herself at the beginning of the call. Carol is pleased to receive the call and appreciates the gesture. The nurse asks whether there was a memorial service for the child. She also asks about Carol's husband's reactions to the death of his child and if the couple is having problems sleeping or eating. Carol shares that she looks at the baby's photo taken in the hospital every day and has shown it to her friends and family members. Carol talks about the support she has been getting from her friends and family. She tells the nurse she still feels spiritually and emotionally connected to her baby. The nurse assures Carol it is normal to maintain the bond between her and her child. Carol shares that her friend recommended a support group for bereaved parents and she and her husband have decided to attend the group.

Questions

1. What should the nurse say as she offers the patient bereavement support?

2. What phases of mourning is the patient experiencing?

3. How is the patient continuing the bond with her infant?

4. What tasks of mourning does the patient need to complete?

5. Why would a bereavement support group for bereaved parents help her and her husband cope with the loss of their child?

6. What will the patient feel if she gets pregnant again and has an ultrasound?

Discussion

The delivery of the stillborn child is handled effectively by Mary Lou, the nurse assigned to Carol. The couple receives spiritual support and is allowed to grieve in private and spend time with the baby. Mementos that the couple can have to remember their child are prepared and given to them. Mary Lou takes time to be with the couple and express her compassionate concern.

Carol was left alone in her room with her door open as three babies were brought to another patient. Upon realizing that the bereaved mother was distressed, the nurse caring for the patient across the hall from Carol enters her room and immediately offers support. This incident could have been avoided if the nurse had closed the patient's door after the first triplet was brought to his mother's room. Carol's nurse, Mary Lou, should have asked another nurse or volunteer to stay with Carol until her husband returned. Also, being that it was a high-risk floor, perhaps Carol should have been moved to another room where there was no chance of her seeing other mothers with their infants.

Mary Lou's follow up call to Carol was well received. Carol was receiving adequate support from friends and family and was grieving appropriately.

SUMMARY

This chapter highlighted the bereavement and mourning of adults, recognizing that, although each person mourns in an unique way, there are commonalities, theories, and models that can direct the nurse's understanding and related interventions. Although nurses are overworked and don't always have the time to offer effective bereavement support, they can learn of valuable resources for the bereaved and make appropriate referrals.

WEB RESOURCES

The American Academy of Bereavement
   http://www.cmieducation.org/AAB.aspx

National Center for Death Education
   http://www.mountida.edu/sp.cfm?pageid=307

The Compassionate Friends
   http://www.compassionatefriends.org

National Sudden and Unexpected Infant/Child Death & Pregnancy Loss Resource Center
   http://www.sidscenter.org

EXAM QUESTIONS

CHAPTER 9
Questions 73-83

Note: Choose the one option that BEST answers each question.

73. Bereavement refers to the

    a. personalized response to loss.

    b. period after death in which the survivor grieves the loss.

    c. explicit expression of grief.

    d. customary response to mourning.

74. Grieving parents should be allowed to

    a. touch and be with the deceased child.

    b. attempt another pregnancy as soon as possible.

    c. avoid discussing the death with the child's siblings.

    d. return to their normal routine as soon as possible.

75. Mourning refers to the

    a. personalized response to loss.

    b. time period following a loss.

    c. explicit expression of grief and the customary response to bereavement.

    d. time to minimize expression of feelings.

76. According to Rando, during the initial process of mourning, the bereaved

    a. reinvest their grief.

    b. recognize loss has occurred.

    c. relinquish attachment.

    d. react to the separation.

77. The Dual Process Model of mourning is seen in the context of coping with which of the following two types of stressors?

    a. Restoration and practical skills

    b. Loss and continuing the bond

    c. Restoration and accepting the reality of loss

    d. Loss and restoration

78. According to Worden (2002), the bereaved who are unable to complete the four tasks of mourning experience

    a. acceptance.

    b. normal grief reactions.

    c. restoration reactions.

    d. abnormal grief reactions.

79. A strength-based model that focuses on practical skills, empowerment, education, relationships, and growth during bereavement is known as

    a. meaning reconstruction.

    b. "companioning" the mourner.

    c. the OTHERS(S) model.

    d. the Dual Process model.

80. What percentage of bereaved individuals experience complicated grief?

    a. 5% to 20%

    b. 25% to 50%

    c. 50% to 60%

    d. 70% to 80%

81. According to Wolfelt, "companioning" the bereaved is a philosophy of caregiving focused upon

    a. giving expert advice.

    b. directing the bereaved through specific tasks of mourning.

    c. being totally present.

    d. using one's expertise to direct the grieving process.

82. Support groups are most beneficial for

    a. persons experiencing complicated grief.

    b. those without Internet access.

    c. grievers who want to express their losses with similarly bereaved persons.

    d. bereaved parents experiencing PTSD.

83. Internet bereavement support

    a. should be discouraged.

    b. contributes to feelings of isolation.

    c. has proven helpful to survivors of suicide.

    d. is usually ineffective.

CHAPTER 10

HELPING BEREAVED CHILDREN AND ADOLESCENTS

CHAPTER OBJECTIVE

After completing this chapter, the reader will be able to describe how bereaved children and adolescents express their grief and cope with the death of significant people in their lives.

LEARNING OBJECTIVES

After studying this chapter, the reader will be able to

1. identify children's emotional, physical, cognitive, behavioral, and spiritual reactions to loss.

2. describe the chronological development of a child's understanding of death.

3. list age-appropriate grief responses for children and adolescents.

4. identify supportive interventions to help grieving children.

INTRODUCTION

One of the most challenging dimensions of nursing is helping children cope with death, dying, and bereavement. Recent research in this area is lacking. This chapter will help nurses understand grief reactions in children and adolescents and their developmental conceptions of death.

One goal of this chapter is to emphasize the significance of effective adult coping and commu-nication with children about death. Kalter et al. (2002-2003) found that parental adjustment to the death of a spouse was a predictor of how well bereaved children 6 to 16 years of age would adjust to the death of a parent. The authors found that parents experiencing a difficult time adjusting to the loss were less likely to communicate with children in the family. Children's adjustment to loss is nega-tively affected if parents are not communicating with them about their own grief, bereavement, and mourning. A parent's distress and sadness may interfere with effective parenting (Kwok et al., 2005) and, as a result, increase complicated grief.

Factors complicating the grief process in children and adolescents, the significance of bereavement support, and what to say to grieving children will also be topics explored in this chapter.

BEREAVED CHILDREN

Common Grief Reactions

Children's reactions to grief are most often dif-ferent from adult reactions. Children respond to their grief emotionally, physically, cognitively, behaviorally, and spiritually, and these reactions depend upon their ages and developmental levels. Their grief responses are dependent on their under-standing of death and comprehension that death is final. Although some of their reactions are compara-ble to the adults in their lives (i.e., crying, inability to sleep, loss of appetite, sadness, withdrawal), children express their grief in less direct ways. They may also move in and out of their grief. Children grieve the loss of their grandparents, parents, siblings, friends, and significant others in their lives. Common emotional reactions in grieving children include feeling numb, sad, withdrawn, angry, guilty, relieved, unreal, and helpless. Cognitive reactions include inability to concentrate, preoccupation, and low self-image. Some common physical reactions are changes in appetite, stomachaches, bladder and/or bowel changes, rashes, headaches, and breathing disturbances. Behavioral reactions include clinging, hoarding toys, withdrawal, having nightmares, acting silly, defiance, fighting, and self-destructive behaviors. Aggressive behaviors, not usually expected in grieving children, might mask depression. Depressed grieving children can be aggressive, hyperactive, and inattentive. A sizeable percentage of children experience significant depressive symptoms, social withdrawal, and academic difficulties long after the death of a significant person in their lives (Cerel, Fristad, Verducci, Weller, & Weller, 2006). Bereaved children may also experience spiritual reactions, such as feeling judged by God, disconnected, lost, and empty. It is not unusual for them to feel the presence of the one who died.

CHILDREN'S DEVELOPMENTAL UNDERSTANDINGS OF DEATH

Birth to Two Years Old

From birth to about 2 years, children have no understanding of death, but they are aware of separation. They may react to that separation with increased crying and fussiness. They may also look around the room waiting for the adult to come back. Although young children lack an understand-

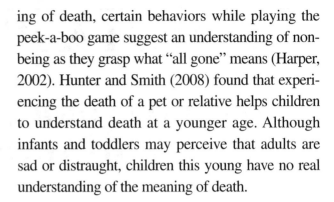

ing of death, certain behaviors while playing the peek-a-boo game suggest an understanding of non-being as they grasp what "all gone" means (Harper, 2002). Hunter and Smith (2008) found that experiencing the death of a pet or relative helps children to understand death at a younger age. Although infants and toddlers may perceive that adults are sad or distraught, children this young have no real understanding of the meaning of death.

Two to Three Years Old

The perceptions of children between 2 and 4 years of age are modeled after their parents' behaviors. Children understand the concept of death by the age of 3; to them, death is a separation and not a permanent situation. Death is temporary to preschool aged children because they frequently watch cartoon characters who are killed and come right back to life again. Being that children understand the concept of separation and abandonment, they may react to the death by wetting the bed, sucking their thumbs, feeling sad, and clinging to adults. From birth to 3 years of age, the most important functions of the adult are providing a sense of security and attempting to maintain schedules.

Three to Five Years Old

Between 3 and 5 years of age, children focus on their own needs first. They want to know who will take care of them. If a child's mother was killed in a car accident, one might assume there would be questions about the accident. However, one of the child's first questions might be, "Who is going to make me peanut butter sandwiches?" Denial is likely and the child may believe his or her loved one is going to come back to life.

When explaining death to children in this age group, it is best to explain the death in physical terms (i.e., the heart stopped beating, the body stopped working). Death is confusing and children may be scared. Adults may see feelings expressed through play and art. Although children between 3 and 5 years of age are fascinated with dead things, such as dead insects or dead animals on the side of the road, they may act as if their loved one did not die. It is common for children between 3 and 5 years of age to think of a person who has died as a ghost. This may reflect cultural beliefs. Fear of separation can be addressed by helping children continue the bond with their loved ones. Although significant persons are dead, children can form a spiritual bond with the deceased.

Prior to 5 years of age, children view death as reversible. In their minds, the dead person continues to exist. Children may even wonder what the deceased is doing. This is why the nurse should never say the persons are "sleeping," as it can confuse children into thinking that they will wake up. At this age, spiritual reactions to death include loss of trust in God's protection, viewing God as a mean old man, and feeling anger at God (McPherson, 2004).

Five to Nine Years Old

Children 5 to 9 years of age give death a personality. The term "boogeyman" is a common euphemism for death in this age group. As children ask questions about death, adults should be open and honest when they attempt to answer the often-difficult questions. Children fluctuate from showing no emotion and playing as usual to showing a great deal of emotion as they seek answers. If family members die at home, it is not uncommon for children in this age group to not want to go into the room where their loved one died. Children may feel sad, anxious, or withdrawn, and may experience nightmares as they attempt to understand death. Children may regress and demonstrate behaviors from an earlier time in their lives. For instance, children may revert to bed-wetting and thumb-sucking after years of not doing so.

Just thinking about talking to children about death can make some nurses nervous. Effective communication about death is prompt and accurate. Age-appropriate language and clear explana-

tions should be used. Consider, for example, a female patient who died at the hospital. Immediately after her death, her 7-year-old daughter was told by an aide that her mother was "at rest." The child walked over to her mother's nurse and asked if her mother was sleeping. The nurse told her that after a person sleeps, they feel rested, but that when a person dies, the body does not work anymore. The nurse gently explained that some people say "at rest" or "at peace" when they really mean "dead." The nurse offered emotional support, explaining to her that her mother was not resting and that she would not wake up. The nurse also spoke with the child's father focusing on the child's needs and reviewing what happens to the body when a person dies. He could then model the dialogue and share the same information with his daughter if she should ask him the same question.

Children depend on their family members and nurses for support because often their friends and classmates simply don't understand what they are going through. Yang and Chen (2002) found that some children reported feeling anxious about the pain their loved one might feel as they approach imminent death. Some children report being afraid the dead will come back as ghosts. The authors found that most children's fear of death is related to their fear of being permanently separated from their loved ones. The children reported feeling anxious because of the separation and being unable to finish what they wanted to do after their loved ones died. Adults can alleviate fears by discussing pain management, explaining what happens to the body as it dies, talking about beliefs in an afterlife, and exploring irrational fears. Hyslop-Christ (2000) found that grieving children 6 to 11 years of age, who were dealing with the death of a parent due to terminal illness, understood the reality of death better than classmates who had no such experience.

Nine to Ten Years Old

By 9 or 10 years of age, children begin to understand death as a final, irreversible, universal event and as the end of the body's functioning. Bereaved children between 9 and 10 years old may become defiant, aggressive, and possessive. Children in this age group may act out and find it difficult to concentrate or sleep. They may feel lonely and/or abandoned, act as if the death never happened, or believe they caused their special person to die. Children may experience nightmares and behave aggressively as they cope. Spiritual reactions in children may include resentment at God, a sense of being abandoned by God, blaming God, and feeling guilty about bad feelings toward God (McPherson, 2004).

Over 25 years have passed since professionals first inquired about children's understanding of the death concept. The four components of children's understanding of death are nonfunctionality, irreversibility, universality, and causality (Speece & Brent, 1984). Most children understand these four components by the age of 9 or 10. The four components are explained as follows:

1. *Nonfunctionality:* All life-sustaining functions cease with death.

2. *Irreversibility:* Death is final and, once dead, a person cannot become alive again.

3. *Universality:* Death is inevitable for living things, including the children themselves.

4. *Causality:* Certain events and conditions cause death. Hunter and Smith (2008) maintain that a child's age, cognitive ability, and exposure to death are major factors affecting the formation of a mature death concept.

Children are better able to adjust to death if their parents communicate effectively with them. Though children understand the finality of death by 9 or 10 years of age, it is still difficult to discuss. Parents who are having a difficult time adjusting to the death are less likely to communicate openly about the loss with their child. Kalter et al. (2002-2003) found that parental adjustment to the death of a spouse was a predictor of their children's adjust-

ment to the death of the parent. Although adults should reinforce that the death was not caused by something the children did or did not do, they should always focus on what brings the children to that conclusion.

Lisa Murphy, a staff nurse at Blessing Hospital in Illinois, was caring for a female in her 30s who was dying of cancer. The nurse attempted to explain to the patient's 9-year-old son that his mother was dying. The nurse knelt down to his eye level for the initial, gentle explanation:

> "This is what dying is, Jay. Your mommy is dying. She doesn't want to, but she can't help it and she can't stop it…Your mommy can't talk with you now, but she can hear you…She can't reach out and hug you, but she can feel you touch her." The nurse put the child on the bed next to his mother and held his hand. He cried and asked, "Mommy are you sleeping?… Mommy, Mommy don't leave me. I promise I'll be a good boy. I promise I'll do better in school." His mother could not respond and before jumping off the bed and running out of the room into his father's arms, he said, "Mommy, I love you" (Murphy, 2001, p. 62).

This nurse understood the child's concept of death and his difficulty comprehending such an event at his young age. The nurse used the word "dying" and assured him that his mother did not want to leave him. She also spoke to him at his eye level and reassured him that his mother could hear what he needed to tell her. Because of what the nurse said, this child would always know that his mother heard him.

Adolescent

This text shall refer to adolescence as the period from 14 to 19 years of age. Early adolescence (roughly 10 to 14 years of age) is a monumental time when youth are worrying about their appearance, experiencing hormonal changes, and asserting their independence. During this time, most adolescents experience the onset of puberty. Friends become very important and they want to identify as closely as possible with their peers. Their siblings are also significant; losing a sibling during this time can shatter the adolescent's world.

Middle adolescent (roughly 15 to 16 years of age) boys and girls will change their appearance frequently, become more sociable, and spend less time with family and more time with friends. Although they have an understanding of the concept of death, middle adolescents usually do not have the life experiences needed to cope effectively with loss. Late adolescence (roughly 17 to 19 years of age) brings the teenager into relationships that may become sexual in nature. Whether in early, middle, or late adolescence, young people will rely on relationships with friends to help them cope with issues related to loss. Spiritual reactions to death during adolescence include a questioning of basic beliefs, sense of isolation from God, and becoming more or less involved in religious activities (McPherson, 2004).

Forward and Garlie (2003) studied bereaved adolescent siblings and found the most important variable in grief was the need to continue the bond with the deceased. The study found adolescents believed the deceased sibling was watching over them. Bereaved adolescents wanted to keep memories alive and to know their purpose in life and how to make meaning in the loss, which for many took years to discover. Horsley and Patterson (2006) found a sibling's death has profound and long-lasting effects on the surviving siblings, and their grief is compounded by witnessing their parents' distress. These grieving adolescents often became overwhelmed and impatient with their parents' grief reactions.

> *Personal Insight*
> *What are your earliest memories of death?*
>
> *Was it a friend, pet, or family member who died?*
>
> *What did people say to you after the death?*

Loss of a Parent

If a parent dies, children are faced with many changes, including decreased economic resources, changes in residence, less contact with friends and neighbors, and increased responsibilities (Wolchik, Ma, Tein, Sandler, & Ayers, 2008). Although some research has found that children report more psychiatric problems in the first 2 years after the parent's death (Cerel et al., 2006), research is limited about the range of grief reactions and when the reactions become pathological. Several factors may complicate grief, including the type of death, the child's characteristics, social support, and multiple losses (Williams, Hackworth, & Cradock, 2002). If the death was sudden or stigmatized, as in the case of suicide, children may not feel comfortable talking about the loss. Factors that may complicate grief include multiple losses, death of both parents, and deaths of other significant people in their lives. Significantly higher complicated grief scores were reported in those children who believed that others were responsible for the death of their parent or that others blamed them for the death of their parent (Melham, Moritz, Walker, Shear, & Brent, 2007). Children who lose a parent due to terrorism or natural disaster are also faced with the risk of traumatic bereavement (Pfeffer, Karus, Siegel, & Jiang, 2000). These children are at a higher risk for depression (Dowdney, 2000; Pfeffer et. al., 2000) and posttraumatic stress disorder (Cohen & Mannarino, 2004). More violent causes of death make the grieving process of children qualitatively more difficult and prolonged (Brown et al., 2008).

Children and Traumatic Deaths

Research is currently being gathered to examine childhood traumatic grief in children (Brown, et al., 2008). Childhood traumatic grief may occur when children become bereaved after their loved ones die in traumatic circumstances and they develop trauma symptoms, which impinge on their abilities to engage in typical grief tasks (Brown et al., 2008; Cohen, Mannarino, Greenberg, Padlo, & Shipley, 2002). Although children are vulnerable to trauma (Fremont, 2004), there is continuing evidence that primary care and health systems are not fully trained to diagnose or treat symptoms of children's distress (Laraque et al., 2004). Many children were impacted by the deaths that occurred on September 11th; the repeated broadcast of the events into many children's homes has been reported to have had a significant negative effect on children's mental functioning (Lengua et al., 2005). One year after the September 11th attacks, residents of New York City who experienced more World Trade Center disaster events reported they were more likely to experience lower well-being, suffer from depression and PTSD, and use mental health services and psychotropic medications compared to those less exposed (Adams & Boscarino, 2005; Boscarino et al., 2004). If parents are unable to cope and are experiencing anxiety, they may have difficulty helping their bereaved children. In most instances, parents grieve normally and don't require grief counseling, but a substantial minority experience intense reactions and develop complicated grief. This, in turn, may complicate their children's and adolescents' grief processes. By addressing the anxiety a parent feels, children's and adolescents' anxiety can be lessened.

Following exposure to disasters or traumatic events, the National Mental Health Information Center recommends the following questions to help children talk about their experiences:

- Where were you and what were you doing when the disaster happened?

- What was your first thought when it happened?

- What did other people around you do during and after the disaster?

- Was anyone you know hurt or killed?

- Did you or do you dream about the disaster?

- What reminds you of the disaster?

- What do you do differently since the disaster?

- How do you feel now?

- How have you gotten through rough times before?

- What, if anything, would you do differently if this happened again?

(Substance Abuse and Mental Health Services Administration, 2009, Paragraph 2)

Death in the Military

War is a stressful event. It effects those men and women who are deployed as well as those who have returned home and their families, including children. In the United States, approximately 1.2 million children have a parent on active duty and, since 2001, thousands of military children have had parents killed in combat in Iraq and Afghanistan (National Child Traumatic Stress Network, 2008). Many military service parents and siblings who died were deployed for extended periods prior to the death. If surviving parents are members of the military, children may worry about that parent's possible deployment and death. Mental health problems among those who had been deployed to Iraq are not uncommon, particularly those exposed to combat and life-threatening events (Hall & Hamaoka, 2005). Children may not understand what their parent is experiencing. It is important for military nurses, nurses in pediatrician's offices, and school nurses to recognize the mental health problems of children whose loved ones have served or are serving in the armed forces.

Although many military deaths occur during combat, many have died due to suicide. Rubel (2008) notes that the highest rate of suicide in the armed forces is for enlisted men 20 to 24 years of age who had a recent loss or experienced a catastrophic event. Eaton et al. (2006) notes that the U.S. military is primarily male (85%) and about half of the troops are between 17 and 26 years of age, an age group at high risk for suicide. The U.S. Army confirmed that 115 active-duty soldiers died by suicide in 2007 and 26% of those soldiers had never been deployed to Iraq or Afghanistan (Voice of America, 2008). Military children will experience grief after their parents, siblings, and friends die while servicing their country, whether the death was related to war or suicide.

Students in college may learn of a significant person's death while away at college. Joseph et al. (2005) found that unexpected bereavement is the most distressing event for college students. The National Child Traumatic Stress Network (2008) recommends the following ways to help military bereaved children at school:

- *Provide frequent praise and positive reinforcement* to help students feel connected and stay engaged academically and emotionally.

- *Use teaching strategies* (for example, scaffolding, mapping) to promote concentration, retention, and recall to increase the child's sense of predictability, control, and performance.

- *Maintain normal school routines,* which can benefit a child who feels that life has become chaotic and out of control. It is extremely beneficial for grieving children to have predictable class schedules and routines.

- *Supportively cue or prompt* students who "go blank." Sensitively draw them back into the discussion or project at hand.

- *Be aware of possible trauma reminders,* such as dates or details related to the death that are specific to a student's situation, because these reminders can interfere with his or her ability to focus, think, or behave. This may be especially true on the anniversary of the death.

- *Be sensitive to possible triggers* in the curriculum and either modify them, prepare the bereaved student, or offer alternatives. This is especially true of history, social studies, and current events topics that may have military-related content.

- *Organize activities* in which the child can either actively participate or choose when and how to participate, without feeling put on the spot.

- *Monitor* the child's performance regularly and make additional tutoring available as needed.

- *Avoid or postpone important tests or projects* that require extensive energy and concentration for a while following the death. Rearrange or modify class assignments or homework for a short time.

- *Let the child know that you are available* to talk about the death if he or she wants to, but do not force the child to talk. School personnel can be most helpful by listening calmly to a student's confusing feelings, worries, or problems and by nonjudgmentally accepting his or her reactions to the death.

- *Encourage expression of feelings* through drawing, writing, playing, acting, and talking. Share any concerns with a school mental health professional.

- *If a child appears to be feeling "overwhelmed"* at school, make sure that he or she is allowed to retreat to a "safe person" (for example, a counselor, a nurse, or the principal), and have a "time-out card" system in place when the student needs a break.

- *Be patient and flexible.* A student's behavior and needs may ebb and flow and may at times become more challenging as the child reacts to his or her loss.

- *Address aggressive or self-destructive behavior* with caring discipline. Do not be punitive, but do set limits to unacceptable behavior. Check in with a school mental health professional to discuss the need for additional help in the classroom or outside.

(p. 6)

HOW TO HELP BEREAVED CHILDREN

Focus on the Family

When children and adolescents experience the death of pets, parents, siblings, friends, and grandparents, the deaths and related experiences will affect their understanding of death, dying, and bereavement. In helping children and adolescents develop a healthy orientation toward death, significant adults in their lives should be honest about death and not attempt to conceal their own emotions. A child's self-concept changes after the death of special persons; self-confidence and self-esteem might suffer. Although friends are very significant and can be supportive in their own way, adults, through their honest and open communication and sharing, are most effective in providing support to children. Children will then decide how much information to share with their friends. While identifying grieving children and assessing their needs, professionals must look at how the significant adults in the children's lives are coping, as the modeling of behaviors and responses will influence their grief.

Families are a basic part of children's lives. Bereaved children and adolescents grieve in a family context. Adults need to be aware of normal childhood grief responses in order to help them. Wolchik et al. (2008) found children cope better with uncontrollable and controllable stressors after a death if their caregivers are highly responsive to their needs, offer warmth, and are consistent with discipline. Surviving parents benefit from programs that promote positive parenting after the death of a parent (Haine, Wolchik, Sandler, Millsap, & Ayers, 2006). Surviving parents, as current caregivers, become a protective resource against negative life events and mental health problems. When the focus is on the family, parents can learn how to cope with their own grief, while effectively helping their grieving children. There are simple do's and don'ts for parents as they provide support and comfort to their child (Table 10-1).

It is important to be sensitive to children's culture and family belief systems. Nurses can advise the adults in children's lives to review customs and traditions of their faith and culture. Children can be involved in the planning of the funeral and services.

As families attempt to cope with the loss, children may become depressed and frightened. They may ask the same questions repeatedly. Nurses can advise parents to encourage questions and answer children honestly as they attempt to make sense of the loss.

Packman, Horsley, Davies, and Kramer (2006) studied sibling bereavement and continuing bonds and found that open communication in the family is crucial in the aftermath of sibling death. Children need to talk about their siblings and express their feelings. If adults do not allow them to openly express their grief, they will feel overlooked and alone in their grief.

The four most frequently mentioned phrases of bereaved siblings are, "I hurt inside," "I don't understand," "I don't belong," and "I'm not enough" (Packman et al., 2006). When children say, "I hurt inside," they are talking about the painful experience in their bodies. Nurses can talk about those things that hurt (e.g., stomachache, headache, and heartache). When children say "I don't understand," they are expressing their frustration with not comprehending what happened to the sibling who died. They need adults to guide them in understanding what happened, why it happened, and how to deal with it. When children say, "I don't belong" they are confused and overwhelmed. They don't feel like themselves and adults need to be empathetic and caring while recognizing how children are attempting to cope with their grief. When children say,

TABLE 10-1: DO'S AND DON'TS FOR PROVIDING SUPPORT AND COMFORT TO A CHILD	
What to Do	*What NOT to Do*
• Allow a child, however young, to attend the funeral if they want to do so.	• Don't try to shelter children from the reality of death; it can be a learning experience.
• Convey your spiritual values about life and death.	• Don't give false or confusing messages, like "Grandma is sleeping now."
• Meet regularly as a family to find out how everyone is coping.	• Don't tell a child to stop crying because others might get upset.
• Pray with your child (if that is part of your belief system).	• Don't force a child to publicly mourn if he or she doesn't want to.
• Help children find ways to symbolize and memorialize the deceased person.	• Don't hesitate to cry in the presence of a child; by expressing genuine emotions you are demonstrating that it is acceptable for the child's feelings to be expressed, too.
• Pay attention to the way a child plays; this can be one of a child's primary ways of communicating.	
• Keep the child's daily routine as normal as possible.	• Don't turn your child into your personal confidante; rely on another adult or a support group instead.

Note. From "Supporting a Grieving Person: Helping Others Through Grief, Loss, and Bereavement, by M. Smith & J. Segal, 2009. Retrieved August 23, 2010, from http://www.helpguide.org/mental/helping_grieving.htm. Reprinted with permission from Helpguide.

"I'm not enough" they are stating they believe the deceased sibling was the favored child and they should have died instead of their sibling. Adults could focus on the deceased's relationships shared with the child and the parents.

Many parents do not know how to help their grieving children and may recruit nurses to help them. School nurses and nurses working with children can be comforting guides and role models, teaching parents that each child grieves in a personal way. Bereaved students exhibit grief symptoms that may interfere with learning. Lohan (2006) studied the necessity for extra support for bereaved children and the degree to which school nurses meet their needs. Rural areas, in particular, don't have adequate community bereavement resources, limiting the ability of the nurse to refer families for help. Although nurses want to help bereaved children, results indicated that many school nurses have considerable caseloads, limited resources, and don't have the time for these students (Lohan, 2006).

Nurses can help children cope with a death by understanding how they think about loss, death and, especially, the changes in their lives (Table 10-2). Kaufman and Kaufman (2005) studied childhood mourning and found that adults are better able to assist a bereaved child in expressing emotions when they do so in a manner most appropriate for the child. The researchers identified three types of grieving children: verbal children, introspective (literary) children, and artistic children (Kaufman & Kaufman, 2005). Nurses can respond and offer suggestions accordingly. For example, when helping verbal children, adults can ask if they want to speak at the eulogy. Nurses can offer such children an opportunity to talk about their loved ones. Most conversations can begin by saying, "Tell me about…" to encourage verbal children to talk about the person. When helping introspective or literary children, nurses can ask if they want to write about their thoughts and feelings using modalities such as poetry or journaling. When supporting artistic children, nurses can encourage them to express themselves through visual media such as drawing pictures, creating collages, or making mem-

TABLE 10-2: WAYS TO HELP A CHILD COPE WITH A LOSS

Advice for Parents, Teachers, and Caregivers

To help children cope with a death, parents, caregivers, teachers, and other significant adults in their lives need to understand how children think about loss, death, and especially what has changed for them.

Remember, helping a child cope with a loss is one of the more important skills you can teach.

The following list includes helpful suggestions for helping a child cope with death.

1. When talking to a child about a tragedy, first, find out what the child knows or thinks about what has happened. The child may be aware of more than you think.

2. Answer any question simply and honestly, but only offer the details that the child can absorb. Do not give the child more information than is requested.

3. Let the child know you will be available to listen. When he or she is ready to talk – listen.

4. Let the child have time to grieve, be upset, and talk about his or her fears. Give him or her a chance to talk. Listen, validate the child's feelings, and then provide reassurance.

5. Give the child different ways of expressing his or her loss, grief, and sadness – verbal, written, creative, musical, and physical.

6. Encourage the child to draw, read, write letters or poetry, sing, tell stories, play with clay, build, and use other creative means of expression – all helpful ways for a child to express grief.

7. Letting the child go outside to play and be active can be a good way to run off the anxiety he or she may sense from the adults and feel himself or herself.

8. Try and keep regular routines. Children can grieve a change in behavior and mourn the environment and the predictability of a schedule that existed before the loss or death. Keeping regular routines can help.

9. Be patient and flexible. Children grieve intermittently. They may cry one moment and then play normally the next.

10. Remember that it may take the child a long time to recover from the loss or the death, depending on the child, the type of loss, and the relationship with the lost person (or pet, object, etc.)

Note. From "Help a child cope with loss and grief," by Squidoo, (n.d.). Retrieved on August 23, 2010, from http://www.squidoo.com/children-grief#module3502613

ory boxes and filling them with special mementos that remind the children of their loved ones.

In cases where feelings of ambivalence, guilt, or hostility are expressed in conjunction with feelings of sadness and loss, it might be helpful to coach children in the expression of these feelings and in the expression of words that were never said or questions that were never asked. These questions and feelings can be shared with other family members as well as directly with the deceased. This can be facilitated by asking them to write a letter to the deceased person and to express in it whatever "unfinished" things are still distressing them.

Children at the Funeral

Adults may ask the nurse whether grieving children should be allowed to go to the funeral home. The answer is simple: As long as the children are prepared and want to go, they should attend. Preparing children begins by explaining that after someone dies, the body is taken to a place called a funeral home until the burial. Everything children will see at the funeral home should be described in advance, including the casket, the color of the clothes the deceased will be wearing, the flowers, and the mourners present. If the adult has been to the funeral home before, he or she should explain the color of the rug and the paintings on the wall. Such details familiarize children with what they will see and will comfort them during the stressful time at the funeral home. After such descriptions have been offered, the child should be asked if he or she wants to go. No matter what the age of the children, they should be allowed to make their own choices as to whether they want to attend the funeral. As adults provide information, children will be better able to make their decisions.

Personal Insight
How old were you when you first attended a funeral?

What was the experience like for you?

Tasks for the Grieving Family

In 1991, William Worden first suggested a series of four tasks to help individuals cope with grief (Worden, 1991). Researchers have noted the significance of Worden's four tasks and have continually updated and revised them to focus on helping the entire family. Walsh and McGoldrick (1988) first adapted these four tasks to the larger family system. Rosen (1990) expanded these tasks with methods for family grief resolution, and Walsh and McGoldrick (1991) then refocused the four tasks and the complex nature of the family mourning process. Shapiro (1994) noted that grief is an interpersonal process and the series of four tasks will help children and adults cope with death as a family. Corr and Corr (1996) identified how each task can be applied to the family emotionally and behaviorally. The tasks for the family unit are:

1. to share acknowledgement of the reality of the death

2. to share the experience of the pain of grief

3. to reorganize the family system

4. to redirect the family's relationships and goals.

When acknowledging the reality of death, the grieving family must accept finality of loss and communicate openly while celebrating rites and rit-

uals together. When sharing the pain of grief, the family accepts a wide range of emotions while sharing feelings and allowing for differences. When reorganizing the family system, the grieving family accepts that they will never be the same and realigns old relationships, delegates new roles, and copes with short-term disorganization. When redirecting relationships and goals, families imagine what their futures will be like without the deceased and move forward together.

PROFESSIONAL BEREAVEMENT INTERVENTION

Bereavement Intervention After Anticipatory and Sudden Death

Kennedy, McIntyre, Worth, and Hogg (2008) studied the literature regarding bereavement support of children and families facing the death of a parent due to cancer, and found that bereavement was reported as a normal life event and part of human experience. Although the needs of bereaved children require careful assessment, not all bereaved children require complex, long-term interventions (Kennedy et al., 2008). Although research indicates that children bereaved by the 9/11 terrorist attacks have been underserved (Fairbrother, Stuber, Galea, Pfefferbaum, & Fleischman, 2004), not all children bereaved by sudden death need professional bereavement support. Factors to consider when assessing a child for bereavement care include the child's level of function, grief responses, coping patterns, beliefs about self and the world, self-worth, and fear of abandonment, regardless of the cause of death (Brown et al., 2007). To help grieving children after a sudden death, the focus must first be on the adults in the children's lives. Research indicates that few adult victims of terror seek professional help (Bleich, Gelkopf, & Solomon, 2003). Tuval-Mashiach and Shalev (2005) suggest that the low number of terror victims seeking help is due to the inconvenience of professional services or the stigma emotionally involved to approach them.

Death by suicide has been a frequently suggested indicator of the need for bereavement intervention (Jordan & McMenamy, 2004). However, there is limited research on the effects of programs for adult survivors of suicide and even less research for child survivors. Dyregrov (2009a) studied the need for psychological assistance to cope with suicide among bereaved children. The children in the study reported they found support by speaking with psychologists (52%), teachers (35%), public health nurses (35%), and clergymen (29%). The main ongoing and lingering problem found in a recent study of bereaved children after a suicide was the inability to concentrate at school. A 14-year-old suicide survivor who had lost an older brother reported:

> It's just like you can't even manage the multiplication tables right? It takes me a lot longer, you know, to understand that an arithmetic problem is right. And I need a much better explanation…(Dyregrov, 2009b, p. 152).

Children bereaved by suicide reported what could be improved in their situations at school:

- The schools and teachers should acquire knowledge about the situation of the young bereaved by traumatic death (including suicide) through basic and continuing education for teachers.

- A follow-up strategy in the schools should be created for the young bereaved by suicide.

- The schools and teachers should have the responsibility for contact being made with the pupil and home in connection with necessary adaptations and plans for care. Involve the pupil in the dialog with the school and parents.

- The school should take the initiative or help the pupil to inform the class about what has happened.

- The school and teachers must be prepared for the fact that the pupil may need to return gradually after the funeral.

- Teachers should show sympathy or be empathetic – but expressions of sympathy must be adapted to the individual and the situation so that teachers don't "fall all over" pupils.

- The school should practice flexible attendance rules, enabling the option to stay home from school should the pupil feel the need to do so.

- The school should provide opportunities for "time-outs," especially in the beginning – e.g., permission to go to a separate group room or activities to allow distraction from difficult thoughts such as use of a computer.

- According to need, exemption from (some) tests and exams should be possible – particularly immediately following the death.

- The school should provide adaptation of tests – e.g., in a separate room, more time, or possibly oral exam if this alleviates concentration problems.

- In order to reduce pressure for grades – the school could try to view new tests in relation to the pupil's previous performance and what he or she has experienced when grades are awarded.

- Pupils should be given permission for a period to be more passive in class, without this having repercussions for grades.

- Young persons should be prepared if the subject of suicide is going to be addressed in class, possibly allow them to miss this class (in particular, immediately following the suicide).

- According to need, practical outplacement or leave from school should be considered for short periods of time.

- Teachers must have coordinated strategy measures in relation to the same pupil at the same school.

- Routine contact with social teacher/nurse/ psychologist should be provided; which, in addition to serving as an outreach program, provides fixed appointments for contact throughout the semester.

- Offers of adaptation and help should be repeated if pupils who are clearly falling through the cracks refuse this. The school and teachers must show that they care and understand the difficult situation following the suicide.

- The school must have a realistic time perspective on grief and difficulties and the need for special care; do not expect it to pass after a few months.

(Dyregrov, 2009b, p. 156)

Although bereavement support groups for child survivors of suicide can address themes, including why the parent died by suicide and shame (Jordan, 2001), studies on the efficacy of bereavement interventions for children have reported weak program effects (Brown et al., 2007). Only one study has evaluated an intervention for child survivors (Pfeffer, Jiang, Kakuma, Hwang, & Metsch, 2002). The bereavement group intervention consisted of 10 weekly group sessions where child survivors of suicide met for 1.5 hours in groups according to age (6 to 9, 10 to 12, and 13 to 15 years old) and focused on discussions about death, grief, suicide, and problem-solving skills (Pfeffer et al., 2002). Reductions in anxiety and depressive symptoms were significantly greater in children who received the group intervention than those who did not. However, the research is limited. For the most part, children can be best served by professionals helping parents identify what bereaved children need to cope with loss. Adults can focus on hope, meaning making, and positive aspects of life. Helping children find meaning in their experiences can provide them with hope for the future and allow them to focus on the positive aspect of their lives, as opposed to dwelling on the tragedies (Saxe, Ellis, & Kaplow, 2007).

The Dougy Center

Established in 1982, the Dougy Center was the first center in the United States to provide peer support groups for grieving children. At this center, grieving children, teens, young adults, and their families share their experiences through peer support groups, education, and training. Serving 350 children and their 200 adult family members each month, the open-ended peer support groups meet every other week. The concurrent adult support groups meet at the same time. The Dougy Center has served over 20,000 children, teens, and their families, and has received national and international acclaim for their pioneering peer support model. Through their National Training Program and training materials, thousands have learned how to help grieving children, and 165 programs modeled after the Dougy Center have been established worldwide. The Dougy Center has a directory of programs across the country and internationally that serve grieving children, teens, and their families after anticipatory and sudden deaths, as in the case of suicide and terrorist acts. Nurses can share information about the center with grieving families and also make referrals.

EFFECTIVE COMMUNICATION

"If adults cannot confront and make peace with their own fears about the end of life, how can they possibly consider the reality of death in the lives of children? Many adults refrain from discussing death with children because of their own anxiety of the subject. In addition, they may inadvertently want to avoid distressing the child and having to respond to questions for which they have no answers. Many parents and adults find it easier to talk to children about sex than about death." (Boyd Webb, 2005, p. 3)

When helping the bereaved, nurses may feel at a loss for words. If this should happen, nurses can use the following statements and questions as a guide to assess and provide support to bereaved children and their families (Rubel, 2009).

Death

- Tell me about the person who died.

- Where were you when your special person died?

- What happened when you heard your special person was dead?

- If you had to explain death to someone younger than you, what did you say?

- What does the death of this person mean to you?

- Do you think adults in your family should talk with children about death?

- If your family members talked about the death, did they say anything that scared or confused you?

- Describe the part of your experience that you once thought you would never tell anyone about.

Grief and Bereavement

- What grief reactions have you noticed in your body?

- If you have ever gotten angry at yourself, what was the reason?

- If you ever get angry, what things do you do to deal with your anger?

- Did you ever feel numb, confused, or angry after the person died?

- What do you do to help you with these feelings?

- What are three facts you know about grief?

- What are three facts you know about bereavement?

- What is one question you want answered today concerning grief and bereavement?

Mourning

- How long was your family in mourning?

- What clothes did your family wear during mourning?

- If anyone made special meals for your family while you all were in mourning, what were the meals?

- If you believe in heaven, what do you think it looks like?

Changes

- If you had a certain routine that changed after the person died, explain how it changed for the better or for the worse.

- How has your world changed since this person died?

- Is there anything the person who died used to do for you that another person has to do?

Worries

- Make a list of all the things that worried you after your loved one's death.

- Did anyone in your family worry about the same things you did? If so, describe what that person was worried about and how he or she worked through these worries.

- Create a list of three situations that you are most worried about right now.

Fears

- If you are staying away from a place that reminds you of this person's death, describe the place.

- What would happen if you went to this place?

- What was your biggest fear after this person died?

- How did you cope with your fear?

- Were you ever afraid that someone else you cared about was going to die? If so, please explain.

Dreams

- Have you had any dreams about the person who died? If so, describe your dream.

- If you ever had a dream that made you feel either angry or sad, describe the dream.

Reminders

- Has someone said or done something that reminded you of the person who died? If so, explain what it was.

- Create a scrapbook with special words and pictures that remind you of the person who died.

Feeling Safe

- Does your home feel safe? Explain your answer.

- If you do not feel safe in your home, what can you do about it?

- Where do you feel the safest?

- With whom do you feel the safest?

- Can you describe why you feel safe in this place and with this person?

- List five people in your life who would be there for you if you ever felt really sad or hopeless.

Linking Objects

- If you could have one item that belonged to the person who died, what would it be?

- Why would you choose this item?

- If you already have something that belonged to this person, describe it.

- Why does the object have a special meaning?

- Where do you keep this special object?

- How does the object make you feel connected to the person?

- If you or anyone else threw away or gave away your loved one's belongings, what was the experience like for you?

Sharing the Bad News

- After the person in your family died, who was the first person you told what happened? What was it like sharing the bad news for the first time?

- Write a list of things people said to you since the death that were helpful.

- Write a list of things people said that were mean.

- If you were ever asked to keep a secret, how did it make you feel?

- What was the most difficult thing you ever had to deal with in your life?

The Funeral

- Do you think adults in your family should allow children to attend funerals?

- Think about the person who died. If you did not attend the funeral, how did you feel about not going?

- If you know what the person was wearing in the casket, are you aware of the reasons why the clothing was chosen?

- Did the clothing have any special meaning?

- If you had a member of your clergy at the funeral, what did he or she say that brought you comfort?

- If someone recited a eulogy, what did he or she say?

- How did their special words make you feel?

- If you could recite a eulogy for this person now, what would you say?

- If you saw anyone taking photos at the funeral home, how did it make you feel?

- If photos were taken, what was it like to look at the photos after they were developed?

- What did the casket look like?

- Was the casket open or closed at the funeral home?

- If anything special was placed in the casket, describe it.

- If the person was cremated, describe the type of urn used.

- If you attended the funeral, describe the hardest part for you.

Rituals

- If you created a ritual after the person died, what was it?

- Who helped you create the ritual?

- Explain what it was like to do the ritual.

- On a sheet of paper, draw a picture of how you looked while performing your ritual.

- If you did not have a chance to say good-bye, write a good-bye letter on a sheet of paper and keep it in a special place.

Creative Thinking

- If you woke up after sleeping for 5 years, what would you want to do and whom would you want to see?

- If you could say anything you wanted to the person who died and that person could hear you, what would you say?

- List five things you would have liked to have told the person who died.

Moments in Time

- Describe the saddest moment in your life.

- Describe the happiest moment in your life.

Memories

- What is your favorite memory of the person who died?

- How does talking about the person who died help you to cope with your loss?

- What are three things you miss the most about the person who died?

Having Fun

- In what ways have you had fun since the person died?

- Do you think the person who died would want you to have fun?

CASE STUDY

*E*sther worked as an LPN in an urban hospital and was caring for Faye, a 42-year-old female with heart disease. The patient's 10-year-old daughter, Lori, visited often. She would comb her mother's hair and read to her. Esther overheard Lori's Aunt tell Lori that her mother would be fine, even though Faye was nearing death. Later, the patient's husband mentioned to Esther that he went to the funeral home that morning, made funeral arrangements, and chose his wife's casket. "I know she doesn't have much time," he said.

Lori overheard her father and Esther and asked if she could draw a picture of herself and her mom to put into the casket. Lori's father told her that he thought her mom would appreciate the drawing. Lori's mom had been buying Lori hair ornaments for years. Lori's dad thought placing a few hair ribbons in his wife's hand would be special. Lori was excited about choosing the ones she thought her mom would like the best. Esther commended him for involving Lori in the funeral planning.

Lori's father asked Esther what he should tell Lori after her mother dies. The nurse said, "Be honest with her. She knows what's happening. I have talked with her about her mom's terminal illness and she knows that her mom will die soon. I explained what happens when a person is dying. I also told her what to expect once her mom is dead."

He replied, "Thank you for your honesty. She'll be okay. I don't think kids grieve, anyway." The nurse attempted to explain that children do grieve and as a family they will get through it together.

A few moments later, his wife died. As the father and daughter cried at Faye's bedside, he told his daughter that he loved her and that they would work together to get over the loss. Lori kissed her mother good-bye and told the nurse that her mom was in heaven.

Questions

1. What should the nurse now say to the child to help her cope with her mom's death?

2. What additional information would be helpful to the nurse to be better able to help the grieving child?

3. What are some of the grief reactions Lori may experience?

4. What could the nurse have said to the aunt when she told Lori that her mother would be fine?

5. Where do you think Lori's father learned that children don't grieve?

Discussion

Although Esther worked in a busy hospital, she took the time to comfort the patient's husband and daughter. When Esther overheard Lori's aunt tell Lori that her mother would be fine, even though Faye was dying, she understood that the patient's sister was not ready to let go and was holding onto hope that she would live. The nurse took the time to discuss terminal illness with the child, the dying process, and what happens to the body when people die. She knew that even though the aunt gave her incorrect information, the child knew what was happening. The nurse spoke with the patient's husband about including Lori in the funeral planning, being honest with her, and realizing children grieve. After his wife died, he used the same words that the nurse used to explain how they will cope, as family – together.

SUMMARY

This chapter discussed children's emotional, physical, cognitive, behavioral, and spiritual reactions to loss. Understanding of death is related to the child's age and previous experiences. Children need adults who can communicate with them in an honest and direct, yet compassionate, manner.

WEB RESOURCES

American Academy of Child and Adolescent Psychiatry (AACAP)
http://www.aacap.org

The Dougy Center for Grieving Children & Families
http://www.dougy.org

The Child Trauma Academy
http://www.childtrauma.org

National Center for Children Exposed to Violence; Yale University Child Study Center
http://www.nccev.org/violence/children_terrorism.htm

The Center for Traumatic Stress in Children and Adolescents
http://www.pittsburghchildtrauma.com

Tragedy Assistance Program for Survivors (TAPS)
http://www.taps.org

EXAM QUESTIONS

CHAPTER 10
Questions 84-90

Note: Choose the one option that BEST answers each question.

84. Children's reactions to grief are most often

    a. different from adult reactions.

    b. delayed responses.

    c. similar to those of adults.

    d. indicative of pathology.

85. After the death of a significant loved one, bereaved children

    a. may continue to feel the presence of the one who died.

    b. are not able to react spiritually.

    c. seldom become depressed.

    d. always react emotionally, rather than physically.

86. A child's developmental understanding of death and separation, from birth to about 2 years old, is they

    a. understand death and are aware of separation.

    b. understand death but are not aware of separation.

    c. have no understanding of death and are not aware of separation.

    d. have no understanding of death but are aware of separation.

87. Grieving preschoolers should

    a. never sleep with their parents.

    b. watch television as a distraction from their sadness.

    c. not be expected to return to a normal routine.

    d. be allowed to express their grief through play and art.

88. Children begin to understand the finality of death by

    a. 4 to 8 years old.

    b. 9 to 10 years old.

    c. 11 to 13 years old.

    d. 14 to 17 years old.

89. When coping with issues related to loss, adolescents rely on relationships with

    a. their friends.

    b. sympathetic school teachers.

    c. counselors or therapists.

    d. their grieving parents.

90. An intervention that will help children cope with death is

    a. sharing acknowledgement of the reality of the death.

    b. hiding the experience of the pain of grief.

    c. ignoring the family system and focusing on the individual.

    d. redirecting the family's faith.

CHAPTER 11

WHEN HELPING HURTS: NURSES' RESPONSES TO DEATH AND DYING

CHAPTER OBJECTIVE

After completing this chapter, the reader will recognize the impact of stress on the nurse who cares for the dying and discuss coping strategies to prevent compassion fatigue and burnout.

LEARNING OBJECTIVES

After studying this chapter, the reader will be able to

1. define burnout.

2. describe symptoms of burnout.

3. define compassion fatigue.

4. list self-care strategies for preventing burnout and compassion fatigue.

5. identify the role of compassion in nursing.

6. describe how resiliency can help a nurse cope with a stressful career.

INTRODUCTION

"The road to success is always under construction."

– Anonymous

The preceding chapters familiarized the reader with essential information on providing support to dying individuals and to those who are grieving. The purpose of this chapter is to expand the nurse's ability to cope with personal and professional stress, burnout, and compassion fatigue while responding in death and dying situations. If nurses do not take care of themselves, they will not be able to care for patients. Morrissette (2004) maintains that compassion fatigue has been found in various nursing professions, including child protective services, trauma survivor counseling, school nursing, sexual abuse survivor counseling, criminal victim counseling, and emergency room nursing. This chapter will also familiarize nurses with the significance of resiliency when coping with stress.

STRESS

All persons experience stress in their lives, especially nurses who are often overworked and stressed as they assist those who are facing life and death situations. Hospital nurses working in China, Japan, South Korea, Thailand, and the United States reported workload and dealing with death and dying to be the two most common workplace stressors (Lambert et al., 2004). The first step in understanding burnout, compassion fatigue, and psychological health in nurses is to establish that stress is an important predictor of reductions in well-being (Rossi, Bisconti, & Bergeman, 2007).

Stress refers to a particular physiological response or reaction, regardless of the source or stimulus (Everly & Lating, 2002). Stress is culturally and personally defined, so what is considered stressful to one nurse may not be stressful to another

193

(Goldsmith, 2007). Hans Selye, a pioneer in stress-related disorders, recognized that the stress response might be provoked by emotional, physical, distressing, and also positive events. Selye defined a stressor as anything disrupting the body's homeostatic equilibrium and the necessary alterations in bodily resources to re-achieve homeostasis. Stressors can be life events, chronic situations, or work-related conditions (Orpana & Lenyre, 2004).

> ### *Personal Insight*
> *What were some of the things you hoped for when you first became a nurse?*
>
> *Do you find that those hopes are clouded by the stress you are now feeling?*

Personal Stress

It is almost impossible for nurses to go to work and not think about personal concerns. As they treat dying patients they may be thinking about family issues that are causing personal or family stress. Family stress is an umbrella term referring to a variety of stressors arising from relationships and problems inherent in managing "child care, school events, sports and recreation, elder care, one's own needs and desires, and spouse's needs" (Goldsmith, 2007, p. 160). Family stressors can include major life transitions, medical issues, or money problems. Nurses may also experience self-induced stressors, such as feelings of perfectionism and fear of failure.

Job Stress

Job stress or professional stress in nurses is caused by harmful physical and emotional responses that occur when the job requirements don't match the capabilities, resources, or needs of nurses (Goldsmith, 2005). Miller and Smith (2005) describe three levels of stress in the workplace:

- *Acute stress* is a response to an immediate perceived physical, psychological, or emotional threat in the workplace that makes nursing more complicated during that particular time period. It is the most common form of stress and is exhausting.

- *Episodic acute stress* occurs when nurses frequently suffer acute stress. It can occur when patients are late for appointments or in situations where the crisis is continual.

- *Chronic stress* is ongoing and long term. It can occur when nurses continually work with patients they don't like, incompetent supervisors, and dysfunctional family members. If nurses become accustomed to chronic stress, it feels old, familiar, and almost comfortable.

Nurses can ask themselves the following questions to assess how they can handle stress at work and how they handled stress in the past:

- Do you feel that your input at work makes a difference in how things turn out?

- Do you rely on yourself to figure out how to solve problems that arise at work?

- Do you feel most comfortable with clearly defined work tasks?

- Do you escape work problems by distracting yourself with daydreams and other fun activities?

(Maddi & Khoshaba, 2005, p. 62)

Job stressors include time pressures, excessive caseloads, unsupportive peers, excessive paperwork, and lack of resources. Professional stress can be caused by a frenetic race to coordinate resources, responding to several emergencies at the same time, or working with incompetent colleagues and supervisors. Nursing-specific stress can be caused by variables such as working double shifts, treating deadly diseases, staffing shortages, watching patients suffer, dealing with dysfunctional family members, job insecurity, nursing shortages, and unfair evaluations. Dickinson and Wright (2008) add interprofessional conflicts, workload, and lack of involvement in decision making to the list of stressors. Unfortunately, stress can force nurses to leave the jobs they once loved and further compound the nursing shortage. Garrett

(2008) notes that hospital nursing vacancies are expected to reach 800,000 by the year 2020. Nurse-specific stress can also be experienced by administrators who must maintain budgets at the expense of patients and hospital staff.

Personal Insight
What is the most stressful part of your job?

Compassion Stress

Wada and Park (2009) maintain that cultivation of self-compassion may alleviate self-criticism. Neff (2004) identified components of self-compassion as follows:

(a) extending kindness and understanding to the self in instances of pain or failure, rather than harsh judgment and self-criticism;

(b) seeing one's experiences as part of the larger human experience, rather than seeing them as separating and isolating; and

(c) holding one's painful thoughts and feelings in mindful awareness, rather than over-identifying with them

(p. 30).

Compassion is the caring awareness of another person's anguish along with the desire to lessen it. Nurses' compassionate responses to dying patients and their family members make them vulnerable to compassion stress when working in death and dying situations. Figley (2002) defines compassion stress as the draining of emotional energy, resulting from the empathetic response to suffering and continuing requirements for nurses to act and relieve suffering. Nurses empathize with their traumatized patients. This empathetic engagement (Nelson-Gardell & Harris, 2003) can lead to an empathetic strain that ruptures the nurse's empathy and results in loss of an effective therapeutic role (Jones 2001b). Nurses want to be effective caregivers and support those in need. However, there are times when their roles as nurses cause personal heartbreak. This is especially true when children die.

Nurse's Response After a Child Dies

Although nurses may work with all age groups, it is extremely difficult to accept children dying. Reilly-Smorawski et al. (2002) studied the relationships between nurse caregivers and the families of dying babies. The findings provide a basis for asserting that nurses experience a personal loss reaction when a baby dies, and it is therapeutic for both the nurses and families if the nurses express their grief. If nurses caring for the babies attempt to be objective and professional, without expressing emotions in front of the families, stress levels may increase. Grieving parents who observed a NICU staff member's tears shared that profound recollection with other parents. Some of the grief reactions (e.g. anger, guilt) of the nurses are similar to those of family members. Post-death follow up may help nurses cope with their feelings of sadness, failure, and spiritual distress accompanying the deaths (Reilly-Smorawski et al., 2002).

In a study of nurses and physicians caring for dying children, findings revealed that both physicians (82%) and nurses (94%) were grieving after the child died (Papadatou, Bellali, Papazoglou, & Petraki, 2002). Nurses reported grief reactions, including crying, sadness, anger, and recurring thoughts of the dying conditions and the death. Unlike physicians, nurses reported sharing their experiences with colleagues for emotional support. Nurses reported finding meaning in the death and 75% felt emotionally supported by their colleagues, as the social sharing of grief became a collective experience.

Nurses may experience the death of several patients over a short period of time. Although it is heart wrenching when those patients are children, it is healthy to express feelings. McCreight (2005) conducted interviews with nurses and midwives in Northern Ireland and found that they suffer grief and fear after a patient's miscarriage or stillbirth and may find it difficult to cope with their emotional distress.

The researcher concluded that emotions in nurses should be seen as a resource rather than a weakness.

Professionals with higher violent or human-induced trauma survivor caseloads, especially when children are involved, appear at greater risk for compassion fatigue and secondary traumatic stress disorder (Creamer & Liddle, 2005; Cunningham, 2003). According to Lambie (2005), over 18,000 children a year suffer permanent injuries due to child abuse. Meyers and Cornille (2002) found that nurses may become traumatized themselves as they help traumatized children. In order to be more effective in their roles as health-care professionals, they could benefit from improved learning about both the children's trauma, and secondary traumatic stress symptoms and methods for emotional self-care. Professionals need to recognize family-of-origin patterns that influence their lives, own their personal trauma histories, identify coping strategies, and work in a supportive environment, if secondary traumatization is to be prevented (Meyers & Cornille, 2002).

> ### Personal Insight
> *Think about when you first became a nurse. What were the reasons why you chose your career?*

BURNOUT

Risks and Warning Signs

Job stress can lead to burnout, a state of physical, emotional, and mental exhaustion brought on by unrealistic goals and aspirations and long hours (Goldsmith, 2007). Studies show that high rates of nurse burnout exceed the norm for healthcare workers (Garret, 2008). Burnout results when the cumulative effects of a stressful nursing environment gradually overwhelm nurses' defenses, compelling them to withdraw psychologically (Sahraian, Fazelzadeh, Mehdizadeh, & Toobaee,

2008). Burnout is usually a result of nurses feeling frustrated and not being able to achieve their goals.

Prolonged fatigue and irritability at work may be early warning signs of burnout. Nurses who experience burnout may also become cynical. Burnout contributes to tardiness, feeling hopeless, and an intention to leave the field of nursing (Mimura & Griffiths, 2003). The symptoms are caused by chronic, cumulative stress that nurses experience throughout their careers.

There are two levels of burnout. All medical and nursing professionals experience level 1 burnout at some point; key signs and symptoms include being mentally fatigued at the end of the day and feeling unappreciated, frustrated, and angry as a result of contacts with patients (Wicks, Parsons, & Capps, 2003). Some nurses experience level 2 burnout, when minor stress becomes distress.

Metaphors use comparisons to express ideas and create strong images. In an earlier chapter, metaphors of grief were explored. Metaphors can also describe burnout in nursing. For example, a candle that goes out because the wax has been used up or lawn grass that is burned out in late summer due to the stress of high heat and less rain may be used as metaphors for nursing burnout (McHolm, 2006).

Nurses must recognize the key signs and symptoms of burnout, which include disillusionment about work, a pervasive feeling of boredom, being ruled by schedule, seeing more and more patients while being no longer attuned to them, and viewing patients impersonally and without thought (Wicks et al., 2003). Health professionals are at risk for burnout if they have experienced any of the following during the previous 3 to 6 months:

- Dreaded going to work or stayed late when it wasn't necessary.

- Took long breaks and lunches or no breaks or lunches.

- Experienced chronic backaches, headaches, or other nagging physical symptoms.

- Felt numb and uninterested in everything.

- Slept restlessly.

- Slept more or less than usual.

- Felt dissatisfied with life.

- Used alcohol, drugs, food, or sex to escape feelings.

- Felt irritable, angry, or hostile with patients or colleagues.

- Spent more time alone or felt withdrawn.

- Felt depressed or emotionally drained.

- Felt as though not accomplishing anything with patients.

- Lost interest in or resented patients.

- Felt preoccupied with thoughts, images, or circumstances of death, even during leisure time.

(Furman, 2002, p. 57).

> **_Personal Insight_**
> *What metaphor would you use to describe burnout?*

COMPASSION FATIGUE

Although burnout and compassion fatigue are used interchangeably, they are uniquely defined. The term "compassion fatigue" refers to a state of tension and preoccupation with the individual or cumulative trauma of clients. Charles Figley began focusing on compassion fatigue, also known as secondary victimization or vicarious trauma, in 1982. Over 10 years later, Figley (1995) described compassion fatigue interchangeably with secondary traumatic stress disorder, which he considered to be less stigmatizing. Seven years later, he suggested that secondary traumatic stress is a natural by-product of caring for traumatized people (Figley, 2002).

Compassion fatigue robs nurses of their passion and energy. Compassion fatigue includes maladaptive compassion strain and consists of severe anguish, intense guilt, and distress associated with the perception of not having done enough to avert suffering or death (Figley, 2002). More recently, Figley (2007) noted that the symptoms of compassion fatigue usually show up without any warning, creating a sense of helplessness, shock, and confusion, along with a sense of isolation.

Nelson-Gardell and Harris (2003) consider primary traumatic stress a reaction that individuals experience when something bad happens to them. When nurses hear their patient's traumatic stories, witness their pain, watch them die, or are present for their families as they grieve, they may duplicate the same symptoms as the patients and become exhausted because of it. Nurses can experience recurrent and intrusive distressing recollections of the patient's event and avoid thoughts and feelings associated with the patient's trauma (Figley, 2002). While treating and supporting primary victims of trauma, nurses can experience compassion fatigue and become secondary victims of trauma. They become indirect trauma victims (Sabin-Farrell & Turpin, 2003). Secondary traumatic stress and compassion fatigue are also caused by long work hours or length of assignment, and caseloads with traumatized patients (Boscarino et al., 2004; Creamer & Liddle, 2005; Meyers & Cornille, 2002). In a study by Roberts, Flannelly, Weaver, & Figley (2003), 27% of the responders to trauma were extremely at risk, 11.7% were at high risk, and 15.4% were at moderate risk.

> **_Personal Insight_**
> *Think for a moment of something that brings you joy. Now imagine never experiencing that thought or the feeling it engenders.*

Compassion fatigue symptoms include cognitive, emotional, behavioral, spiritual, personal relation, somatic, and work performance reactions or changes. These include lowered concentration, decreased self-esteem, apathy, powerlessness, anxiety, guilt, impatience, irritability, withdrawal, loss of purpose and faith, loneliness, and low morale and motivation (Figley, 2002). Compassion fatigue may cause a decline in the ability to experience joy. The body becomes exhausted and aches, pains, dizziness, and sweating may be experienced. This can make professionals vulnerable to some of the same psychological turbulence that is experienced by the primary victims whom they support (Racanelli, 2005). Nurses with compassion fatigue may experience hopelessness, blame, anger, physical fatigue, and drug abuse. They may be irritable and unable to fall asleep. Lack of sleep, along with the other symptoms, may put their jobs in jeopardy as well as their patients' lives. There is a risk for depression, anxiety disorders, or total avoidance of others. The most significant by-product of compassion fatigue is when nurses quit the field they were once so passionate about.

McCann and Pearlman (1990) coined the phrase *vicarious trauma,* which occurs over time, to describe disruptions in cognitive schemas (core beliefs about the self, others, and the world).

Nurses who work in child protective services, mental health, trauma, or on disaster teams are at risk for being vicariously traumatized due to their empathetic engagement with those who are traumatized and experiencing distress. Child protective service workers have a high risk for transmission of traumatic stress symptomatology (Pryce, Shackelford, & Pryce, 2007). Meldrum, King, and Spooner (2002) found that 17% of community mental health workers met the criteria for secondary traumatic stress disorder. Disaster response teams also have higher distress levels (Holtz, Salama, Cardozo, & Gotway, 2002). Nurses who provide disaster relief observe fear, anger, prejudice, and hostility in traumatized officials and fellow professionals, and such secondary trauma can magnify the disaster (Parkes, 2003). Whether witnessing patients' deaths or comforting family members, the cost of caring takes its toll. A supportive work environment and adequate supervision can diminish the occurrence of secondary traumatic stress and compassion fatigue (Boscarino et al., 2004; Korkeila et al., 2003).

A number of key variables may influence the development of compassion fatigue in nurses including age, gender, education, personal trauma history, specialized training, work environment, professional experience, and social support (Figley, 2002; Somer, Buchbinder, Peled-Avram, & Ben-Yizhack, 2004; Stamm, 2002; Wee & Myers, 2002). As age increases, the risk for compassion fatigue or burnout decreases (Nelson-Gardell & Harris, 2003). Males are at significantly lower risk for secondary traumatic stress and vicarious trauma than females (Meyers & Cornille, 2002; Sprang, Clark, & Whitt-Woosley, 2007). If nurses have control in their work environments and are well educated, they may be spared the intense stress of compassion fatigue. Being that specialized training is a protective factor for trauma counselors (Ortlepp & Friedman, 2001), workshops and trainings could benefit nurses in the long run.

If nurses experience personal traumas in their lives, it is imperative that they work through those traumas because personal trauma history is associated with increased risk for secondary traumatic stress and vicarious trauma (Cunningham, 2003; Nelson-Gardell & Harris, 2003). Coworkers, supervisors, and nursing directors must support staff in their stressful careers because supportive work environments and adequate supervision were found to mitigate the incidence of secondary traumatic stress and burnout (Boscarino et al., 2004; Korkeila et al., 2003; Ortlepp & Friedman, 2001). Rather than seeing symptoms of compassion fatigue as pathological, nurses can view symptoms as messages about what is good and strong within them, rather than indicators of shameful weakness or sickness (Baranowsky, Gentry, & Schultz, 2005).

HOW NURSES USE SELF-CARE STRATEGIES TO IMPROVE THEIR SOCIAL AND EMOTIONAL FUNCTIONING

Most of the intervention strategies that deal with burnout or compassion fatigue are common sense and represent the same advice and recommendations nurses always give others (Wood, 2005). To address the special needs of nurses who work with dying patients, a number of intervention strategies have been found to improve social and emotional functioning. Such strategies include monitoring their stress levels; feeling as though they have some control over their work; utilizing supervision, training, and support systems; maintaining healthy life styles and senses of humor; and meditating. Figley (2002) notes leisure activities, such as dinner, movies, reading, walking, and making time for hobbies along with family time, are useful self-care strategies to deal with stressful careers in nursing. Wicks (2006) designed a questionnaire to help nurses self-evaluate and identify professional secondary stress that can be used as a springboard for further reflection (Table 11-1).

Monitoring Stress

To better cope with stress, nurses can monitor themselves for stress daily by using a scale of 1 to 10. Once identified and acknowledged, it is critical to find ways to manage stress. To maintain a high level of job performance, nurses must be able to effectively cope with the physical, mental, and emotional stress of their work and personal lives. The goal is to better cope with stress, develop a stronger sense of self, and improve personal boundaries, while remaining safe in their professional roles. Garret (2008) notes that nurses often cope with increased stress and burnout by calling in sick, which can compromise patient safety. Coworkers do not appreciate this particular coping strategy because it puts a strain on an already strained system of care.

Having Control

A nurse's strength comes from the willingness to give to patients; that strength is challenged when patient assignments are overwhelming and unrealistic. Fatigue is a contributing factor for nurse absenteeism, burnout, and job dissatisfaction. It is not uncommon to hear a nurse describe her day off by saying, "All morning, I could still hear my pager going off and the monitors too. I stayed in my pajamas until the afternoon. All I had energy to do was zone out on TV and eat" (*Nurse Advocate,* 2008).

Kanel (2003) maintains that to reduce burnout, workers need to have some control over their time at work and their workload; however, this is very hard to do when there is no control over the high patient-to-nurse ratio (Aiken, Clarke, Sloane, Sochalski, & Silber, 2002). Nurses also need to organize their own work, and have clarity over their roles at work. Nurses should be realistic about what they can control, acknowledge the painful experiences that occur in the workplace, and not allow resentments to build. Many things that take place in the work environment are out of the nurse's control. Rather than becoming stressed out from factors that cannot be controlled in the workplace, nurses can focus on those things that that can be affected by positive action.

Supervision, Training, and Support Systems

Nurses can transcend burnout, workplace stress, and compassion fatigue by utilizing existing hospital professional development processes, supervision, reflective practice, in-service education, and other forms of professional development (Edward & Hercelinskyj, 2007). Easy access to support systems and clinical supervision are also essential (Dickinson & Wright, 2008). In a recent study, higher levels of clinical supervision were associated with lower levels of burnout (Khani, Jaafarpour, & Jamshidbaigi, 2008). Nurses need

continued on page 201

TABLE 11-1: MEDICAL/NURSING PROFESSIONAL SECONDARY STRESS SELF-AWARENESS QUESTIONNAIRE (1 OF 2)

Instructions: Find a quiet, comfortable, and private place. Read each question and respond on a separate sheet of paper by writing the first thing that comes to mind. Once you have completed a page, do not turn back to it or refer to it when working on the other pages. Work as quickly as you can without setting a pace that is too stressful.

1. What is the reason you believe denial is so prevalent in the medical setting as a response to stress for physicians, nurses, and allied health personnel? What are the most common lies you tell yourself about your own stress?

2. At this point, what are the most realistic and helpful steps you can take to prevent, limit, and learn from stress?

3. What are the ways you have heard that are excellent approaches to reducing stress and improving self-care but you feel are unrealistic in your case? What would it take to make them realistic? ("A miracle!" is not an acceptable answer.)

4. When you think of the terms "burnout," "compassion fatigue," and "chronic secondary stress," what do you think of in terms of your own life?

5. What are the issues that make you most anxious? What are the ones you deal with the best?

6. What are the types of situations or interactions from the past that still haunt you?

7. Given the realistic demands of work and family, what would it take to balance these two areas in your life a bit more? (List only those steps that can be realistically taken by you within the next 2 to 3 years).

8. In your own case, what helps you to fall prey to the common masochistic tenet that the only worthy medical or nursing professional is the one involved enough to be on the edge of burnout or physical fatigue?

9. In what ways did your professional schooling, clinical rotations, modeling by supervisors, and initial work after graduation inadvertently teach you that taking care of yourself is a sign of weakness and that an unhealthy lifestyle is the price of being in the field of health care?

10. What are the "bad habits" of the people you observe in your profession that you do not want to emulate? How are you seeking to embrace the wonder, passion, and intense involvement in medicine and nursing without also absorbing the pathological side of the profession?

11. When you are under a great deal of stress, what fantasies do you have? What do you think are healthy fantasies you should act upon someday? What are the unhealthy ones that, if acted upon, would cause you and others harm?

12. What elements that are currently in your self-care protocol have been most beneficial for you? What are the least?

13. What do you struggle with most in your efforts to take care of yourself? Because your presence as a professional in the healthcare field means that de facto you are a bright and accomplished person, you would not think that these struggles should be so hard for you; why are they?

14. How would people describe your attitudes toward work?

15. What should be included in your list of personal doubts and insecurities that most people would be surprised to know about you?

16. In health care, focus on the person and clinical situation that are before you is essential; what do you find are the main sources of external distraction and inner preoccupation that prevent you from doing this?

17. What are the most positive and negative effects your personality style has on the way you interact with patients? With staff?

continued on next page

TABLE 11-1: MEDICAL/NURSING PROFESSIONAL SECONDARY STRESS SELF-AWARENESS QUESTIONNAIRE (2 OF 2)

18. When under extreme stress, what is the style of interacting with others and handling the situation that you would most like to change? What steps are necessary to produce such a change?

19. What would you include in your list of motivations for originally becoming a physician, nurse, or allied health professional? (Make the list as long as you can. Be sure to include any reasons you might now perceive as unrealistic or possibly immature – such as status, power over other people's life and death struggles, financial security, voyeurism – so you have as complete an accounting as possible.)

20. Has the primacy of certain motivations changed for you over time? If so, how? Why do you think this is so? If this is problematic in some way, what might you do about it? For those beneficial changes in priorities, how are you ensuring that they remain in focus for you?

21. What are the most awkward subjects for you to discuss in relationship to your emotional and physical well-being as a health professional?

22. Where do you feel your narcissism comes into play in your role in health care?

23. What would be included in a list of what you like best about being a physician, nurse, or allied health professional? What would be on the list of what you like least?

24. What is most surprising to you about the professional life you now have?

25. What are the most frustrating aspects of your professional life? Your personal life?

26. If you have ever considered changing specialties, moving to a different healthcare setting, or leaving the field, what are the reasons for this?

27. When you think of the profession you are now in, how would you describe it for someone thinking of entering the field now? Suppose someone asked you how you think it would be different in 5 years, what would you say?

28. What are the most important self-care procedures you have put into place in the past 5 years? What has been their impact on you? What ways would you now like to modify your plan?

29. Given your own personality style, what types of patients do you find most challenging? What types of colleagues, subordinates, and supervisors are able to easily elicit an emotional reaction for you? Given this, what ways have you found to most effectively interact with them? (Praying for their early happy death is not a sufficient response.)

30. How would you describe the seemingly beneficial and adverse impacts your professional life has had on your personal life and vice versa?

Note. From *Overcoming Secondary Stress in Medical and Nursing Practice,* by R. Wicks, 2005, New York: Oxford University Press. Reprinted with permission.

managers who foster an open and honest culture where feelings can be expressed and frustrations addressed. Rotating wards to increase personal and professional development and reduce boredom and apathy can be helpful; being provided with, and encouraged to undertake, continuing professional development, including psychosocial interventions training, has also been shown to reduce stress and burnout (Dickinson & Wright, 2008). Nurses treating traumatized children benefit from improved training, owning one's own personal trauma history, and working in a supportive work environment (Meyers & Cornille, 2002).

To combat professional stress, nurses can utilize mentors, participate in groups with similar interests, blog, and join online nursing forums (*Nurse Advocate,* 2008). Nurses can find role models of good self-care and develop self-care practices. Grove and Erickson (2006) found that younger nurses are more likely to experience feelings of agitation and burnout. Utilizing older, more experienced nurses as emotional mentors could be of benefit to the younger nurse new to the profession (Grove & Erickson, 2006).

Healthy Lifestyle

To alleviate stress in their lives, nurses can take action to remain positive and maintain healthy lifestyles. Stress reducing techniques include having a positive attitude and being surrounded by positive people. Healthy stress reducers also include talking to a supportive friend or colleague, taking a long bath, going for a long walk, practicing yoga, or playing with a pet. Nurses can cope with their stressful jobs by doing regular exercise, not smoking, limiting their alcohol use, maintaining a reasonable weight, and living within their means (Flannery, 2004). Nurses can utilize some of the same stress-reducing techniques as psychiatrists, which include seeking support from a colleague and having a hobby (Amos, 2006).

The Power of Positive Thinking

To cope with a stressful career, nurses can replace negative self-talk with positive affirmations (Eubanks, 2007). Affirmations are customarily a sentence or two that reflect a conscious positive thought. Taubman-Ben-Ari and Weintroub (2008) found that a high level of professional self-esteem is an important factor in filtering out threatening aspects of work, especially when routinely exposed to patients' deaths.

Many years ago, the television program *Saturday Night Live* had a character named Stuart Smalley, played by Al Franken, who promoted positive thinking by sharing affirmations while looking into a mirror. Although Al Franken's skits were very funny, they did speak true to what people need to say about themselves and their self-esteem. Some of his comments were:

- I'm good enough, I'm smart enough, and dog-gone it, people like me.

- Whining is anger coming through a very small opening.

- Compare and despair.

- I am a human being, not a human doing.

A Sense of Humor

Although many nurses have a good sense of humor, some have forgotten where they put it!

Goodman and Brown (2008) noted that the most successful teams created after September 11th were those whose staff members were flexible, shared a sense of humor, and had leaders who promoted cohesiveness. Respectful conversations, laughter, and support for each other helped the newly hired, trained, and dedicated clinicians prevent vicarious traumatization and burnout (Goodman & Brown, 2008). Nurses who use humor to cope experience lower levels of emotional exhaustion and depersonalization, and higher levels of personal accomplishment (McCreaddie & Wiggins, 2008).

Nurses can create humor in the workplace. Rubel and McCown (2007) note that appropriate use of humor and fun should be modeled by nursing directors. Those seeking to encourage a happier environment can establish a fun committee, plan structured fun activities, or create a humor bulletin board. Used by crisis nurses to cope with their stressful job, gallows humor (also called dark humor) is a cognitive and behavioral coping strategy as a reaction to stressful events (Maxwell, 2003).

To increase positive emotions, nurses can also focus on how their parents modeled fun, the obstacles in their way to having some fun, their hang-ups about having fun, whom they enjoy having fun with, and how they can integrate some fun into their lives (Spradlin, 2003). To overcome secondary stress in nursing practice, Wicks (2006) recommends retail therapy (shopping) and finding opportunities to laugh as stress relievers. Although retail therapy can be a great deal of fun, watching a comedy or reading a joke book could also alleviate stress in an entertaining way, while not costing anything.

The Internet can also offer nurses humorous medical sites that can alleviate stress. For example, Carenurse.com listed the following humorous quotations taken from documentation in patients' medical records:

- "When she fainted, her eyes rolled around the room."

- "By the time he was admitted, his rapid heart had stopped and he was feeling better."

- "Patient has chest pain if she lies on her left side for over a year."

- "On the second day knee was better; on the third day it had completely disappeared."

- "Patient was released to outpatient department without dressing."

- "Discharge status: Alive but without permission. Patient needs disposition; therefore we will get Dr. Blank to dispose of him."

- "The patient expired on the floor uneventfully."

- "The patient left the hospital feeling much better except for her original complaints."

- "She is numb from her toes down."

- "While in the ER, she was examined, X-rated and sent home."

Personal Insight
What role does your sense of humor play in helping you deal with stress in the workplace?

Meditation

Simple techniques to deal with stress include monitoring daily levels of stress and developing self-care practices such as meditation (the act of pondering or reflecting). Meditation helps nurses focus and regain control of their careers and personal lives, and many nurses experience deep relaxation when meditating. Meditation has a rich, vast history and is one way to engender a relax-

ation response, which can help nurses deal with their stress (Everly & Lating, 2002). Davies (2008) indicated that mindful meditation represents a complementary therapy that has shown promise in the reduction of negative stress in nurses and those extraneous factors that lead to burnout.

Smith (2002) surveyed over 1,000 research participants regarding the benefits of meditating and found the following themes:

(a) Deeper Perspective (Life has a purpose greater than my personal wants and desires)

(b) God (God guides, loves, and comforts me; I put myself in God's hands)

(c) Inner Wisdom (I trust the body's wisdom and healing powers; there are sources of strength and healing deep within me)

(d) Taking It Easy (Sometimes it is important to know when to stop trying, let go, and relax)

(e) Acceptance (Sometimes it is important to accept things that cannot change)

(f) Optimism (I believe in being optimistic, both in general and about how well I will deal with current hassles)

(p. 235).

According to Everly and Lating (2002), there are four general forms of meditative technique: (1) *mental repetition,* in which the focal device is a word or phrase repeated over and over again (e.g., chanting); (2) *physical repetition,* in which the focal device is focusing awareness on a physical act (e.g., yoga); (3) *problem contemplation,* in which the focal device is attempting to solve a challenging problem and the response to the problem is found in the wisdom and life experience of the person; and (4) *visual concentration,* in which the focal device is an image (e.g., a relaxing scene or candle flame).

Personal Insight
What advice might you offer a new nurse
about managing stress in the workplace?

Measuring Compassion Satisfaction as Well as Fatigue

As defined earlier, compassion is the caring awareness of another person's anguish and, at the same time, a need to lessen it. If a health professional experiences compassion satisfaction, they may not experience compassion fatigue. Wee and Myers (2003) found that experience, knowledge, and maturity play a role in compassion satisfaction. Growing older might counter the effects of burnout, perhaps due to the wisdom and experience gained through the years. Perhaps through their own experience, older nurses realize they are simply doing the best they can. As an experienced critical care nurse noted, "I say, 'I am only one person' to remind others or myself that it takes many people many days to achieve a difficult goal" (Figley, 2002, p. 217).

Nurses can personally address stress and possible burnout (Table 11-2).

RESILIENT NURSES

Resiliency is the ability to withstand and rebound from disruptive life challenges. Resilience involves key processes over time that foster the ability to struggle well, surmount obstacles, and go on to live and love fully (Walsh, 2003, p. 1).

Resilience can be defined as the capacity to overcome life challenges and become more resourceful. Resilience is the ability to return to original form after being stretched out of shape. The hallmark of resilient objects is that they can bend under stress and then bounce back, rather than break.

Resiliency is a protective factor against compassion fatigue. Resilient individuals are optimistic about their futures, have strong beliefs in themselves, have unusually ambitious dreams and aspirations that motivate them to succeed, and are able to feel less emotionally trapped due to positive identities (Glicken, 2006). Although many nurses struggle with the stressors of their jobs, they overcome the daily obstacles and continue to love nursing and working in death and dying situations.

Edward and Hercelinskyj (2007) propose that using knowledge of resilient behaviors is a means to rise above burnout and nursing stress. To have a resilient mindset, nurses should know their strengths and vulnerabilities, feel in control, and be realistic, empathetic problem solvers who are able to manage their feelings while maintaining balance (Brooks & Goldstein, 2004). Resilient nurses have a broad capacity to cope creatively and to adjust flexibly to difficulties by maintaining a positive image of themselves and others and investing in caregiving relationships with transformed energy and commitment (International Work Group on Death, Dying, and Bereavement, 2006).

According to Milne (2007), the following behaviors can help nurses increase their resiliency:

1. Be optimistic.
2. Have cognitive flexibility.
3. Clarify your personal beliefs.
4. Be altruistic.
5. Have a role model.
6. Face fears.
7. Develop positive coping skills.
8. Have a social network in place.
9. Keep fit.
10. Have a sense of humor.

continued on page 208

TABLE 11-2: PROFESSIONAL QUALITY OF LIFE SCALE (PROQOL) (1 OF 3)

Compassion Satisfaction and Compassion Fatigue (ProQOL) Version 5 (2009)

When you *help* people you have direct contact with their lives. As you may have found, your compassion for those you *help* can affect you in positive and negative ways. Below are some questions about your experiences, both positive and negative, as a *helper*. Consider each of the following questions about you and your current work situation. Select the number that honestly reflects how frequently you experienced these things in the *last 30 days*.

0=Never	1=Rarely	2=A Few Times	3=Somewhat Often	4=Often	5=Very Often

_____ 1. I am happy.

_____ 2. I am preoccupied with more than one person I [*help*].

_____ 3. I get satisfaction from being able to [*help*] people.

_____ 4. I feel connected to others.

_____ 5. I jump or am startled by unexpected sounds.

_____ 6. I feel invigorated after working with those I [*help*].

_____ 7. I find it difficult to separate my personal life from my life as a [*helper*].

_____ 8. I am not as productive at work because I am losing sleep over traumatic experiences of a person I [*help*].

_____ 9. I think that I might have been affected by the traumatic stress of those I [*help*].

_____ 10. I feel trapped by my job as a [*helper*].

_____ 11. Because of my [*helping*], I have felt "on edge" about various things.

_____ 12. I like my work as a [*helper*].

_____ 13. I feel depressed because of the traumatic experiences of the people I [*help*].

_____ 14. I feel as though I am experiencing the trauma of someone I have [*helped*].

_____ 15. I have beliefs that sustain me.

_____ 16. I am pleased with how I am able to keep up with [*helping*] techniques and protocols.

_____ 17. I am the person I always wanted to be.

_____ 18. My work makes me feel satisfied.

_____ 19. I feel worn out because of my work as a [*helper*].

_____ 20. I have happy thoughts and feelings about those I [*help*] and how I could help them.

_____ 21. I feel overwhelmed because my case work load seems endless.

_____ 22. I believe I can make a difference through my work.

_____ 23. I avoid certain activities or situations because they remind me of frightening experiences of the people I [*help*].

_____ 24. I am proud of what I can do to [*help*].

_____ 25. As a result of my [*helping*], I have intrusive, frightening thoughts.

_____ 26. I feel "bogged down" by the system.

_____ 27. I have thoughts that I am a "success" as a [*helper*].

_____ 28. I can't recall important parts of my work with trauma victims.

_____ 29. I am a very caring person.

_____ 30. I am happy that I chose to do this work.

continued on next page

TABLE 11-2: PROFESSIONAL QUALITY OF LIFE SCALE (PROQOL) (2 OF 3)

What is my score and what does it mean?

In this section, you will score your test and then you can compare your score to the interpretation below.

Scoring

1. Be certain you respond to all items.

2. Go to items 1, 4, 15, 17 and 29 and reverse your score. For example, if you scored the item 1, write a 5 beside it. We ask you to reverse these scores because we have learned that the test works better if you reverse these scores.

You Wrote	Change to
1	5
2	4
3	3
4	2
5	1

To find your score on **Compassion Satisfaction,** add your scores on questions 3, 6, 12, 16, 18, 20, 22, 24, 27, 30.

The sum of my Compassion Satisfaction questions was	So My Score Equals	My Level of Compassion Satisfaction
22 or less	43 or less	Low
Between 23 and 41	Around 50	Average
42 or more	57 or more	High

To find your score on **Burnout,** add your scores questions 1, 4, 8, 10, 15, 17, 19, 21, 26 and 29. Find your score on the table below.

The sum of my Burnout questions	So My Score Equals	My Level of Burnout
22 or less	43 or less	Low
Between 23 and 41	Around 50	Average
42 or more	57 or more	High

To find your score on **Secondary Traumatic Stress,** add your scores on questions 2, 5, 7, 9, 11, 13, 14, 23, 25, 28. Find your score on the table below.

The sum of my Secondary Traumatic Stress questions	So My Score Equals	My Level of Secondary Traumatic Stress
22 or less	43 or less	Low
Between 23 and 41	Around 50	Average
42 or more	57 or more	High

Your Scores on the ProQOL: Professional Quality of Life Screening

Based on your responses, your personal scores are below. If you have any concerns, you should discuss them with a physical or mental health care professional.

continued on next page

TABLE 11-2: PROFESSIONAL QUALITY OF LIFE SCALE (PROQOL) (3 OF 3)

Compassion Satisfaction _____

Compassion satisfaction is about the pleasure you derive from being able to do your work well. For example, you may feel like it is a pleasure to help others through your work. You may feel positively about your colleagues or your ability to contribute to the work setting or even the greater good of society. Higher scores on this scale represent a greater satisfaction related to your ability to be an effective caregiver in your job.

The average score is 50 (SD 10; alpha scale reliability .88). About 25% of people score higher than 57 and about 25% of people score below 43. If you are in the higher range, you probably derive a good deal of professional satisfaction from your position. If your scores are below 40, you may either find problems with your job, or there may be some other reason – for example, you might derive your satisfaction from activities other than your job.

Burnout _____

Most people have an intuitive idea of what burnout is. From the research perspective, burnout is one of the elements of compassion fatigue. It is associated with feelings of hopelessness and difficulties in dealing with work or in doing your job effectively. These negative feelings usually have a gradual onset. They can reflect the feeling that your efforts make no difference, or they can be associated with a very high workload or a non-supportive work environment. Higher scores on this scale mean that you are at higher risk for burnout.

The average score on the burnout scale is 50 (SD 10; alpha scale reliability .75). About 25% of people score above 57 and about 25% of people score below 43. If your score is below 18, this probably reflects positive feelings about your ability to be effective in your work. If you score above 57 you may wish to think about what at work makes you feel like you are not effective in your position. Your score may reflect your mood; perhaps you were having a "bad day" or are in need of some time off. If the high score persists or if it is reflective of other worries, it may be a cause for concern.

Secondary Traumatic Stress _____

The second component of Compassion Fatigue (CF) is secondary traumatic stress (STS). It is about your work-related, secondary exposure to extremely or traumatically stressful events. Developing problems due to exposure to other's trauma is somewhat rare but does happen to many people who care for those who have experienced extremely or traumatically stressful events. For example, you may repeatedly hear stories about the traumatic things that happen to other people, commonly called Vicarious Traumatization. You may see or provide treatment to people who have experienced horrific events. If your work puts you directly in the path of danger, due to your work as a soldier or civilian working in military medicine personnel, this is not secondary exposure; your exposure is primary. However, if you are exposed to others' traumatic events as a result of your work, such as providing care to casualties or for those in a military medical rehabilitation facility, this is secondary exposure. The symptoms of STS are usually rapid in onset and associated with a particular event. They may include being afraid, having difficulty sleeping, having images of the upsetting event pop into your mind, or avoiding things that remind you of the event.

The average score on this scale is 50 (SD 10; alpha scale reliability .81). About 25% of people score below 43 and about 25% of people score above 57. If your score is above 57, you may want to take some time to think about what at work may be frightening to you or if there is some other reason for the elevated score. While higher scores do not mean that you do have a problem, they are an indication that you may want to examine how you feel about your work and your work environment. You may wish to discuss this with your supervisor, a colleague, or a health care professional.

Note. © B. Hudnall Stamm, 2009. *Professional Quality of Life: Compassion Satisfaction and Fatigue Subscales, R-V (ProQOL).* http://www.isu.edu/~bhstamm. This test may be freely copied as long as (a) author is credited, (b) no changes are made other than those authorized below, and (c) it is not sold. You may substitute the appropriate target group for [*helper*] if that is not the best term. For example, if you are working with teachers, replace [*helper*] with teacher. Word changes may be made to any word in italicized square brackets to make the measure read more smoothly for a particular target group.

Disclaimer This information is presented for educational purposes only. It is not a substitute for informed medical advice or training. Do not use this information to diagnose or treat a health problem without consulting a qualified health or mental health care provider. If you have concerns, contact your health care provider, mental health professional, or your community health center.

As nurses acknowledge personal and professional losses, recognize their most difficult working situations, and identify sources of stress, burnout, and compassion fatigue, they must simultaneously seek out ways to remain resilient (Table 11-3).

Glozier, Hough, Henderson, and Holland-Elliot (2006) studied attitudes of nurses toward coworkers returning to work following a psychiatric or physical illness and found that staff members suffering from mental conditions were much more likely to

TABLE 11-3: 10 WAYS TO BUILD RESILIENCE

Make connections. Good relationships with close family members, friends, or others are important. Accepting help and support from those who care about you and will listen to you strengthens resilience. Some people find that being active in civic groups, faith-based organizations, or other local groups provides social support and can help with reclaiming hope. Assisting others in their time of need also can benefit the helper.

Avoid seeing crises as insurmountable problems. You can't change the fact that highly stressful events happen, but you can change how you interpret and respond to these events. Try looking beyond the present to how future circumstances may be a little better. Note any subtle ways in which you might already feel somewhat better as you deal with difficult situations.

Accept that change is a part of living. Certain goals may no longer be attainable as a result of adverse situations. Accepting circumstances that cannot be changed can help you focus on circumstances that you can alter.

Move toward your goals. Develop some realistic goals. Do something regularly – even if it seems like a small accomplishment – that enables you to move toward your goals. Instead of focusing on tasks that seem unachievable, ask yourself, "What's one thing I know I can accomplish today that helps me move in the direction I want to go?"

Take decisive actions. Act on adverse situations as much as you can. Take decisive actions, rather than detaching completely from problems and stresses and wishing they would just go away.

Look for opportunities for self-discovery. People often learn something about themselves and may find that they have grown in some respect as a result of their struggle with loss. Many people who have experienced tragedies and hardship have reported better relationships, greater sense of strength even while feeling vulnerable, increased sense of self-worth, a more developed spirituality, and heightened appreciation for life.

Nurture a positive view of yourself. Developing confidence in your ability to solve problems and trusting your instincts helps build resilience.

Keep things in perspective. Even when facing very painful events, try to consider the stressful situation in a broader context and keep a long-term perspective. Avoid blowing the event out of proportion.

Maintain a hopeful outlook. An optimistic outlook enables you to expect that good things will happen in your life. Try visualizing what you want, rather than worrying about what you fear.

Take care of yourself. Pay attention to your own needs and feelings. Engage in activities that you enjoy and find relaxing. Exercise regularly. Taking care of yourself helps to keep your mind and body primed to deal with situations that require resilience.

Additional ways of strengthening resilience may be helpful. For example, some people write about their deepest thoughts and feelings related to trauma or other stressful events in their life. Meditation and spiritual practices help some people build connections and restore hope.

The key is to identify ways that are likely to work well for you as part of your own personal strategy for fostering resilience.

Note. From "The Road to Resilience," by L. Comas-Diaz et al., n.d. Retrieved on May 29, 2010 from http://www.apa.org/helpcenter/road_resilience.aspx#

be viewed negatively than those suffering from physical conditions. Such stigmatization makes it very difficult for nurses to share their stress with co-workers. According to Maddi and Khoshaba (2005), resilient nurses accurately and courageously face stressors, rather than use avoidant coping strategies, and are more effective at using social support, rather than isolating themselves. Resilience is emerging as a pattern of attitudes and actions that transforms nursing stressors from potential disasters in the workplace into growth opportunities (Maddi & Khoshaba, 2005).

CASE STUDY

Charlie, Eileen, and Debbie met at an annual nursing conference. They decided to have lunch and spent the next hour and a half getting to know one another. Charlie, a nephrology nurse for 8 years, is married with a 3-year-old daughter, Abbey. Though Abbey often asks her dad to play with her, Charlie is too tired. He mentioned that he has not enjoyed the outdoors in years.

Charlie was once enthusiastic about his work. Through the years he overidentified with his patients and invested much of his own energy in their care. Charlie spends a great deal of time with each of his patients and feels exhausted by their pain, their stories, their hopes, and their challenges. He complained to the other nurses about not having enough power over his workload, having to work many hours of overtime, and feeling resentful toward his patients, even those whom he has treated for years. Charlie is so exhausted after work that he usually eats dinner, has a couple of beers, watches a few television shows, and goes to sleep by 10 p.m. His wife complains that he is ignoring her.

Eileen commended Charlie for his hard work and acknowledged the difficult and exhausting job he has as a nephrology nurse. Debbie recommended that he find the time to play with his

daughter after work, even if only for a short time after dinner, and suggested that he and his wife take her to the park together so he can appreciate nature and enjoy his family. She also shared that she attends the circus annually and recommended that Charlie and his wife take Abbey the next time the circus visits town.

Eileen has been a psychiatric nurse for the past 3 years and has witnessed significant violence in the workplace. Many of her patients are verbally and physically abusive and she is constantly on guard in the workplace. She made a point of sharing her feelings with Charlie and Debbie during lunch. She told them that if she finds herself obsessing about certain thoughts, she will talk about them with members of her team. She keeps a journal and tries to write in it every few days to help her reframe and solve problems, and she finds it reduces her stress. She loves being a psychiatric nurse and cares deeply for her patients. Eileen mentioned that although she feels at times just as stressed as her patients, like Charlie, she believes she makes a difference in the lives of her patients.

Debbie has been an emergency room nurse for 6 years and has helped save countless patients but also has witnessed many deaths. She mentioned that last month, three children were brought in from a school bus crash caused by a drunk driver. Although the staff worked on the children, all three died in the emergency room. Debbie told them that she is a religious person. She also copes by speaking with her supervisor when she feels overwhelmed. Eileen also recommended talking with coworkers or lighting a candle at home in memory of the patients who died.

Debbie mentioned that having a sense of humor and laughing whenever she can helps her to cope. Charlie mentioned that he can't remember the last time he had a good laugh. Eileen told them she recently joined an online discussion group that focuses on laughter and offered Charlie the website information. Eileen selects comedies when she goes to the movies, and rents a comedy once a week. Debbie explained that as a nursing director she supervises many nurses and tries to keep it light whenever possible. She shared her belief that humor should be modeled by supervisors and told the other nurses that she established a fun committee several years ago in her hospital, and members plan structured fun activities throughout the year. A few months ago, Debbie created a humor bulletin board and nurses are always adding cartoons and pictures of themselves as babies.

As the nurses shared their meals and their stories, they talked about their jobs, their coworkers, and their struggles. Though they could only spend an hour and a half together before attending the afternoon general session, they took the time to brainstorm and figure out ways to cope with their stressful careers in nursing. Debbie took a rubber band from around her wrist and asked each nurse to describe the rubber band. Their answers included "It stretches," "It bounces back," and "It's flexible." Debbie said that each of them needs to be like the rubber band, flexible and able to bounce back. She explained that if rubber bands are stretched too far, they will snap. Each of the nurses understood they had to be like Debbie's rubber band. If they stretch themselves too far they will, in the long run, snap! As they walked back to the conference, Debbie told them that they all make a difference and that's what they have to hold onto when job stress gets to them.

Questions

1. What concerns do you have for these nurses?

2. Do you have the same concerns for yourself?

3. What additional information would be useful to these nurses when they return home from the conference?

4. What can you suggest to prevent burnout and compassion fatigue in these nurses?

Discussion

The three nurses were able to use a window of opportunity to share their concerns and problems. As they ate, they shared stories about their families, their hobbies, and their stressful jobs. Eileen, a psychiatric nurse, asked both Charlie and Debbie what they thought was most rewarding about their jobs and what was most stressful. All three agreed that what was most stressful was not having enough time in the day to adequately treat their patients. Little (2002) indicated that emergency nurses witness cruel and malicious acts of inhumanity that sometimes result in human suffering. Debbie has probably witnessed many brutal acts in her 6 years as an emergency department nurse. She felt comfortable sharing with Charlie, a nephrology nurse, and Eileen, a psychiatric nurse. Antai-Ontong (2001) reported that psychiatric nurses are more likely to come across workplace violence than nurses in other settings and must be prepared to use proactive health-promoting activities. Eileen can also debrief at the end of the day with a supervisor and coworkers to deal with her stressful job. Debbie's idea about the rubber band is a good one as it keeps her mindful to bounce back and be flexible on the job. Both women were able to empathize with Charlie and offer suggestions for self-care. The three nurses would benefit from keeping in touch through e-mail and continuing to encourage and support each other.

SUMMARY

This chapter explored the scope of professional stress. Strategies for preventing burnout and compassion fatigue while working with dying patients were suggested. The significance of resiliency while working with patients was noted. Nurses have chosen a career that is inherently stressful, but they can also choose stress relievers that will help them to cope. Patients stressed by their health conditions rely on nurses to alleviate their concerns and provide support and compassion. To do so, nurses must first have self-care practices that effectively offset the daily stresses that can lead to burnout and compassion fatigue.

WEB RESOURCES

American Academy of Experts in Traumatic Stress
  http://www.aaets.org

NurseWeek: "Sudden Impact" article on stress
  http://www.nurseweek.com/news/features/
  01-11/stress.html

Sidran Traumatic Stress Education & Advocacy
  Institute:
  http://www.sidran.org/index.cfm

Physician Heal Thyself: Thoughts, Links, and
  Readings on Caregiver Stress & Burnout for
  Medical and Psychological Professionals,
  Family Caregivers, and Clergy
  http://www.synspectrum.com/healself.html

EXAM QUESTIONS

CHAPTER 11
Questions 91-100

Note: Choose the one option that BEST answers each question.

91. A physiological response or reaction, regardless of the source or stimulus, is known as

    a. a flash-back.

    b. secondary traumatic stress.

    c. stress.

    d. compassion fatigue.

92. The caring awareness of another person's anguish and, at the same time, a desire to lessen it is known as

    a. mindful meditation.

    b. inner wisdom.

    c. resiliency.

    d. compassion.

93. A state of physical, emotional, and mental exhaustion brought on by unrealistic goals and aspirations and long work hours is known as

    a. compassion stress.

    b. compassion fatigue.

    c. burnout.

    d. balance.

94. An indication of a level 2 burnout is

    a. being mentally fatigued at the end of the day.

    b. feeling frustrated and angry after patient contact.

    c. feeling unappreciated for your work effort.

    d. when minor stress becomes distress.

95. A state of tension and preoccupation with the individual or cumulative trauma of patients is known as

    a. compassion stress.

    b. compassion fatigue.

    c. burnout.

    d. vicarious trauma.

96. When looking at compassion fatigue, research has shown that the incidence of secondary traumatic stress and burnout can be diminished by

    a. a supportive work environment and adequate supervision.

    b. taking frequent "mental health days."

    c. an increase in pay and responsibility.

    d. changing ones specialty area and position.

97. A strategy professionals may employ to prevent compassion fatigue is to

    a. maintain a strong support network.

    b. give up a hobby.

    c. avoid other professionals.

    d. isolate oneself.

98. A healthy way to deal with stress in the workplace is to

    a. call in sick when you anticipate a tough day at work.

    b. drink wine after work to calm your nerves.

    c. plan frequent, regular exercise.

    d. avoid your supervisor.

99. The ability to withstand and rebound from disruptive life challenges is

    a. mindful meditation.

    b. inner wisdom.

    c. resiliency.

    d. compassion.

100. Behaviors that are associated with resiliency include

    a. rigidity and determination.

    b. optimism, a sense of humor, and altruism.

    c. perfectionism and perseverance.

    d. introversion, fear avoidance, and control.

This concludes the final examination.

Please answer the evaluation questions found on page v of this workbook.

APPENDIX

A NATIONAL FRAMEWORK AND PREFERRED PRACTICES FOR PALLIATIVE AND HOSPICE CARE QUALITY

1. Provide palliative and hospice care by an interdisciplinary team of skilled palliative care professionals, including, for example, physicians, nurses, social workers, pharmacists, spiritual care counselors, and others who collaborate with primary healthcare professional(s).

2. Provide access to palliative and hospice care that is responsive to the patient and family 24 hours a day, 7 days a week.

3. Provide continuing education to all healthcare professionals on the domains of palliative care and hospice care.

4. Provide adequate training and clinical support to assure that professional staff are confident in their ability to provide palliative care for patients.

5. Hospice care and specialized palliative care professionals should be appropriately trained, credentialed, and/or certified in their areas of expertise.

6. Formulate, utilize, and regularly review a timely care plan based on a comprehensive interdisciplinary assessment of the values, preferences, goals, and needs of the patient and family and, to the extent that existing privacy laws permit, ensure that the plan is broadly disseminated, both internally and externally, to all professionals involved in the patient's care.

7. Ensure that upon transfer between healthcare settings, there is timely and thorough communication of the patient's goals, preferences, values, and clinical information so that continuity of care and seamless follow-up are assured.

8. Healthcare professionals should present hospice as an option to all patients and families when death within a year would not be surprising and should reintroduce the hospice option as the patient declines.

9. Patients and caregivers should be asked by palliative and hospice care programs to assess physicians'/healthcare professionals' ability to discuss hospice as an option.

10. Enable patients to make informed decisions about their care by educating them on the process of their diseases, prognoses, and the benefits and burdens of potential interventions.

11. Provide education and support to families and unlicensed caregivers based on the patient's individualized care plan to assure safe and appropriate care for the patient.

12. Measure and document pain, dyspnea, constipation, and other symptoms using available standardized scales.

13. Assess and manage symptoms and side effects in a timely, safe, and effective manner to a level that is acceptable to the patient and family.

14. Measure and document anxiety, depression, delirium, behavioral disturbances, and other common psychological symptoms using available standardized scales.

15. Manage anxiety, depression, delirium, behavioral disturbances, and other common psychological symptoms in a timely, safe, and effective manner to a level that is acceptable to the patient and family.

16. Assess and manage the psychological reactions of patients and families (including stress, anticipatory grief, and coping) in a regular, ongoing fashion in order to address emotional and functional impairment and loss.

17. Develop and offer a grief and bereavement care plan to provide services to patients and families prior to and for at least 13 months after the death of the patient.

18. Conduct regular patient and family care conferences with physicians and other appropriate members of the interdisciplinary team to provide information, to discuss goals of care, disease prognosis, and advance care planning and to offer support.

19. Develop and implement a comprehensive social care plan that addresses the social, practical, and legal needs of the patient and caregivers, including but not limited to relationships, communication, existing social and cultural networks, decision making, work and school settings, finances, sexuality/intimacy, caregiver availability/stress, and access to medicines and equipment.

20. Develop and document a plan based on an assessment of religious, spiritual, and existential concerns using a structured instrument, and integrate the information obtained from the assessment into the palliative care plan.

21. Provide information about the availability of spiritual care services, and make spiritual care available either through organizational spiritual care counseling or through the patient's own clergy relationships.

22. Specialized palliative and hospice care teams should include spiritual care professionals appropriately trained and certified in palliative care.

23. Specialized palliative and hospice spiritual care professionals should build partnerships with community clergy and provide education and counseling related to end-of-life care.

24. Incorporate cultural assessment as a component of comprehensive palliative and hospice care assessment, including but not limited to locus of decision making; preferences regarding disclosure of information; truth telling and decision making; dietary preferences; language; family communication; desire for support measures, such as palliative therapies and complementary and alternative medicine; perspectives on death, suffering, and grieving; and funeral/burial rituals.

25. Provide professional interpreter services and culturally sensitive materials in the patient's and family's preferred language.

26. Recognize and document the transition to the active dying phase, and communicate to the patient, family, and staff the expectation of imminent death.

27. Educate the family on a timely basis regarding the signs and symptoms of imminent death in an age-appropriate, developmentally appropriate, and culturally appropriate manner.

28. As part of the ongoing care planning process, routinely ascertain and document patient and family wishes about the care setting for the site of death, and fulfill patient and family preferences when possible.

29. Provide adequate dosage of analgesics and sedatives as appropriate to achieve patient comfort during the active dying phase, and address concerns and fears about using narcotics and of analgesics hastening death.

30. Treat the body after death with respect according to the cultural and religious practices of the family and in accordance with local law.

31. Facilitate effective grieving by implementing in a timely manner a bereavement care plan after the patient's death, when the family remains the focus of care.

32. Document the designated surrogate/decision maker in accordance with state law for every patient in primary, acute, and long-term care and in palliative and hospice care.

33. Document the patient/surrogate preferences for goals of care, treatment options, and setting of care at first assessment and at frequent intervals as conditions change.

34. Convert the patient treatment goals into medical orders, and ensure that the information is transferable and applicable across care settings, including long-term care, emergency medical services, and hospital care, through a program such as the Physician Orders for Life-Sustaining Treatment (POLST) program.

35. Make advance directives and surrogacy designations available across care settings, while protecting patient privacy and adherence to HIPAA regulations, for example, by using Internet-based registries or electronic personal health records.

36. Develop healthcare and community collaborations to promote advance care planning and the completion of advance directives for all individuals, for example, the Respecting Choices and Community Conversations on Compassionate Care programs.

37. Establish or have access to ethics committees or ethics consultation across care settings to address ethical conflicts at the end of life.

38. For minors with decision making capacity, document the child's views and preferences for medical care, including assent for treatment, and give them appropriate weight in decision making. Make appropriate professional staff members available to both the child and the adult decision maker for consultation and intervention when the child's wishes differ from those of the adult decision maker.

Note. From "A National Framework and Preferred Practices for Palliative and Hospice Care Quality," National Quality Forum, 2006. Washington, DC. Retrieved on February 5, 2010, from http://www.qualityforum.org/publications/2006/12A_National_Framework_and_Preferred_Practices_for_Palliative_and_Hospice_Care_Quality.aspx

GLOSSARY

active euthanasia (assisted suicide or assisted death): Self-administration of a death-causing agent facilitated by individuals (typically physicians) who provide the means.

acute phase: Period of illness initiated by diagnosis, during which individuals attempt to understand disease, maximize health, develop coping strategies, explore effect of diagnosis, express feelings, and integrate present reality into their senses of past and future.

acute stress: Response to an immediate perceived physical, psychological, or emotional threat in the workplace that impacts the ability to perform one's responsibilities.

active voluntary euthanasia: A patient's voluntary request of the physician to administer a lethal dose of medication.

advance directive: An oral or written document detailing a person's future preferences regarding medical treatment should he or she become incapacitated.

altruistic suicide: Suicide committed in the name of peace, without selfish motives.

anomic suicide: Suicide resulting when major changes in society create a crisis for the individual.

anticipatory grief: Grief response prior to the actual death in anticipation of the future loss(es).

bereavement: Time period after a death that encompasses adjustment to living without the person who died.

bereavement self-help group: A support group facilitated by the bereaved that offers mutual aid to other bereaved individuals.

brain death: Termination of all brain activity indicated by a flat electroencephalogram, no muscular movement, complete unresponsiveness, and no spontaneous breathing.

cardiac death: Termination of heart beat.

burnout: A state of physical, emotional, and mental exhaustion brought on by unrealistic goals and aspirations and long hours.

causality: Reason death occurs.

celebrants: Life-cycle ceremony specialists with a background in the history of ritual, ceremony, and funeral traditions.

cell death: Death of individual body cells; during this process, respiration, heartbeat, and brain activity stop.

chronic phase: Time period of an illness when the focus is upon managing symptoms and side effects while carrying out health regimes, normalizing life, maximizing social support, expressing feelings, and finding meaning in suffering.

chronic stress: Ongoing, long-term stress.

closed awareness: Everyone but patient is aware that patient is dying.

compassion: Caring awareness of another person's anguish, combined with a desire to lessen it.

compassion fatigue: Depletion of emotional energy from the empathetic response when expectation is for the nurse to act and relieve suffering.

compassion stress: State of tension and preoccupation with the individual or cumulative trauma of clients.

complicated grief disorder: Intense grief response by mourner devastated by the death.

complementary therapies: Nonpharmacological treatments focusing on relaxation and/or distraction and reduction of suffering, including massage, aroma therapy, reflexology, yoga, acupuncture, music, and art.

cremation: Process of reducing the deceased human body to bone fragments using high heat and flame.

culture: Shared beliefs, values, and practices that structure behaviors and the way people act at end of life.

death anxiety: Stressful condition that occurs when individuals are unable to cope with the reality of death.

death certificate: Form documenting a death, including the time and cause of death, considered to be legal proof of death.

death notification: The compassionate and supportive act of informing significant others their loved one is dead.

determinants of grief: Factors influencing the individual's grief experience.

discussed assisted suicide: Patient and physician discussion of alternatives to suicide.

disenfranchised grief: Grief which cannot be openly acknowledged, publicly mourned, or socially supported.

disillusionment phase: Period beginning approximately two months after a disaster and lasting from 1 to 2 years, during which resources are seen as too little, too late, and people work through their grief and come to terms with loss.

do not resuscitate (DNR) order: Physician's order not to conduct cardiopulmonary resuscitation (CPR) should the patient die.

egotistical suicide: Suicide resulting from under-involvement or under-integration, disintegration, and isolation of an individual from society.

encouraged assisted suicide: Physician encourage suicide and provides the means to end the individual's life.

episodic acute stress: Frequent, recurrent experience of stress.

ethics: Systems of moral values that guide professionals in their conduct and treatment of patients.

euphemism: Verbal symbols that replace the words "death," "dead," and "dying" in an effort to use a more pleasant word or phrase.

euthanasia: Administration of drugs by a physician, with the explicit intention of ending a patient's life at his or her request.

family stress: An umbrella term referring to a variety of stressors arising from relationships and problems inherent in family functioning, including managing child care, school events, sports and recreation, elder care, one's own needs and desires, and spouse's needs.

fatalistic suicide: Suicide committed by individuals who believe they have no future.

final arrangements: Care and disposition of a human body and the ceremony following death.

Five Wishes: An easy-to-understand form used to communicate medical, personal, and spiritual preferences should one become seriously ill and unable to communicate.

functional death: End to all vital functions.

grief: Blending of physical, emotional, cognitive, spiritual, and behavioral reactions resulting from the experience of loss.

heroic phase: Period immediately post-disaster when services are disrupted; people watch out for one another and risk their own safety to save strangers.

home hospice care: Hospice care provided in the patient's home setting.

homicide: Criminal death resulting from an intentional action of the murderer.

honeymoon phase: Period occurring 1 week to 6 months after a disaster, when individuals help each other and collaborate in recovery efforts.

hospice care: A comprehensive program of palliative and supportive care services providing physical, psychological, social, and spiritual care for dying persons and their families.

hospital-based palliative care: Holistic care focused on symptom management provided to seriously ill hospital patients.

hospital/hospice partnerships in hospital-based palliative care: Hospice interdisciplinary team partners with hospital to provide palliative care expertise and assist the hospital in providing patients with pain and symptom management and counseling.

impact phase: Initial impact or actual onset of a disaster, during which survivors take inventory and the focus is on rescue, food, warmth, and safety.

informed consent: Process whereby physicians inform patients about procedures and treatments and the risks and benefits involved, verify patient understanding, and secure the patient's agreement to proceed.

instrumental pattern of grief: Grief expression characterized by thinking rather than feeling, less intense feelings, and a reluctance to talk about feelings.

interdisciplinary hospice team: The group of clinical care providers who provide care to the hospice patient; disciplines represented include medicine, nursing, social work, pastoral care, and home health aides, plus additional therapies (such as occupational, speech, or physical therapy) as indicated by the hospice interdisciplinary plan of care. Volunteers also serve as team members, providing additional assistance and support to the patient and family.

intuitive pattern of grief: Grief expression characterized by intensive emotions; expressions such as crying and lamenting, which mirror the inner experience; and successful adaptive strategies.

irreversibility: Understanding that death is final and, once dead, a person cannot become alive again.

job stress: Harmful physical and emotional responses that occur when the job requirements don't match the capabilities, resources, or needs of the worker.

linking objects: Objects of the deceased that bring comfort to the bereaved.

living wills (also known as instruction directives): Legal document indicating preferences for medical treatments should one become unable to communicate.

local death: Death of a part of the body.

mass trauma: Events that are extremely frightening, possibly life threatening, and experienced by a large number of people at the same time.

meditation: The act of pondering or reflecting.

mental health counselors: Professionals with extensive education and training in individual and group therapy.

moral dilemmas: Discord between rightness or wrongness of actions and goodness or badness of the cost of those actions.

mourning: Public expression of grief and the customary response to bereavement.

medical power of attorney (health care proxy): Document appointing a representative to make healthcare decisions about one's medical care should he or she become incapacitated.

metaphors: Use of comparisons to express ideas and create strong images.

mutual pretense: Patient, family members, and professionals pretend they do not know prognosis; unless patient initiates conversation about impending death, no one talks about it.

near-death experience: Lucid experience occurring at the time of death that is associated with perceived consciousness apart from body and is reported by individuals who have come back to life.

nonfunctionality: Termination of all life-sustaining functions.

no-suicide contracts (no-harm contracts): Detailed contract including commitment to goal of living a long life, seeking ways to reduce emotional stress, agreeing not to kill oneself and, if suicidal, agreement to call for help.

open awareness: Patient is aware of impending death and is preparing for and discussing it.

organ donation: Act of giving one's physical organs or tissue to someone else.

palette of grief: Metaphor that captures the blending of physical, emotional, cognitive, behavioral, and spiritual grief reactions after a final separation.

palliative care: Care focused on improving the quality of life for seriously ill patients by offering prevention and control of distressing symptoms, relief of suffering, early identification, assessment and treatment of pain, and support for physical, psychosocial, and spiritual issues.

palliative care and hospice in long term care: Provision of palliative and/or hospice care in nursing homes; often provided through a partnership with a hospice organization.

passive euthanasia: Withholding or withdrawing life-sustaining treatment (such as ventilator support or necessary medications); therefore, contributing to the patient's death.

palliative sedation: Intentional sedation of patients, rendering them unconscious when, despite aggressive management of pain and symptoms associated with terminal disease, patients continue to suffer.

perinatal loss: Stillbirths and deaths occurring in the first week of life.

physician-assisted suicide: Suicide in which the physician provides the means, such as giving the patient information on how to end his or her life, prescribing medication, or giving the patient equipment.

physician orders for life-sustaining treatment (POLST) document: Physician's orders for an individual's treatment preferences regarding life-sustaining treatments, such as resuscitation, provision of nutrition, pain management, CPR, medical interventions, and antibiotics. The form is honored by all healthcare settings and during emergency transports.

postvention: Actions taken after an attempted suicide or when someone dies by suicide that serve to mollify aftereffects of the event or to deal with the adverse effects on survivors and bereaved.

predisaster phase: Period preceding a disaster, when warning systems and preparedness plans are established and mental health liaisons and responders are recruited and trained.

postmortem care: Care of the body immediately after death, usually performed by nurses, sometimes with the assistance of bereaved family members.

posttraumatic stress disorder (PTSD): Intense physical and emotional response to thoughts and reminders of a traumatic event that lasts for many weeks or months after the traumatic event.

prediagnostic phase: Period before the diagnosis, when individuals suspect an illness and seek out medical attention.

pronouncement of death: Actual declaration of death, which includes examining the patient to determine death, notifying the family and loved ones, and proper documentation.

psychache: Psychological and emotional pain, which reaches intolerable intensity and may lead to suicide.

psychiatric clinical nurse specialists: Nurses with education and training in psychiatric illness and treatment at the graduate school level.

psychiatrist: Medical doctor specializing in mental disorders and related treatment, including medication management.

psychoanalyst: Psychiatrist or psychologist with special training in psychoanalysis.

psychological autopsy: Evaluation of a suicide aimed at reconstructing the person's psychological makeup, including lifestyle, thoughts, feelings, behaviors, intentions, risk factors, motivations, psychodynamics, life circumstances, and mode and details of the suicide.

psychologist: Professional trained in psychological assessment and intervention techniques but not licensed to prescribe medications.

public tragedy: Tragic event resulting in substantial impact on many individuals.

reconstruction phase: Phase after a disaster, during which recovery and rebuilding takes place.

recovery phase: Period in which disease has been ameliorated or is in remission.

resiliency: Ability to adapt to adversity and rebound from disruptive life challenges through effective coping strategies.

rigor mortis: Partial contraction of skeletal muscles and stiffening of joints after death.

rituals: Ceremonial actions that have meaning and significance to the individual performing or observing the act in response to a loss situation.

social support: Amount of emotional or instrumental assistance a person receives.

social worker: Professional trained to counsel those with emotional problems and arrange for needed resources and social services.

spiritual death: Time when the soul, as defined by various religions, departs the body.

stress: Physical, mental, and/or emotional strain or tension in reaction to an event or situation.

sudden infant death syndrome (SIDS): Most common cause of death in infants who die suddenly of no immediately obvious cause.

suicide: Death by self-inflicted means in which there is evidence that the intent was to cause death.

suicide hotlines: A 24-hour, toll-free suicide prevention service available to anyone in suicidal crisis.

suspected awareness: Reaction to illness in which a patient suspects what others know and attempts to find out more information about prognosis as he or she becomes increasingly ill.

terminal phase: Phase of illness in which the individual copes with dying by managing pain, symptoms, health procedures, and institutional stress. Individual may prepare for death by saying good-bye and finding meaning in life and death.

terrorism: Form of psychological warfare in which the goal is to coerce, instill a state of fear, punish, blame its victims, and induce psychological toxicity by targeting a large number of people.

thanatology: A discipline devoted to the study of death and dying; term is derived from Greek mythology.

thanatophobia: Fear of death. Freud believed that it was not death that people feared and that fear of death is a disguise for a deeper source of concern.

transgender: Individual self-identities or gender expressions that are different from sex at birth; includes transsexuals, cross-dressers, and gender benders.

trauma: Any experience that produces psychological injury or pain. Trauma may result from: (1) direct personal experience involving actual or threatened death or serious injury or other threat to one's physical integrity; (2) witnessing an event that involves death, injury, or threat to physical integrity of another person; (3) learning about unexpected or violent death, serious harm, or threat of death or injury experienced by family member or other close associate.

traumatic brain injury (TBI): Head injury that disrupts normal function of brain. Can range from "mild," which is a brief change in mental status or consciousness, to "severe," which is an extended period of unconsciousness or amnesia that results in disturbance of behavioral or emotional functioning.

universality: Child's understanding that death is inevitable to living things, including oneself.

warning signs for suicide: Observable behavioral manifestations of precipitating conditions that reflect the current state of the individual and indicate the presence of a suicidal crisis.

werther effect: Imitative suicidal behavior resulting from knowledge of another's successful suicide.

REFERENCES

Adams, R.E. & Boscarino, J.A. (2005). Stress and well-being in the aftermath of the World Trade Center attack: The continuing effects of a communitywide disaster. *Journal of Community Psychology, 33*(2), 175–190.

Ai, A.L., Cascio, T., Santangelo, L.K., & Evans-Campbell, T. (2005). Hope, meaning, and growth following the September 11, 2001, terrorist attacks. *Journal of Interpersonal Violence, 20*(5), 523–548.

Aiken, L.H., Clarke, S.P., Sloane, D.M., Sochalski, J., & Silber, J.H. (2002). Hospital nurse staffing and patient mortality, nurse burnout, and job dissatisfaction. *Journal of the American Medical Association (JAMA), 288*(16), 1987–1993.

Alberta Mental Health Board. (2008). *What's in a word: The language of suicide.* Retrieved August 19, 2008, from http://www.amhb.ab.ca/ Publications/reports/Documents/AMHB%20SPS %20_%20Language%20of%20Suicide_1p.pdf

Allchin, L. (2006). Caring for the dying: Nursing student perspectives. *Journal of Hospice and Palliative Nursing, 8*(2), 118–119.

Almedom, A.M. & Glandon, D. (2007). Resilience is not the absence of PTSD any more than health is the absence of disease. *Journal of Loss and Trauma, 12*(2), 127–143.

Al-Sabwah, M.N. & Abdel-Khalek, A.M. (2006). Religiosity and death distress in Arabic college students. *Death Studies, 30*(4), 365–375.

Amella, E.J. (2003). Geriatrics and palliative care: Collaboration for quality of life until death. *Journal of Hospice and Palliative Nursing, 5*(1), 49–50.

American Academy of Child and Adolescent Psychiatry. (2008). *Facts for families: Children and grief.* Retrieved September 12, 2008, from http://www.aacap.org/galleries/FactsForFamilies/ 08_children_and_grief.pdf

American Association of Colleges of Nursing. (2009). *Fact sheet: End-of-life nursing education consortium.* Retrieved August 14, 2009, from http://www.aacn.nche.edu/elnec/fact sheet.htm

American Association of Suicidology (AAS). (n.d.a). *Suicide in the U.S.A. based on current (2006) statistics.* Retrieved August 20, 2009, from http://www.suicidology.org/c/document _library/get_file?folderId=232&name=DLFE-159.pdf

American Association of Suicidology (AAS). (n.d.b). *Understanding and helping the suicidal individual.* Retrieved August 7, 2009, from http://www.suicidology.org/c/document_library /get_file?folderId=232&name=DLFE-30.pdf

American Association of Suicidology (AAS). (2008). *Survivors of suicide fact sheet.* Retrieved May 17, 2010, from http://www. suicidology.org/c/document_library/get_file? folderId=232&name=DLFE-23.pdf

American Association of Suicidology (AAS). (2009a). *Elderly suicide fact sheet.* Retrieved February 5, 2010, from http://www.suicidology. org/c/document_library/get_file?folderId=232 &name=DLFE-158.pdf

American Association of Suicidology (AAS). (2009b). *Some facts about suicide and depression.* Retrieved February 5, 2010, from http://www.suicidology.org/c/document_library /get_file?folderId=232&name=DLFE-157.pdf

American Bar Association (ABA) Commission on Law and Aging. (2005). How to select your health care agent or proxy. In *Consumer's tool kit for health care advance planning* (2nd ed.). Washington, DC: Author.

American College of Obstetricians and Gynecologists (ACOG). (2008). *ACOG Committee Opinion: End-of-life decision making.* Retrieved September 10, 2008, from http://www.acog.org/from_home/public ations/ethics/co403.pdf

American Foundation for Suicide Prevention (AFSP). (n.d.a). *Facts and figures.* Retrieved August 22, 2009, from http://www.afsp.org/ index.cfm?page_id=04EA1254-BD31-1FA 3-C549D77E6CA6AA37

American Foundation for Suicide Prevention (AFSP). (n.d.b). *For the media: Reporting on suicide: Recommendations for the media.* Retrieved August 22, 2009, from http://www. afsp.org/index.cfm?fuseaction=home.viewpage &page_id=7852EBBC-9FB2-6691-54 125A1AD4221E49

American Foundation for Suicide Prevention (AFSP). (n.d.c). *Risk factors for suicide.* Retrieved August 21, 2009, from http://www. afsp.org/index.cfm?fuseaction=home.viewPage &page_id=05147440-E24E-E376BDF 4BF8BA6444E76

American Foundation for Suicide Prevention (AFSP). (n.d.d). *When you fear someone may take their life.* Retrieved August 22, 2009, from http://www.afsp.org/index.cfm?page_id=F2F2 5092-7E90-9BD4-C4658F1D2B5D19A0

American Psychiatric Association. (2000). *Diagnostic and statistical manual of mental disorders* (4th ed., text revision). Washington, DC: Author.

American Psychological Association. (2007). *SAMHSA (Garrett Lee Smith Memorial Act) Suicide Prevention Programs FY 08 Funding - July 2007.* Retrieved August 23, 2010 from http://www.apa.org/about/gr/education/news/ 2007/glsma-funding.aspx

Amos, J. (2006). Stress and the psychiatrist: An introduction. *Psychiatric Times, 23*(7). Retrieved December 28, 2008, from http://www.psychiatrictimes.com/display/ article/10168/51486

Anderson, A.L., Lester, D., & Rogers, J.R. (2008). A psychometric investigation of the suicide opinion questionnaire. *Death Studies, 32*(10), 924–936.

Anderson-Butcher, D., Khairallah, A.O., & Race-Bigelow, J. (2004). Mutual support groups for long-term recipients of TANF. *Social Work, 49*(1), 131–140.

Anglin, D.M., Gabriel, K.O.S., & Kaslow, N.J. (2005). Suicide acceptability and religious well-being: A comparative analysis in African American suicide attempters and non-attempters. *Journal of Psychology and Theology, 33*(2), 140–150.

Antai-Otong, D. (2001). Critical incident stress debriefing: A health promotion model for workplace violence. *Perspectives in Psychiatric Care, 37*(4), 125–132, 139.

Arber, S., Vandrevala, T., Daly, T., & Hampson, S. (2008). Understanding gender differences in older people's attitudes towards life-prolonging medical technologies. *Journal of Aging Studies, 22*(4), 366–375.

Ardelt, M. (2003). Effects of religion and purpose in life on elders' subjective well-being and attitudes toward death. *Journal of Religious Gerontology, 14*(4), 55–77.

Armour, M. (2003). Meaning making in the aftermath of homicide. *Death Studies, 27*(6), 519–540.

Arnold, J. & Gemma, P.B. (2008). The continuing process of parental grief. *Death Studies, 32*(7), 658–673.

Astrow, A.B., Wexler, A., Texeira, K., He, M.K., & Sulmasy, D.P. (2007). Is failure to meet spiritual needs associated with cancer patients' perceptions of quality of care and their satisfaction with care? *Journal of Clinical Oncology, 25*(36), 5753–5757.

Attig, T. (1996). *How we grieve: Relearning the world.* New York, NY: Oxford University Press.

Baier, R.R., Gifford, D.R., Patry, G., Banks, S.M., Rochon, T., DeSilva, D., & Teno, J.M. (2004). Ameliorating pain in nursing homes: A collaborative quality-improvement project. *Journal of the American Geriatrics Society, 52*(12), 1988–1995.

Balk, D.E. (2004). Recovery following bereavement: An examination of the concept. *Death Studies, 28*(4), 361–374.

Baranowsky, A.B., Gentry, J.E., & Schultz, D.F. (2005). *Trauma Practice: Tools for stabilization and recovery.* Cambridge, MA: Hogrefe & Huber Publishers.

Barr, P. (2004). Guilt- and shame-proneness and the grief of perinatal bereavement. *Psychology and Psychotherapy, 77*(Pt 4), 493–510.

Barr, P. & Cacciatore, J. (2008). Problematic emotions and maternal grief. *Omega: Journal of Death and Dying, 56*(4), 331–348.

Barrera, M., O'Connor, K., D'Agostino, N.M., Spencer, L., Nicholas, D., Jovcevska, V., … Schneiderman G. (2009). Early parental adjustment and bereavement after childhood cancer death. *Death Studies, 33*(6), 497–520.

Bassett, J.F., McCann, P.A., & Cate, K.L. (2008). Personifications of personal and typical death as related to death attitudes. *Omega: Journal of Death and Dying, 57*(2). 163–172.

Bateman, K., Hansen, L., Turkington, D., & Kingdon, D. (2007). Cognitive behavioral therapy reduces suicidal ideation in schizophrenia: Results from a randomized controlled trial. *Suicide & Life-Threatening Behavior, 37*(3), 284–290.

Beaudin, C.L., Vigil, V.J., & Weber, S. (2004). Suicide risk assessment in an MCO. *Managed Care Interface, 17*(5), 39–44.

Beck, A.T., Brown, G.K., & Steer, R.A. (1997). Psychometric characteristics of the Scale for Suicide Ideation with psychiatric outpatients. *Behavior Research and Therapy, 35*(11), 1039–1046.

Bedikian, S.A. (2008). The death of mourning: From Victorian crepe to the little black dress. *Omega: Journal of Death and Dying, 57*(1) 35–52.

Benight, C.C. & McFarlane, A.C. (2007). Challenges for disaster research: Recommendations for planning and implementing disaster mental health studies. *Journal of Loss and Trauma, 12*(5), 419–434.

Berry, S.R. (2008). The art of oncology: When the tumor is not the target: Just say die. *Journal of Clinical Oncology, 26*(1), 157–159.

Berzoff, J. & Silverman, P.R. (Eds.). (2004). *Living with dying: A handbook for end-of-life practitioners.* New York, NY: Columbia University Press.

Bharucha, A.J., Pearlman, R.A., Back, A.L., Gordon, J., Starks, H., & Hsu, C. (2003). The pursuit of physician-assisted suicide: Role of psychiatric factors. *Journal of Palliative Medicine, 6*(6), 873–883.

Black, K. (2007). Health care professionals' death attitudes, experiences, and advance directive communication behavior. *Death Studies, 31*(6), 563–572.

Bleich, A., Gelkopf, M., & Solomon, Z. (2003). Exposure to terrorism, stress-related mental health symptoms, and coping behaviors among nationally representative sample in Israel. *Journal of the American Medical Association, 290*(5), 612–620.

Blood, R.W., Pirkis, J., & Holland, K. (2007). Media reporting of suicide methods: An Australian perspective. Crisis. *The Journal of Crisis Intervention and Suicide Prevention, 28*(Supplement 1), 64–69.

Bluck, S., Dirk, J., Mackay, M.M., & Hux, A. (2008). Life experience with death: Relation to death attitudes and to the use of death-related memories. *Death Studies, 32*(6), 524–549.

Boelen, P.A. & Van Den Bout, J. (2002–2003). Gender differences in traumatic grief symptom severity after the loss of a spouse. *Omega: Journal of Death and Dying, 46*(3), 183–198.

Bonanno, G.A. (2004). Loss, trauma, and human resilience: Have we underestimated the human capacity to thrive after extremely aversive events? *American Psychologist, 59*(1), 20–28.

Bonanno, G.A., Galea, S., Bucciarelli, A., & Vlahov, D. (2006). Psychological resilience after disaster: New York City in the aftermath of the September 11th terrorist attack. *Psychological Science, 17*(3), 181–186.

Bonanno, G.A., Moskowitz, J.T., Papa, A., & Folkman, S. (2005). Resilience to loss in bereaved spouses, bereaved parents, and bereaved gay men. *Journal of personality and social psychology, 88*(5), 827–843.

Bonanno, G.A., Wortman, C.B., & Nesse, R.M. (2004). Prospective patterns of resilience and maladjustment during widowhood. *Psychology and Aging 19*(2), 260–271.

Boscarino, J.A., Adams, R.E., & Figley, C.R. (2004). Mental health service use 1-year after the World Trade Center disaster: Implications for mental health care. *General Hospital Psychiatry, 26*(5), 346–358.

Botega, N.J., Silva, S.V., Reginato, D.G., Rapeli, C.B., Cais, C.F., Mauro, M.L., & Cecconi, J.P. (2007). Maintained attitudinal changes in nursing personnel after a brief training on suicide prevention. *Suicide and Life-Threatening Behavior, 37*(2) 145–153.

Botella, C., Osma, J., Palacios, A.G., Guillén, V., & Baños, R. (2008). Treatment of complicated grief using virtual reality: A case report. *Death Studies, 32*(7), 674–692.

Boyd Webb, N. (2004). The impact of traumatic stress and loss on children and families. In N. Boyd Webb (Ed.), *Mass trauma and violence: Helping families and children cope* (pp. 3–22). New York, NY: Guilford Press.

Boyd Webb, N. (Ed.). (2005). *Helping bereaved children: A handbook for practitioners* (2nd ed.). New York, NY: Guilford Press.

Boyle, J. (2004). Medical ethics and double effect: The case of terminal sedation. *Theoretical Medicine and Bioethics, 25*(1), 51–60.

Brandt, H.E., Deliens, L., Ooms, M.E., van der Steen, J.T., van der Wal, G., & Ribbe, M.W. (2005). Symptoms, signs, problems, and diseases of terminally ill nursing home patients: A nationwide observational study in the Netherlands. *Archives of Internal Medicine, 165*(3), 314–320.

Brausch, A.M. & Gutierrez, P.M. (2009). The role of body image and disordered eating as risk factors for depression and suicidal ideation in adolescents. *Suicide and Life-Threatening Behavior, 39*(1), 58–71.

Brazil, K., Bedard, M., Krueger, P., Abernathy, T., Lohfeld, L., & Willison, K. (2005). Service preferences among family caregivers of the terminally ill. *Journal of Palliative Medicine, 8*(1), 69–78.

Bregman, L. (2006). Spirituality: A glowing and useful term in search of a meaning. *Omega: Journal of Death and Dying, 53*(1–2), 5–26.

Breitbart, W., Gibson, C., Poppito, S.R., & Berg, A. (2004). Psychotherapeutic interventions at the end of life: A focus on meaning and spirituality. *Canadian Journal of Psychiatry, 49*(6), 366–372.

Briller, S.H., Meert, K.L., Myer Schim, S., Thurston, C.S., & Kabel, A. (2008). Implementing a triangulation protocol in bereavement research: A methodological discussion. *Omega: Journal of Death and Dying, 57*(3), 245–260.

Brodsky, B.S., Groves, S.A., Oquendo, M.A., Mann, J.J., & Stanley, B. (2006). Interpersonal precipitants and suicide attempts in borderline personality. *Suicide and Life-Threatening Behavior, 36*(3), 313–322.

Bromet, E.J. & Havenaar, J.M. (2002). Mental health consequences of disasters. In N. Sartorius, W. Gaebel, J.J. López-Ibor, & M. Maj (Eds.), *Psychiatry in Society* (241–261). West Sussex, UK: John Wiley & Sons.

Brooks, R. & Goldstein, S. (2004). *The power of resilience: Achieving balance, confidence, and personal strength in your life.* New York, NY: McGraw Hill.

Brown, A.B., Buchan, A.B., Copeland, S.C., Dempster, P., Grundy, M., Ramage, F.R., ... Work, F. (2006) *Literature review on bereavement and bereavement care.* Available at http://www.crusebereavementcare.org.uk/BPP papers/BCLitReview.pdf

Brown, A.C., Sandler, I.N., Tein, J.Y., Liu, X., & Haine, R.A. (2007). Implications of parental suicide and violent death for promotion of resilience of parentally-bereaved children. *Death Studies, 31*(4), 301–335.

Brown, E.J., Amaya-Jackson, L., Cohen, J., Handel, S., Thiel De Bocanegra, H., Zatta, E., ... Mannarino, A. (2008). Childhood traumatic grief: A multi-site empirical examination of the construct and its correlates. *Death Studies, 32*(10), 899–923.

Brown, S.L., Nesse, R.M., House, J.S., & Utz, R.L. (2004) Religion and emotional compensation: Results from a prospective study of widowhood. *Personality and Social Psychology Bulletin, 30*(9), 1165–1174.

Bull, M.A., Clark, S., & Duszynski, K. (2002–2003). Lessons from a community's response to the death of Diana, Princess of Wales. *Omega: Journal of Death and Dying, 46*(1), 35–49.

Byock, I. (1996). The nature of suffering and the nature of opportunity at the end of life. *Clinics in Geriatric Medicine, 12*(2), 237–252.

Byock, I. (2004). *The four things that matter most: A book about living.* New York, NY: Free Press.

Byrne, J.P. (2004). *The black death.* Westport, CT: Greenwood Press.

Cadell, S. & Marshall, S. (2007). The (re)construction of self after the death of a partner to HIV/AIDS. *Death Studies 31*(6), 537–548.

Cantor, J. (2001). The Media and Children's Fears, Anxieties, and Perceptions of Danger. In D.G. Singer & J.L. Singer (Eds.), *Handbook of children and the media* (207–307). Thousand Oaks, CA: Sage.

Caring Connections, a program of the National Hospice and Palliative Care Organization (2007). *Talking with your child about his or her illness.* Retrieved July 29, 2008, from http://careprodcc.belmonsterexpress.com/User Files/File/PDFs/PediatricResources/Talking_ with_Your_Child_about_His_or_Her_Illness.pdf

Carlson, M.D., Morrison, R.S., & Bradley, E.H. (2008). Improving access to hospice care: Informing the debate. *Journal of Palliative Medicine, 11*(3), 438-443.

Carr, J.R., Hoge, C.W., Gardner, J., & Potter, R. (2004). Suicide surveillance in the U.S. military – Reporting and classification biases in rate calculations. *Suicide and Life-Threatening Behavior, 34*(3), 233–241.

Carter, P.J. (2008). *Lippincott's textbook for nursing assistants: A humanistic approach to caregiving* (2nd ed.). Philadelphia, PA: Lippincott Williams & Wilkins.

Caserta, M.S. & Lund, D.A. (2007) Toward the development of an inventory of daily widowed life (IDWL): Guided by the dual process model of coping with bereavement. *Death Studies 31*(6), 505–535.

Center for Ethics in Health Care, Oregon Health & Science University. (2008). Physician orders for life-sustaining treatment paradigm (POLST). Retrieved August 16, 2008, from http://www.ohsu.edu/polst/index.htm

Center to Advance Palliative Care. (2008). *New analysis shows hospitals continue to implement palliative care programs at rapid pace: New medical subspecialty fills gap for aging population.* Retrieved May 29, 2010, from http://www.capc.org/news-and-events/ releases/news-release-4-14-08

Centers for Disease Control and Prevention (CDC). (n.d.a). *Coping with a traumatic event.* Retrieved August 23, 2010, from http://cdc. gov/masstrauma/factsheets/public/coping.pdf

Centers for Disease Control and Prevention (CDC). (n.d.b). *Helping Patients Cope with a traumatic event.* Retrieved February 4, 2010, from http://www.cdc.gov/masstrauma/factsheets/ professionals/coping_professional.pdf

Centers for Disease Control and Prevention (CDC). (2003). *U.S. Standard Certificate of Death.* Available from http://www.cdc.gov/nchs/data/ dvs/DEATH11-03final-ACC.pdf

Centers for Disease Control and Prevention (CDC). (2005). *Coping with a traumatic event: Information for health professionals.* Retrieved August 23, 2010, from http://emergency. cdc.gov/masscasualties/copingpro.asp

Centers for Disease Control and Prevention (CDC). (2007). *Suicide prevention: Scientific information: Consequences.* Retrieved February 5, 2010, from http://www.cdc.gov/ncipc/dvp/ Suicide/Suicide-conque.htm

Centers for Disease Control and Prevention (CDC). (2008a). *Emergency preparedness and response: Blast injuries: Bombings & mental health.* Retrieved December 15, 2008, from http://www.bt.cdc.gov/masscasualties/blast injury-bombings-mentalhealth.asp

Centers for Disease Control and Prevention (CDC). (2008b). *New estimates of U.S. HIV prevalence, 2006.* Retrieved December 14, 2008, from http://www.cdc.gov/hiv/topics/sur veillance/resources/factsheets/prevalence.htm

Centers for Disease Control and Prevention (CDC). (2008c) *Youth Risk Behavior Surveillance – United States, 2007.* MMWR Surveillance Summaries, 57(SS-4). Available at http://www.cdc.gov/mmwr/PDF/ss/ss5704.pdf

Centers for Disease Control and Prevention (CDC). (2009a). *Sudden infant death syndrome (SIDS) and sudden unexpected infant death (SUID): Home.* Retrieved February 5, 2010, from http://www.cdc.gov/SIDS/index.htm

Centers for Disease Control and Prevention (CDC). (2009b). *Suicide: Facts at a glance.* Retrieved February 4, 2010, from http://www.cdc.gov/violenceprevention/pdf/Suicide-Data Sheet-a.pdf

Centers for Disease Control and Prevention (CDC). (2010). *Unintentional Drowning: Fact Sheet.* Retrieved June 30, 2010, from http://www.cdc.gov/HomeandRecreationalSafety/Water-Safety/waterinjuries-factsheet.html

Centers for Disease Control and Prevention (CDC). (2010a). *FastStats: Deaths and mortality.* Retrieved November 8, 2010, from http://www.cdc.gov/nchs/fastats/deaths.htm

Centers for Disease Control and Prevention (CDC): National Center for Health Statistics (NCHS). (n.d.). *10 leading causes of injury death by age group highlighting violence-related injury deaths, United States–2007.* Retrieved August 23, 210, fromhttp://web appa.cdc.gov/cgi-bin/broker.exe

Centers for Disease Control and Prevention (CDC): National Center for Health Statistics (NCHS). (2008). *U.S. mortality drops sharply in 2006, latest data show.* Retrieved May 29, 2010, from http://www.cdc.gov/nchs/pressroom/08newsreleases/mortality2006.htm

Centers for Disease Control and Prevention (CDC): National Center for Health Statistics (NCHS). (2010). *National home and hospice care survey.* Retrieved May 29, 2010, from http://www.cdc.gov/nchs/nhhcs/nhhcs_hospice_highlights.htm

Centers for Disease Control and Prevention (CDC): National Center for Injury Prevention and Control (NCIPC). (2008). *Understanding suicide: Fact sheet.* Retrieved December 15, 2008, from http://www.cdc.gov/ncipc/pub-res/suicide_factsheet2008.pdf

Centers for Disease Control and Prevention (CDC): National Center for Injury Prevention and Control (NCIPC). (2009). *10 leading causes of death, United States 2006: All races, both sexes.* Retrieved August 5, 2009, from http://webappa.cdc.gov/sasweb/ncipc/leadcaus10.html

Centers for Disease Control and Prevention (CDC): National Center for Injury Prevention and Control (NCIPC). (2010a). *Injury prevention & control: Data & statistics (WISQARS).* Retrieved from http://www.cdc.gov/injury/wisqars/index.html

Centers for Disease Control and Prevention (CDC): National Center for Injury Prevention and Control (NCIPC). (2010b). *WISQARS leading causes of death reports, 1999 – 2006: Homicide.* Retrieved March 19, 2010, from http://webappa.cdc.gov/sasweb/ncipc/leadcaus10.html

Cerel, J., Fristad, M.A., Verducci, J., Weller, R.A., & Weller, E.B. (2006) Childhood bereavement: Pychopathology in the 2 years postparental death. *Journal of the American Academy of Child and Adolescent Psychiatry, 45*(6), 681–690.

Chochinov, H.M. (2006). Dying, dignity, and new horizons in palliative end-of-life care. *Cancer Journal for Clinicians, 56*(2), 84–103.

Chochinov, H.M., Hack, T., Hassard, T., Kristjanson, L.J., McClement, S., & Harlos, M. (2005). Dignity therapy: A novel psychotherapeutic intervention for patients near the end of life. *Journal of Clinical Oncology, 23*(24), 5520–5525.

Chow, A.Y., Chan, C.L., & Ho, S.M. (2007). Social sharing of bereavement experience by Chinese bereaved persons in Hong Kong. *Death Studies, 31*(7), 601–618.

Cicirelli, V.G. (2001). Personal meanings of death in older adults and young adults in relation to their fears of death. *Death Studies, 25*(8), 663–683.

Cigularov, K., Chen, P.Y., Thurber, B.W., & Stallones, L. (2008). What prevents adolescents from seeking help after a suicide education program? *Suicide and Life-Threatening Behavior, 38*(1), 74–86.

Clark, S., Burgess, T., Laven, G., Bull, M., Marker, J., & Browne, E. (2004). Developing and evaluating the GriefLink web site: Process, protocols, dilemmas and lessons learned. *Death Studies, 28*(10), 955–970.

Cohen J.A., Mannarino A.P., Greenberg, T.A., Padlo S., & Shipley, C. (2002). Childhood traumatic grief: Concepts and controversies. *Trauma, Violence and Abuse 3*(4), 307-327.

Cohen, J.A. & Mannarino, A.P. (2004). Treatment of childhood traumatic grief. *Journal of Clinical Child and Adolescent Psychology, 33*(4), 819–831.

Cohen, L., Ganzini, L., Mitchell, C., Arons, S., Goy, E., & Cleary, J. (2005). Accusations of murder and euthanasia in end-of-life care. *Journal of Palliative Medicine, 8*(6), 1096–1104.

Comas-Diaz, L., Luthar, S.S., Maddi, S.R., O'Neill, H.K., Saakvitne, K.W., & Tedeschi, R.G. (n.d.). *The Road to Resilience.* Retrieved on May 29, 2010, from http://www.apa.org/helpcenter/road-resilience.aspx#

Committee for Disaster Medicine Reform. (2008). *Pou defense fund event a huge success.* Retrieved February 4, 2010, from http://www.cdmr.org

Conwell, Y. (2001). Suicide in later life: A review and recommendations for prevention. *Suicide and Life-Threatening Behavior, 31*(suppl), 32–47.

Cooperman, N.A. & Simoni, J.M. (2005). Suicidal ideation and attempted suicide among women living with HIV/AIDS. *Journal of Behavioral Medicine, 28*(2), 149–156.

Corr, C.A. (1991–1992). A task-based approach to coping with dying. *Omega: Journal of Death and Dying 24*(2), 81–94.

Corr, C.A. & Corr, D.M. (Eds.). (1996). *Handbook of childhood death and bereavement.* New York, NY: Springer.

Corr, C.A., Nabe, C.M., & Corr, D.M. (2000). *Death and dying, life and living* (3rd ed). Belmont, CA: Wadsworth.

Corr, C.A., Nabe, C.M., & Corr, D.M. (2003). *Death and dying, life and living* (4th ed.). Belmont, CA: Wadsworth.

Corr, C.A., Nabe, C.M., & Corr, D.M. (2006). *Death and dying, life and living* (5th ed.). Belmont, CA: Thompson Wadsworth.

Corrigan, J.D., Whiteneck, G., & Mellick, D. (2004). Perceived needs following traumatic brain injury. *Journal of Head Trauma Rehabilitation, 19*(3), 205–216.

Cort, M.A. (2004). Cultural mistrust and use of hospice care: Challenges and remedies. *Journal of Palliative Medicine, 7*(1), 63–71.

Cotter, R.P. (2003). High risk behaviors in adolescence and their relationship to death anxiety and death personifications. *Omega: Journal of Death and Dying, 47*(2), 119–137.

Cowan, J.D. & Walsh, D. (2001). Terminal sedation in palliative medicine: Definition and review of the literature. *Support Cancer Care 9*(6), 403-407.

Cox, B.J., Enns, M.W., & Clara, I.P. (2004). Psychological dimensions associated with suicidal ideation and attempts in the National Comorbidity Survey. *Suicide and Life-Threatening Behaviors, 34*(3), 209–219.

Creamer, T.L. & Liddle, B.J. (2005). Secondary traumatic stress among disaster mental health workers responding to the September 11 attacks. *Journal of Traumatic Stress, 18*(1), 89–96.

Cunningham, M. (2003). Impact of trauma work on social work clinicians: Empirical findings. *Social Work, 48*(4), 451–459.

Currier, J.M., Holland, J.M., & Neimeyer, R.A. (2006). Sense-making, grief, and the experience of violent loss: Toward a mediational model. *Death Studies, 30*(5), 403–428.

Currier, J.M., Holland, J.M., & Neimeyer, R.A. (2008). Making sense of loss: A content analysis of end-of-life practitioners' therapeutic approaches. *Omega: Journal of Death and Dying, 57*(2), 121–141.

Cuvala, A.H. (2008). Ethical issues surround the under treatment of pain. *ONS Pain Management: Special Interest Group Newsletter, 18*(2). Retrieved August 18, 2008, from http://onsopcontent.ons.org/Publications/SIGNewsletters/pm/pm18.2.html

Daaleman, T.P., Usher, B.M., Williams, S.W., Rawlings, J., & Hanson, L.C. (2008). An Exploratory Study of Spiritual Care at the End of Life. *Annals of Family Medicine 6*(5), 406-411.

Dahlberg, L.L., Ikeda, R.M., & Kresnow, M. (2004). Guns in the home and risk of violent death in the home: Findings from a national study. *American Journal of Epidemiology, 160*(10), 929–936.

Dannemiller. H.C. (2002). The parents' response to a child's murder. *Omega: Journal of Death and Dying, 45*(1), 1–21.

D'Augelli, A.R., Hershberger, S.L., & Pilkington, N.W. (2001). Suicidality patterns and sexual orientation-related factors among lesbian, gay, and bisexual youths. *Suicide and Life-Threatening Behavior, 31*(3), 250–264.

Davey, J.D., Obst, P.L., & Sheehan, M.C. (2000). The use of AUDIT as a screening tool for alcohol use in the police workplace. *Drug and Alcohol Review, 19*(1), 49–54.

Davies, R. (2004). New understanding of parental grief: Literature review. *Journal of Advanced Nursing, 46*(5), 506–513.

Davies, W.R. (2008). Mindful meditation: Healing burnout in critical care nursing. Holistic Nursing Practice, 22(1), 32–36.

Dean, M., McClement, S., Bond, J.B., Jr., Daeninck, P., & Nelson, F. (2005). Parental experiences of adult child death from cancer. *Journal of Palliative Medicine, 8*(4), 751–765.

de Graeff, A. & Dean, M. (2007): Palliative sedation therapy in the last weeks of life: A literature review and recommendations for standards. *Journal of Palliative Medicine, 10*(1), 67–85.

Deichmann, R.E. (2007). *Code blue: A Katrina physician's memoir.* Bloomington, IN: Rooftop.

Demmer, C. (2003). Use of complementary therapies with terminally ill patients: The need for more research. *Illness, Crisis, & Loss, 11*(3), 281–291.

Deng, G. & Cassileth, B.R. (2005). Integrative oncology: Complementary therapies for pain, anxiety, and mood disturbance. *Cancer Journal for Clinicians, 55*(2), 109–116.

Dennis, D. (2009). *Living, dying, grieving.* Sudbury, MA: Jones & Bartlett.

DePaola, S.J., Griffin, M., Young, J., & Neimeyer, R.A. (2003). Death anxiety and attitudes toward the elderly among older adults: The role of gender and ethnicity. *Death Studies, 27*(4), 335–354.

Department of Health and Human Services (HHS): Centers for Medicare and Medicaid Services. (2008). *Federal Register: 42 CFR Part 418: Medicare and Medicaid programs: Hospice: Conditions of participation; Final rule.* Retrieved August 9, 2008, from http://edocket.access.gpo.gov/2008/pdf/08-1305.pdf

DeSpelder, L.A. & Strickland, A.L. (2005). *The last dance: Encountering death and dying* (7th ed.). Boston, MA: McGraw-Hill.

de Vries, B., Blieszner, R., & Blando, J.A. (2002). Faces of grief and intimacy in later life. In K.J. Doka (Ed.), *Living with grief: Loss in later life* (pp. 225–242). Washington, DC: Hospice Foundation of America.

DeWolfe, D.J. (2000). *Training manual for mental health and human service workers in major disasters* (2nd ed.). DHHS Publication No. ADM 90-538. Washington, DC: Department of Health and Human Services, Substance Abuse and Mental Health Services Administration, Center for Mental Health Services.

Dezutter, J., Soenens, B., Luyckx, K., Bruyneel, S., Vansteenkiste, M., Duriez, B., & Hutsebaut, D. (2009). The role of religion in death attitudes: Distinguishing between religious belief and style of processing religious contents. *Death Studies, 33*(1), 73–92.

Diaz-Cabello, N. (2004). The Hispanic way of dying: Three families, three perspectives, three cultures. *Illness, Crisis, & Loss, 12*(3), 239–255.

Dickinson, G.E. (2006). Teaching end-of-life issues in U.S. medical schools: 1975–2005. American *Journal of Hospice & Palliative Medicine, 23*(3), 197–204.

Dickinson, G.E. (2007). End-of-life and palliative care issues in medical and nursing schools in the United States. *Death Studies, 31*(8), 713–726.

Dickinson, T. & Wright, K.M. (2008). Stress & burnout in forensic mental health nursing: A literature review. *British Journal of Nursing, 17*(2), 82–87.

DiGiovanni, C., Jr., Reynolds, B., Harwell, R. Stonecipher, E.B., & Burkle, F.M., Jr. (2003). Community reaction to bioterrorism: Prospective study of simulated outbreak. *Emerging Infections Diseases, 9*(6), 708–712.

Doka, K.J. (1995–1996). Coping with life-threatening illness: A task model. *Omega: Journal of Death and Dying, 32*(2), 111–122.

Doka, K.J. (Ed.). (2002). *Disenfranchised grief: New directions, challenges, and strategies for practice.* Champaign, IL: Research Press.

Doka, K.J. (2003). What makes a tragedy public? In M. Lattanzi-Licht & K.J. Doka (Eds.), Living with grief: Coping with public tragedy (3–14). Washington, DC: Hospice Foundation of America.

Doka, K.A. & Martin, T. (2001). Take it like a man: Masculine response to loss. In D.A. Lund (Ed.), *Men coping with grief* (37–47). Amityville, NY: Baywood.

Donatelle, R.J. (2003). *Health: The basics* (5th Ed.). San Francisco, CA: Benjamin Cummings.

Dowdney, L. (2000). Annotation: Childhood bereavement following parental death. *Journal of Child Psychology and Psychiatry and Allied Disciplines, 41*(7), 819–830.

Duffy, S.A., Jackson, F.C., Schim, S.M., Ronis, D.L., & Fowler, K.E. (2006). Racial/ethnic preferences, sex preferences, and perceived discrimination related to end-of-life care. *Journal of the American Geriatrics Society, 54*(1), 150–157.

Dunne, K. (2004). Grief and its manifestations. *Nursing Standard, 18*(45), 45–51.

Durkheim, E. (1897a). Il suicidio dal punto di vista sociologico. *Rivista italiana di sociologia 1,* 17-27.

Durkheim, E. (1897b). *Le Suicide. Paris: Presses Universitaires de France.* Reissued in 1981.

Durkheim, E. (1951). *Suicide: A study in suicidology.* J.A. Spaulding & G. Simpson, Trans. New York: Free Press of Glenco. (Originally published in 1897).

Dyer, K. (2001) *Dealing with death & dying in medical education and practice.* Retrieved June 22, 2010, from http://www.journeyofhearts. org/kirstimd/AMSA/pronounce.htm

Dyregrov, K. (2002). Assistance from local authorities versus survivors' needs for support after suicide. *Death Studies, 26*(8), 647–668.

Dyregrov, K. (2003–2004). Micro-sociological analysis of social support following traumatic bereavement: Unhelpful and avoidant responses from the community. *Omega: Journal of Death and Dying, 48*(1), 23–44.

Dyregrov, K. (2009a). How do the young suicide survivors wish to be met by psychologists? A user study. *Omega: Journal of Death and Dying, 59*(3), 221–238.

Dyregrov, K. (2009b). The important role of the school following suicide in Norway. What support do young people wish that school could provide? *Omega: Journal of Death and Dying, 59*(2), 147–161.

Dyregrov, K., Nordanger, D., & Dyregrov, A. (2003). Predictors of psychosocial distress after suicide, SIDS, & accidents. *Death Studies, 27*(2), 143–165.

Eaton, K.M., Messer, S.C., Garvey Wilson, A.L., & Hoge, C.W. (2006). Strengthening the validity of population-based suicide rate comparisons: An illustration using U.S. military and civilian data. *Suicide and Life-Threatening Behavior, 36*(2), 182–191.

Edward, K.L. & Hercelinskyj, G. (2007). Burnout in the caring nurse: Learning resilient behaviors. *British Journal of Nursing, 16*(4), 240–242.

Emanuel, E.J. (2008). Bioethics in the practice of medicine. In L. Goldman & D. Ausiello (Eds.), *Cecil Medicine* (23rd ed., pp. 6–10). Philadelphia, PA: Saunders Elsevier.

Encyclopedia of Death and Dying. (n.d.a). *Definitions of death.* Retrieved June 30, 2010, from http://www.deathreference.com/ Da-Em/Definitions-of-Death.html

Encyclopedia of Death and Dying. (n.d.b). *Rigor mortis and other postmortem changes.* Retrieved March 19, 2010, from http://www.deathreference.com/Py-Se/Rigor-Mortis-and-Other-Postmortem-Changes.html

Engström, J., Bruno, E., Holm, B., & Hellzén, O. (2007). Palliative sedation at end of life – a systematic literature review. *European Journal of Oncology Nursing 11*(1), 26–35.

Ersek, M. & Wilson, S.A. (2003). The challenges and opportunities in providing end-of-life care in nursing homes. *Journal of Palliative Medicine, 6*(1), 45–57.

Etzersdorfer, E. & Sonneck, G. (1998). Preventing suicide by influencing mass-media reporting: The Viennese experience 1980–1996. *Archives of Suicide Research, 4*(1), 67–74.

Eubanks, K.A. (2007). *October is positive attitude month: Tips for maintaining a positive attitude.* Retrieved August 28, 2008, from http://www.selfgrowth.com/articles/October_is _Positive_Attitude_Month_Tips_for_Maintaining _a_Positive_Attitude.html

Everly, G.S., Jr. (2003). Pastoral crisis intervention in response to terrorism. *International Journal of Emergency Mental Health, 5*(1), 1–2.

Everly, G.S., Jr. & Lating, J.M. (2002). *A clinical guide to the treatment of the human stress response* (2nd Ed.). New York, NY: Kluwer Academic/Plenum.

Exline, J.J. (2003). Belief in heaven and hell among Christians in the United States: Denominational differences and clinical implication. *Omega: Journal of Death and Dying, 47*(2), 155–168.

Fairbrother, G., Stuber, J., Galea, S., Pfefferbaum, B., & Fleischman, A.R. (2004). Unmet need for counseling services by children in New York City after the September 11th attacks on the World Trade Center: Implications for pediatricians. Pediatrics, 113(5), 1367–1374.

Fallowfield, J.L., Jenkins, V.A., & Beveridge, H.A. (2002). Truth may hurt but deceit hurts more: Communication in palliative care. *Palliative Medicine, 16*(4), 297–303.

Fast, J.D. (2003). After Columbine: How people mourn sudden death. *Social Work, 48*(4), 484–491.

Fazio, R.J. & Fazio, L.M. (2005). Growth through loss: Promoting healing and growth in the face of trauma, crisis, and loss. *Journal of Loss and Trauma, 10*(3), 221–252.

Federation of Texas Psychiatry. (2005). Texas psychiatrists respond to hurricane disasters. *Texas Psychiatrist.* Retrieved from http://www.tx psych.org/newsoctnov2005.pdf

Feifel, H. & Branscomb, A.B. (1973). Who's Afraid of Death? *Journal of Abnormal Psychology, 81*(3), 282–288.

Feigelman, W., Gorman, B.S., Beal, K.C., & Jordan, J.R. (2008). Internet support groups for suicide survivors: A new mode for gaining bereavement assistance. *Omega: Journal of Death and Dying, 57*(3), 217–243.

Feigelman, W., Gorman, B.S., & Jordan, J.R. (2009). Stigmatization and suicide bereavement. *Death Studies, 33*(7), 591-608.

Feigelman, W., Jordan, J.R., & Gorman, B.S. (2008–2009). How they died, time since loss, and bereavement outcomes. *Omega: Journal of Death and Dying, 58*(4), 251–273.

Federal Emergency Management System (FEMA). (2010). *Get disaster information.* Retrieved from http://www.fema.gov/hazard/index.shtm

Fenton, W.S. (2000). Depression, suicide, and suicide prevention in schizophrenia. *Suicide and Life-Threatening Behavior, 30*(1), 34–49.

Ferrell, B., Virani, R., Grant, M., Coyne, P., & Uman, G. (2000). End-of-life care: Nurses speak out. *Nursing, 30*(7), 54–57.

Field, M.J. & Cassel, C.K. (Eds.). (1997). *Approaching death: Improving care at the end of life.* Washington DC: National Academy Press. Retrieved August 15, 2009, from http://www.nap.edu/openbook.php?record_id=5801

Figley, C.R. (Ed.). (1995). *Compassion fatigue: Coping with secondary traumatic stress disorder in those who treat the traumatized.* New York, NY: Brunner-Routledge.

Figley, C.R. (2002). Epilogue. In C.R. Figley (Ed.), *Treating compassion fatigue* (213–218). New York, NY: Routledge.

Figley, C.R. (2007). *Gift from within – PTSD: Resources for survivors and caregivers: The art and science of caring for others without forgetting self-care.* Retrieved September 12, 2008, from http://www.giftfromwithin.org/html/art scien.html

Fiske, A. & Arbore, P. (2000–2001). Future directions in late life suicide prevention. *Omega: Journal of Death and Dying, 42*(1), 37–53.

Flannery, R.B. (2004). Managing stress in today's age: A concise guide for emergency services personnel. *International Journal of Emergency Mental Health, 6*(4), 205–209.

Foliart, D.E., Clausen, M., & Siljestrom, C. (2001). Bereavement practices among California hospices: Results of a statewide survey. *Death Studies, 25*(5), 461–467.

Forward, D.R. & Garlie, N. (2003). Search for new meaning: Adolescent bereavement after the sudden death of a sibling. *Canadian Journal of School Psychology, 18*(1–2), 23–53.

Foster, M. (2008). *Doctor cleared in patient deaths recounts Katrina scene.* Retrieved June 22, 2010, from http://www.usatoday.com/weather/hurricane/2008-07-20-Katrina-hospital-horror_N.htm

Fowler, K.L. (2008). The wholeness of things: Infusing diversity and social justice into death education. *Omega: Journal of Death and Dying 57*(1), 53–91.

Fox, J.A. & Zawitz, M.W. (2010). *Homicide trends in the U.S.* Retrieved January 27, 2010, from http://bjs.ojp.usdoj.gov/content/homicide/homtrnd.cfm

Fox, S. (2005). *Health information online.* Retrieved June 22, 2010, from http://www.pewinternet.org/Reports/2005/Health-Information-Online.aspx

Fremont, W.P. (2004). Childhood reactions to terrorism-induced trauma: A review of the past 10 years. *Journal of the American Academy of Child and Adolescent Psychiatry, 43*(4), 381–392.

Freud, E.L. (Ed.). (1961). *Letters of Sigmund Freud.* New York, NY: Basic Books.

Freud, S. (1953). Thoughts for the Times on War and Death. In *The Standard Edition of the Complete Psychological Works of Sigmund Freud,* Vol. 4. London, UK: Hogarth Press.

Furman, J. (2001). Living with dying: How to help the family caregiver. *Nursing, 31*(4), 37–42.

Furman, J. (2002). What you should know about chronic grief: Learning to deal with your own lingering emotions when a patient dies. *Nursing, 32*(2), 56–57.

Gadberry, J.H. (2000). When is a funeral not a funeral? *Illness, Crisis, & Loss, 8*(2), 166–180.

Gajdos, K.C. (2002). The intergenerational effects of grief and trauma. *Illness, Crisis, & Loss, 10*(4), 304–317.

Gamino, L.A., Hogan, N.S., & Sewell, K.W. (2002). Feeling the absence: A content analysis from the Scott and White Grief Study. *Death Studies, 26*(10), 793–813.

Gamino, L.A., Sewell, K.W., & Easterling, L.W. (2000). Scott and White Grief Study – phase II: Toward an adaptive model of grief. *Death Studies, 24*(7), 633–660.

Garces-Foley, K. (2002–2003). Funerals of the unaffiliated. *Omega: Journal of Death and Dying, 46*(4), 287–302.

Garrett, C. (2008). The effect of nurse staffing patterns on medical errors and nurse burnout. *AORN Journal, 87*(6), 1191–1204.

Gelfman, L.P. & Morrison, R.S. (2008). Research funding for palliative medicine. *Journal of Palliative Medicine, 11*(1), 36–43.

Genevro, J.L., Marshall, T., & Miller, T. (2004). Report on bereavement and grief research. *Death Studies, 28*(6), 491–575.

Gensch, B.K. & Midland, D. (2000). When a baby dies: A standard of care. *Illness, Crisis, & Loss, 8*(3), 286–295.

Gerber-Epstein, P., Leichtentritt, R.D., & Benyamini, Y. (2009). The experience of miscarriage in first pregnancy: *The women's voices. Death Studies, 33*(1), 1–29.

Geron, Y., Ginzburg, K., & Solomon, Z. (2003). Predictors of bereaved parents' satisfaction with group support: An Israeli perspective. *Death Studies, 27*(5), 405–426.

Gillick, M.R. (2004). Adapting advance medical planning for the nursing home. *Journal of Palliative Medicine, 7*(2), 357–361.

Gillies, J. & Neimeyer, R.A. (2006). Loss, grief and the search for significance: Toward a model of meaning reconstruction in bereavement. *Journal of Constructivist Psychology, 19*(1), 31–65.

Ginzburg, K., Geron, Y., & Solomon, Z. (2002). Patterns of complicated grief among bereaved parents. *Omega: Journal of Death and Dying, 45*(2), 119–132.

Glaser, B. & Strauss, A. (1968). *Time for dying.* Chicago, IL: Aldine.

Glicken, M.D. (2006). *Learning from resilient people: Lessons we can apply to counseling and psychotherapy.* Thousand Oaks, CA: Sage.

Glozier, N., Hough, C., Henderson, M., & Holland-Elliot, K. (2006). Attitudes of nursing staff towards co-workers returning for psychiatric and physical illnesses. *International Journal of Social Psychiatry, 52*(6), 525–534.

Goin, M. (2003). *The "Suicide Prevention Contract": A dangerous myth.* Retrieved May 29, 2010, from http://pn.psychiatryonline.org/content/38/14/3.full

Goldsmith, B., Morrison, R.S., Vanderwerker, L.C., & Prigerson, H.G. (2008). Elevated rates of prolonged grief disorder in African Americans. *Death Studies, 32*(4), 352–365.

Goldsmith, E. (2005). *Resource management for individuals and families* (3rd ed.). Belmont, CA: Wadsworth.

Goldsmith, E. (2007). Stress, fatigue, and social support in the work and family context. *Journal of Loss and Trauma, 12*(2), 155–169.

Goldsmith, S.K., Pellmar, T.C., Kleinman, A.M., & Bunney, W.E. (Eds.). (2002). *Reducing suicide: A national imperative.* Washington, DC: National Academies Press. Retrieved July 12, 2008, from http://www.nap.edu/books/0309083214/html

Goodkin, K., Lee, D., Molina, R., Zheng, W., Frasca, A., O'Mellan, S., ... Khamis, I. (2005–2006). Complicated bereavement: Diseased state or state of being? *Omega: Journal of Death and Dying, 52*(1), 21–36.

Goodman, R.F. & Brown, E.J. (2008). Service and science in times of crisis: Developing, planning, and implementing a clinical research program for children traumatically bereaved after 9/11. *Death Studies, 32*(2), 154–180.

Gould, M.S. (2001). Suicide and the media. In H. Hendin & J.J. Mann (Eds.), *The clinical science of suicide prevention* (pp. 200–224). New York, NY: New York Academy of Sciences.

Gould, M.S., Kalafat, J., Harrismunfakh, J.L., & Kleinman, M. (2007). An evaluation of crisis hotline outcomes part 2: Suicidal callers. *Suicide and Life-Threatening Behavior, 37*(3), 338–352.

Green, B.L. (2000). Traumatic loss: Conceptual and empirical links between trauma and bereavement. *Journal of Personal and Interpersonal Loss, 5*(1), 1–17.

Greene, M.V. (2006). *Safety & health around the clock.* Retrieved August 11, 2009, from http://downloads.nsc.org/pdf/otj/OTJ_Mar06.pdf

Gross, D. (2004). *Missing: Death education for nursing facilities; Staff need to be trained in comforting dying residents, their families, and themselves.* Retrieved December 12, 2008, from http://www.thefreelibrary.com/Missing:+death+education+for+nursing+facilities%3B+Staff+need+to+be...-a0122914283

Grossman, A.H. & D'Augelli, A.R. (2007). Transgender youth and life-threatening behaviors. *Suicide and Life-Threatening Behavior, 37*(5), 527–537.

Grossman, A.H., D'Augelli, A.R., Howell, T.J., & Hubbard, S. (2005). Parents' reactions to transgender youth' gender nonconforming expression and identity. *Journal of Gay & Lesbian Social Services, 18*(1), 3–16.

Grove, W. & Erickson, R. (2006). *The role of emotion in reducing burnout among registered nurses.* Paper presented at the annual meeting of the American Sociological Association, Montreal Convention Center, Montreal, Quebec, Canada.

Gutierrez, P.M., Rodriguez, P.J., & Garcia, P. (2001). Suicide risk factors for young adults: Testing a model across ethnicities. *Death Studies, 25*(4), 319–340.

Haine, R.A., Wolchik, S.A., Sandler, I.N., Millsap, R.E., & Ayers, T.S. (2006). Positive parenting as a protective resource for parentally bereaved children. *Death Studies, 30*(1), 1–28.

Hale, B. (2007). Culpability and blame after pregnancy loss. *Journal of Medical Ethics, 33*(1), 24–27.

Hall, M.J. & Hamaoka, D. (2005). *Terrorism and Disaster: What clinicians need to know.* Psychiatric Sequelae in a Survivor of 9/11. Retrieved May 29, 2010, from http://www.cstsonline.org/csts_items/CSTS_CME_RUSH_USU_survivor_9_11_attack.pdf#search="disasters world trauma"

Harper, J.M. (2002). What should they know of death. *Trauma Response, 8,* 18–19.

Hartley, B. (2004). Bereavement groups soon after traumatic death. In N. Boyd Webb (Ed.), *Mass trauma and violence: Helping families and children cope* (pp. 167–190). New York, NY: Guilford Press.

Harvey, J. (2001). *Debunking myths about post-mortem care.* Retrieved August 2, 2008, from http://findarticles.com/p/articles/mi_qa3689/is_200107/ai_n9002202

Hatton, R. (2003). Homicide bereavement counseling: A survey of providers. *Death Studies, 27*(5), 427–448.

Hawton, K., Houston, K., Malmbergand, A., & Simpkin, S. (2003). Psychological autopsy interviews in suicide research: The reactions of informants. *Archives of Suicide Research, 7*(1), 73–82.

Hedtke, L. (2002). Reconstructing the language of death and grief. *Illness, Crisis, & Loss, 10*(4), 285–293.

Heidenreich, C. & Weissman, D.E. (2000). *Death pronouncement and death notification: What the resident needs to know.* Available at http://www.journeyofhearts.org/kirstimd/AMSA/pronounce.htm

Heron, M., Hoyert, D., Murphy, S., Xu, J., Kochanek, K., & Tejada-Vera, B. (2009). *Deaths: Final data for 2006.* Retrieved January 11, 2010, from http://www.cdc.gov/NCHS/data/nvsr/nvsr57/nvsr57_14.pdf

Herrin Allen, C. (2008). Providing compassionate end-of-life care. *Nursing Made Incredibly Easy, 6*(4), 46–53.

Hinton, J. (2003). Exploring and mapping a borderland. *Illness, Crisis, & Loss, 11*(1), 25–36.

Hirschfeld, R. & Russell, J. (1997). Assessment and treatment of suicidal patients. *New England Journal of Medicine, 337*(13), 910–915.

Ho, S.W. & Brotherson, S.E. (2007). Cultural influences on parental bereavement in Chinese families. *Omega: Journal of Death and Dying, 55*(1), 1–25.

Hogan, N.S., Greenfield, D.B., & Schmidt, L.A. (2001). Development and validation of the Hogan grief reaction checklist. *Death Studies, 25*(1), 1–32.

Hogan, N.S. & Schmidt, L.A. (2002). Testing the grief to personal growth model using structural equation modeling. *Death Studies, 26*(8), 615–634.

Hogan, N.S., Worden, J.W., & Schmidt, L.A. (2005–2006). Considerations in conceptualizing complicated grief. *Omega: Journal of Death and Dying, 52*(1), 81–85.

Holkup, P.A. (2003). Evidence-based protocol elderly suicide: Secondary prevention. *Journal of Gerontological Nursing, 29*(6), 6–17.

Holland, J., Neimeyer, R., Currier, J., & Berman, J. (2007). The efficacy of personal construct therapy: A comprehensive review. *Journal of Clinical Psychology, 63*, 93–107.

Holland, K., Jenkins, J., Solomon, J., & Whittam, S. (Eds.). (2008). *Applying the Roper-Logan-Tierney Model in practice.* Philadelphia, PA: Churchill Livingstone/Elsevier.

Holtz, T.H., Salama, P., Lopes Cardozo, B., & Gotway, C.A. (2002). Mental health status of human rights workers, Kosovo, June 2000. *Journal of Traumatic Stress, 15*(5), 389–395.

Hoover, J.H., Markell, M.A., & Wagner, P. (2004–2005). Death and grief as experienced by adults with developmental disabilities: Initial explorations. *Omega: Journal of Death & Dying, 50*(3), 181–196.

Hopp, F.P. & Duffy, S.A. (2000). Racial variations in end of life care. *Journal of the American Geriatrics Society, 48*(6), 658–663.

Horne-Thompson, A. & Grocke, D. (2008). The effect of music therapy on anxiety in patients who are terminally ill. *Journal of Palliative Medicine, 11*(4), 582–590.

Horowitz, M. (2005–2006). Meditating on complicated grief disorder as a diagnosis. *Omega: Journal of Death and Dying, 52*(1), 87–89.

Horowitz, M.J., Siegel, B., Holen, A., Bonnano, G.A., Milbrath, C., & Stinson, C.H. (1997). Diagnostic criteria for complicated grief disorder. *American Journal of Psychiatry, 154*(7), 904–910.

Horsley, H. & Patterson, T. (2006). The effect of a parent guidance intervention on communication among adolescents who have experienced the sudden death of a sibling. *American Journal of Family Therapy, 34*(2), 119–137.

Hosay, C.K. (2003). State long-term care ombudsman knowledge of state laws concerning nursing home conscience policies. *Illness, Crisis, & Loss, 11*(4), 305–317.

Hospice Foundation of America. (n.d.). *What is hospice?* Retrieved January 28, 2010, from http://www.hospicefoundation.org/pages/page.asp?page_id=47055

Hossain, M.S. & Siddique, M.Z. (2008). Does religiosity help Muslims adjust to death? A research note. *Omega: Journal of Death and Dying, 57*(1), 113–119.

Hsu, C.Y., O'Connor, M., & Lee, S. (2009). Understandings of death and dying for people of Chinese origin. *Death Studies, 33*(2), 153–174.

Hudnall Stamm, B. (2009). *Professional quality of life: Compassion satisfaction and fatigue Version 5 (ProQOL)*. Retrieved June 22, 2010, from http://www.proqol.org/uploads/ProQOL_5_English_Selfscore.pdf

Hui, V.K. & Fung, H. (2009). Mortality anxiety as a function of intrinsic religiosity and perceived purpose in life. *Death Studies, 33*(1), 30–50.

Hunter, E.G. (2007–2008). Beyond death: Inheriting the past and giving to the future, transmitting the legacy of one's self. Omega: *Journal of Death and Dying, 56*(4), 313–329.

Hunter, S.B. & Smith, D.E. (2008). Predictors of children's understandings of death: Age, cognitive ability, death experience and maternal communicative competence. *Omega: Journal of Death and Dying, 57*(2), 143–162.

Hyslop-Christ, G. (2000). *Healing children's grief: Surviving a parent's death from cancer.* New York, NY: Oxford University Press.

Ilgen, M.A., Zivin, K., McCammon, R.J., & Valenstein, M. (2008) Mental illness, previous suicidality, and access to guns in the United States. Psychiatric Services, 59(2), 198–200.

Ingram, K.M., Jones, D.A., & Smith, N.G. (2001). Adjustment among people who have experienced AIDS-related multiple loss: The role of unsupportive social interactions, social support, and coping. *Omega: Journal of Death and Dying, 43*(4), 287–309.

International Work Group on Death, Dying, and Bereavement. (2002). Assumptions and principles about psychosocial aspects of disasters. *Death Studies, 26*(6), 449–462.

International Work Group on Death, Dying, and Bereavement. (2006). Caregivers in death, dying, and bereavement situations. *Death Studies, 30*(7), 649–663.

Iserson, K.V. (1999). *Grave words: Notifying survivors about sudden, unexpected deaths.* Tucson, AZ: Galen Press.

Jacobs, D. & Brewer, M. (2004). *APA practice guideline: Provides recommendations for assessing and treating patients with suicidal behaviors.* Retrieved December 15, 2008, from http://med.umich.edu/depression/suicide_assessment/Psych%20Annals%20Summary%20and%20Review%20APA%20Suicide%20Guidelines%20Review%20PDF.pdf

Janzen, L., Cadell, S., & Westhues, A. (2003–2004). From death notification through the funeral: Bereaved parents' experiences and their advice to professionals. *Omega: Journal of Death and Dying, 48*(2), 149–164.

Jayasinghe, N., Spielman, L., Cancellare, D., Difede, J., Klausner, E.J., & Giosan, C. (2005). Predictors of treatment utilization in World Trade Center attack disaster workers: Role of race/ethnicity and symptom severity. *International Journal of Emergency Mental Health, 7*(2), 91–99.

Jenkins, C., Lapelle, N., Zapka, J.G., & Kurent, J.E. (2005). End of life care and African Americans: Voices from the community. *Journal of Palliative Medicine, 8*(3), 585–692.

Joe, S., Romer, D., & Jamieson, P.E. (2007). Suicide acceptability is related to suicide planning in U.S. adolescents and young adults. *Suicide and Life-Threatening Behavior, 37*(2), 165–178.

Joffe, P. (2008). An empirically supported program to prevent suicide in a college student population. *Suicide and life-Threatening Behavior, 38*(1), 87–103.

Johnson, J.G., First, M.B., Block, S., Vanderwerker, L.C., Zivin, K., Zhang, B., & Prigerson, H.G. (2009). Stigmatization and receptivity to mental health services among recently bereaved adults. *Death Studies, 33*(8), 691–711.

Johnson, J.G., Zhang, B., & Prigerson, H.G. (2008). Investigation of a developmental model of risk for depression and suicidality following spousal bereavement. *Suicide and Life-Threatening Behavior, 38*(1), 1–12.

Johnson, K., Elbert-Avila, K., & Tulsky, J. (2005). The influence of spiritual beliefs and practices on the treatment preferences of African Americans: A review of the literature. *Journal of the American Geriatrics Society, 53*(4), 711–719.

Jones, K. (2001a). Sharing last touch. *Nursing, 31*(10), 44–45.

Jones, K.D. (2001b). Counselor reactions to clients traumatized by violence. In D. Sandhu (Ed.), *Faces of violence: Psychological correlates, concepts and intervention strategies* (379–388). Huntington, NY: Nova Science.

Jordan, J.R. (2001). Is suicide bereavement different? A reassessment of the literature. *Suicide and Life-Threatening Behavior, 31*(1), 91–102.

Jordan, J.R. & McMenamy, J. (2004). Interventions for suicide survivors: A review of the literature. *Suicide and Life-Threatening Behavior, 34*(4), 337–349.

Jordan, J.R. & Neimeyer, R. (2003). Does grief counseling work? *Death Studies, 27*(9), 765–786.

Joseph, S., Linley, P.A., Andrews, L., Harris, G., Howle, B., Woodward, C., & Shevlin, M.. (2005). Assessing positive and negative changes in the aftermath of adversity: Psychometric evaluation of the changes in outlook questionnaire. *Psychological Assessment, 17*(1), 70–80.

Kalafat, J., Gould, M.S., Munfakh, J.L., & Kleinman, M. (2007). An evaluation of crisis hotline outcomes. Part 1: Nonsuicidal crisis callers. *Suicide and Life-Threatening Behavior, 37*(3), 322–337.

Kalter, N., Lohnes, K.L., Chasin, J., Cain, A.C., Dunning, S., & Rowan, J. (2002–2003). The adjustment of parentally bereaved children: Factors associated with short-term adjustment. *Omega: Journal of Death and Dying, 46*(1), 15–34.

Kanel, K. (2003). *A guide to crisis intervention* (2nd ed.). Pacific Grove, CA: Brooks/Cole.

Karch, D.L., Dahlberg, L.L., Patel, N., Davis, T.W., Logan, J.E., Hill, H.A., & Ortega, L. (2009). *Surveillance for Violent Deaths; National Violent Death Reporting System, 16 States, 2006.* MMWR Surveillance Summaries. Retrieved February 5, 2010, from http://www.cdc.gov/mmwr/preview/mmwrhtml/ss5801a1.htm

Kastenbaum, R. (2000a). *The psychology of death* (3rd ed.). New York, NY: Springer.

Kastenbaum, R.J. (2000b). *Death, society, and human experience* (7th ed.). Boston, MA: Allyn & Bacon.

Kastenbaum, R.J. (2004). *Death, society, and human experience* (8th ed.). Boston, MA: Pearson/Allyn & Bacon.

Kastenbaum, R.J. (2009). *Death, society, and human experience* (10th ed.). Boston, MA: Allyn & Bacon.

Kastenbaum, R. & Herman, C. (1997). Death personification in the Kevorkian era. *Death Studies, 21*(2), 115–130.

Kauffman, J. (2008). What is no recovery? *Death Studies, 32*(1), 74–83.

Kaufman, K.R. & Kaufman, N.D. (2005). Childhood mourning: Prospective case analysis of multiple losses. *Death Studies, 29*(3), 237–249.

Kennedy, C., McIntyre, R., Worth, A., & Hogg, R. (2008). Supporting children and families facing the death of a parent: Part 1. *International Journal of Palliative Nursing, 14*(4), 162–168.

Kenyon, G.M., Clark, P., & de Vries, B. (Eds.). (2001). *Narrative gerontology: Theory, research, and practice.* New York, NY: Springer.

Khani, A., Jaafarpour, M., Jamshidbeigi, Y. (2008). The relationship between clinical supervision and burnout in the nurse's job – An Iranian study. *Journal of Clinical and Diagnostic Research, 2*(4), 913–918. Retrieved August 30, 2008, from http://www.jcdr.net/articles/PDF/304/280_E(c)_F(P)_R(p)_Pf_p.pdf

Kim, B.H. & Choi, P.S. (2000). The experiences of the spouse whose parent has a terminal cancer [In Korean]. *Qualitative Study, 1,* 60–73.

Kinzbrunner, B.M. (2002). How to help patients access end-of-life care. In B.M. Kinzbrunner, N.J. Weinreb, & J.S. Policzer (Eds.). *Twenty common problems in end-of-life care* (pp. 29–45). New York, NY: McGraw Hill.

Kipnis, K. (2007). Forced abandonment and euthanasia: A question from Katrina. *Social Research 74*(1), 79–100.

Klass, D., Silverman, P.R., & Nickman, S.L. (1996). *Continuing bonds: New understanding of grief.* Washington, DC: Taylor & Francis.

Knight, K.H., Elfenbein, M.H., & Capozzi, L. (2000). Relationship of recollections of first death experience to current death attitudes. *Death Studies, 24*(3), 201–221.

Kolski, T.D., Avriette, M., & Jongsma, A.E., Jr. (2001). *The crisis counseling and traumatic events treatment planner.* New York, NY: John Wiley & Sons.

Komiti, A., Judd, F., Grech, P., Mijch, A., Hoy, J., Lloyd, J.H., & Street, A. (2001). Suicidal behavior in people with HIV/AIDS: A review. *Australian & New Zealand Journal of Psychiatry, 35*(6), 747–57.

Korkeila, J.A., Töyry, S., Kumpulainen, K., Toivola, J.M., Räsänen, K., & Kalimo, R. (2003). Burnout and self-perceived health among Finnish psychiatrists and child psychiatrists: A national survey. *Scandinavian Journal of Public Health, 31*(2), 85–91.

Kübler-Ross, E. (1969). *On death and dying.* New York, NY: MacMillan.

Kuebler, K.K., Davis, M.P., Moore, C.D. (2005). *Palliative Practices: An interdisciplinary approach.* St. Louis, MO: Mosby/Elsevier.

Kuhn Timby, B. (2009). *Fundamental nursing skills and concepts.* Philadelphia, PA: Wolters Kluwer Health/Lippincott Williams & Wilkins.

Kwak, J. & Haley, W.E. (2005). Current research findings on end-of-life decision making among racially or ethnically diverse groups. *Gerontologist, 45*(5), 634–641. Retrieved July 1, 2010, from http://gerontologist.oxford journals.org/content/45/5/634.abstract

Kwok, O., Haine, R.A., Sandler, I.N., Ayers, T.S., Wolchik, S.A., & Tein, J. (2005). Positive parenting as a mediator of the relations between parental psychological distress and mental health problems of parentally bereaved children. *Journal of Clinical Child and Adolescent Psychology, 34*(2), 260–271.

LaGrand, L.E. (2005). The nature and therapeutic implications of the extraordinary experiences of the bereaved. *Journal of Near Death Studies, 24*(1), 3–20.

Lambert, V., Lambert, C., Itano, J., Inouye, J., Kim S., Kuniviktikul, W., … Ito, M. (2004). Cross-cultural comparison of workplace stressors, ways of coping and demographic characteristics as predictors of physical and mental health among hospital nurses in Japan, Thailand, South Korea and the USA (Hawaii). *International Journal of Nursing Studies, 41*(6), 671–684.

Lambie, G.W. (2005). Child abuse and neglect: A practical guide for professional school counselors. *Professional School Counseling, 8*(3), 249–259.

Langhinrichsen-Rohling, J., Arata, C., Bowers, D., O'Brien, N., & Morgan A. (2004). Suicidal behavior, negative affect, gender, and self-reported delinquency in college students. *Suicide and Life-Threatening Behavior, 34*(3), 255–66.

Laraque, D., Boscarino, J.A., Battista, A., Fleischman, A.R., Casalino, M., Hu, Y.Y., … Chemtob, C. (2004). Reactions and needs of tristate-area pediatricians after the events of September 11th: Implications for children's mental health services. *Pediatrics, 113*(5), 1357–1366.

Larson, D.G. & Tobin, D.R. (2000). End-of-life conversations: Evolving practice and theory. *Journal of American Medical Association, 284*(12), 1573–1578.

Laszlo, E. & Currivan, J. (2008). *CosMos: A co-creator's guide to the whole world.* Carlsbad, CA: Hay House, Inc.

Laurie, A. & Neimeyer, R.A. (2008). African Americans in bereavement: Grief as a function of ethnicity. *Omega: Journal of Death and Dying, 57*(2), 173–193.

Lee, D., Chan, K., Lee, S., & Yip, P.S. (2002). Burning charcoal: A novel and contagious method of suicide in Asia. *Archives of General Psychiatry, 59*(3), 293–294.

Lee, J.B. & Bartlett, M.L. (2005). Suicide prevention: Critical elements for managing suicidal clients and counselor liability without the use of a no-suicide contract. *Death Studies, 29*(9), 847–865.

Lee, N.P. & Washington, G. (2008). Management of common symptoms at end of life in acute care settings. *Journal for Nurse Practitioners, 4*(8), 610–615. Retrieved August 14, 2009, from http://www.npjournal.org/article/S1555-4155(08)00305-X/abstract

Lengua, L.J., Long, A.C., Smith, K.I., & Meltzoff, A.N. (2005). Pre-attack symptomology and temperament as predictors of children's responses to the September 11 terrorist attacks. *Journal of Childhood Psychology and Psychiatry, 46*(6), 631–645.

Leong, F.T.L. & Leach, M.M. (2007). Ethnicity and suicide in the United States: Guest editors' introduction. *Death Studies, 31*(5), 393–398.

Lester, D. (1999–2000). The social causes of suicide: A look at Durkheim's Le Suicide one hundred years later. *Omega: Journal of Death and Dying, 40*(2), 307–321.

Lester, D., Aldridge, M., Aspenberg, C., Boyle, K., Radsniak, P., & Waldron, C. (2001-2002). What is the afterlife like? Undergraduate beliefs about the afterlife. *Omega: Journal of death and dying, 44*(2), 113-126.

Levetown, M., Barnard, M.U., Hellsten, M.B., Byock, I.R., Carter, B.S., Connor, S.R., … Solomon-Jowiak, S. (2001). *A call for change: Recommendations to improve the care of children living with life-threatening conditions.* Retrieved June 22, 2010, from www.nhp co.org/files/public/ChIPPSCallforChange.pdf

Linehan, M.M., Goodstein, J.L., Nielsen, S.L., & Chiles, J.A. (1983). Reasons for staying alive when you are thinking of killing yourself: The Reasons for Living Inventory. *Journal of Consulting and Clinical Psychology, 51*(2), 276–286.

Little, S. (2002). Vicarious traumatisation. *Emergency Nurse, 10*(6), 27–30.

Lo, B. & Rubenfeld, G. (2005). Palliative sedation in dying patients: We turn to it when everything else hasn't worked. *Journal of the American Medical Association (JAMA), 294*(14), 1810–1816.

Lohan, J.A. (2006). School nurses' support for bereaved students: A pilot study. *Journal of School Nursing, 22*(1), 48–52.

Lohan, J.A. & Murphy, S.A. (2002). Exploring family functioning and family typology after an adolescent or young adult's sudden violent death. *Journal of Family Nursing, 8*(1), 32–49.

Long, J. (2003). *Emotions and the near-death experience, part 3: Soulmates.* Retrieved August 3, 2008, from www.nderf.org/emotions.htm

Loo, R. (2003). A meta-analysis of police suicide rates: Findings and issues. *Suicide and Life-Threatening Behavior, 33*(3), 313–325.

Loprinzi, C.L., Johnson, M.E., & Steer, G. (2000). Doc, how much time do I have? *Journal of Clinical Oncology, 18*(3), 699–701.

Lowey, S.E. (2008) Communication between the nurse and family caregiver in end-of-life care: A review of the literature. *Journal of Hospice and Palliative Nursing, 10*(1), 35–45.

Lund, D.A. & Caserta, N.S. (2002). Facing life alone: Loss of a significant other in later life. In K.J. Doka (Ed.), *Living with grief: Loss in later life* (pp. 207–224). Washington, DC: Hospice Foundation of America.

Maddi, S.R. & Khoshaba, D.M. (2005). *Resilience at work: How to succeed no matter what life throws at you.* New York, NY: American Management Association.

Mandrusiak, M., Rudd, M.D., Joiner, T.E., Jr., Berman, A.L., Van Orden, K.A., & Witte, T. (2006). Warning signs for suicide on the Internet: A descriptive study. *Suicide and Life-Threatening Behavior, 36*(3), 263–271.

Mann, J.J., Apter, A., Bertolote, J., Beautrais, A., Currier, D., Haas, A., … Hendin, H. (2005). Suicide prevention strategies: A systematic review. *Journal of the American Medical Association, 294*(16), 2064–2074.

Marion, M.S. & Range, L.M. (2003). African-American college women's suicide buffers. *Suicide and Life-Threatening Behavior, 33*(1), 33–43.

Marsh, J. (2004). Social work in a multicultural society. *Social Work, 49*(1), 1, 5–6.

Marshall, R. (2005). *End of life issues guide: Public opinion; Poll: No majority for assisted suicide.* Retrieved August 13, 2009, from http://www.all.org/article.php?id=10685

Martin, G. (1998). Media influence to suicide: The search for solutions. *Archives of Suicide Research, 4*(1), 51–66.

Martin, T. & Doka, K. (2000). *Men don't cry…women do: Transcending gender stereotypes of grief.* Philadelphia, PA: Brunner/Mazel.

Martino, C. (2002). Psychological consequences of terrorism. *International Journal of Emergency Mental Health, 4*(2), 105–111.

Marwit, S.J. & Datson, S.L. (2002). Disclosure preferences about terminal illness: An examination of decision-related factors. *Death Studies, 26*(1), 1–20.

Mastrogianis, L. & Lumley, M.A. (2002). Aftercare services from funeral directors to bereaved men: Surveys of both providers and recipients. *Omega: Journal of Death and Dying, 45*(2), 167–185.

Matakas, F. & Rohrbach, E. (2007). Suicide prevention in the psychiatric hospital. *Suicide and Life-Threatening Behavior, 37*(5), 507–517.

Maxwell, W. (2003). The use of gallows humor and dark humor during crisis situations. *International Journal of Emergency Mental Health, 5*(2), 93–98.

McCabe, O.L., Everly, G.S., Siegel, E.R., Heitt, M.C., & Kaminsky, M.J. (2004). Psychiatry and terrorism: The profession's role in disaster response planning. International Journal of Emergency Mental Health, 6(4), 197–204.

McCann, I.L. & Pearlman, L.A. (1990). Vicarious traumatization: A framework for understanding the psychological effects of working with victims. *Journal of Traumatic Stress 3*(1), 131-149.

McConnell Lewis, L. (2007). No-harm contracts: A review of what we know. *Suicide and Life-Threatening Behavior, 37*(1), 50–57.

McCreaddie, M. & Wiggins, S. (2008). The purpose and function of humour in health, health care and nursing: A narrative review. *Journal of Advanced Nursing, 61*(6), 584–595.

McCreight, B. (2005). Emotion as a resource rather than a weakness. *Nursing Standard, 20*(13), 18.

McCreight, B.S. (2008). Perinatal loss: A qualitative study in northern Ireland. *Omega: Journal of Death and Dying, 57*(1), 1–19.

McHolm, F. (2006). RX for compassion fatigue. *Journal of Christian Nursing, 23*(4), 12–19.

McIntosh, J.L. (2010). *U.S.A. suicide 2007: Official final data.* Retrieved June 22, 2010, from http://www.suicidology.org/c/document_library/get_file?folderId=232&name=DLFE-232.pdf

McMenamy, J.M., Jordan, J.R., & Mitchell, A.M. (2008). What do suicide survivors tell us they need? Results of a pilot study. *Suicide and Life-Threatening Behavior, 38*(4), 375–389.

McPherson, K.F. (2004). Pastoral crisis intervention with children: Recognizing and responding to the spiritual reaction of children. *International Journal of Emergency Mental Health, 6*(4), 223–233.

Meert, K.L., Briller, S.H., Myers Schim, S., Thurston, C., & Kabel, A. (2009). Examining the needs of bereaved parents in the pediatric intensive care unit: A qualitative study. *Death Studies, 33*(8), 712–740.

Meldrum, L., King, R., & Spooner, D. (2002). Secondary traumatic stress in case managers working in community mental health services. In C.R. Figley (Ed.), *Treating compassion fatigue* (85–106). New York, NY: Routledge.

Melham, N.M., Moritz, G., Walker, M., Shear, M.K., & Brent, D. (2007). Phenomenology and correlates of complicated grief in children and adolescents. *Journal of the American Academy of Child & Adolescent Psychiatry, 46*(4), 493–499.

Merriam Webster Dictionary. (2010). *Attitude.* Retrieved August 23, 2010, from http://www.merriam-webster.com/dictionary/attitude

Metzger, P.L. & Gray, M. (2008). End-of-life communication and adjustment: Pre-loss communication as a predictor of bereavement-related outcomes. *Death Studies, 32*(4), 301–325.

Meyers, T.W. & Cornille, T.A. (2002). The trauma of working with traumatized children. In C.R. Figley (Ed.), *Treating compassion fatigue* (39–55). New York, NY: Brunner-Routledge.

Milam, J. (2006). Posttraumatic growth and HIV disease progression. *Journal of Consulting and Clinical Psychology, 74*(5), 817–827.

Miller, J.S., Segal, D.L., & Coolidge, F.L. (2001). A comparison of suicidal thinking and reasons for living among younger and older adults. *Death Studies, 25*(4), 357–365.

Miller, L. (2004). Good cop – bad cop: Problem officers, law enforcement culture, and strategies for success. *Journal of Police and Criminal Psychology, 19*(2), 30–48.

Miller, L. (2005). Police officer suicide: Causes, prevention, and practical intervention strategies. *International Journal of Emergency Mental Health, 7*(2), 101–114.

Miller, L. (2008). Death notification for families of homicide victims: Healing dimensions of a complex process. *Omega: Journal of Death and Dying, 57*(4), 367–380.

Miller, L.H. & Smith, A.D. (2005). *Stress: The different kinds of stress.* Retrieved September 12, 2008, from http://www.apa.org/helpcenter/stress-kinds.aspx

Miller, S.C. (2007). *Nursing home/hospice partnerships: A model for collaborative success – through collaborative solutions.* Retrieved July 1, 2010, from http://www.nhpco.org/files/public/nhhp-final-report.pdf

Milne, D. (2007). Professional news: People can learn markers on road to resilience. *Psychiatric News, 42*(2), 5.

Mimura, C. & Griffiths, P. (2003). The effectiveness of current approaches to workplace stress management in the nursing profession: An evidence based literature review. *Occupational and Environmental Medicine, 60*(1), 10–15.

Miniño, A.M., Heron, M.P., Murphy, S.L., & Kochanek, K.D. (2007). Deaths: Final data for 2004. *National Vital Statistics Reports, 55*(19), 1–119.

Monk, T.H., Houck, P.R., & Shear, M.K. (2006). The daily life of complicated grief patients – what gets missed, what gets added? *Death Studies, 30*(1), 77–85.

Moody, R., Jr. & Arcangel, D. (2001). *Life after loss: Conquering grief and finding hope.* San Francisco, CA: HarperSanFrancisco.

Mooney, D.C. (2005). Tactical reframing to reduce death anxiety in undergraduate nursing students. *American Journal of Hospice & Palliative Care, 22*(6), 427–432.

Morgan, L. (2008). *New analysis shows hospitals continue to implement palliative care programs at rapid pace: New medical subspecialty fills gap for aging population.* Retrieved May 28, 2010, from http://www.capc.org/news-and-events/releases/news-release-4-14-08

Morrissette, P.J. (2004). *The pain of helping: Psychological injury of helping professionals.* New York, NY: Brunner-Routledge.

Mosenthal, A.C., Murphy, P.A., Barker, L.K., Lavery, R., Retano, A., & Livingston, D.H. (2008). Changing the culture around end-of-life care in the trauma intensive care unit. *Journal of Trauma 64*(6), 1587–1593.

Muramatsu, N., Hoyem, R.L., Yin, H., & Campbell, R.T. (2008). Place of death among older Americans: Does state spending on home- and community-based services promote home death? *Medical Care, 46*(8), 829–838.

Murphy, L.D. (2001). The child left behind. *Nursing, 31*(1), 62–63.

Murphy, S.A. (2000). The use of research findings in bereavement programs: A case study. *Death Studies, 24*(7), 585–602.

Murphy, S.A. & Johnson, L.C. (2003). Finding meaning in a child's violent death: A five-year prospective analysis of parents' personal narratives and empirical data. *Death Studies, 27*(5), 381–404.

Murphy, S.A., Johnson, L.C., Lohan, J., & Tapper, V.J. (2002). Bereaved parents' use of individual, family, and community resources 4 to 60 months after a child's violent death. *Family & Community Health, 25*(1), 71–82.

Murphy, S.A., Johnson. L.C., & Weber, N.A. (2002). Coping strategies following a child's violent death: How parents differ in their responses. *Omega: Journal of Death and Dying, 45*(2), 99–118.

National Child Traumatic Stress Network. (2008). *Military children and families: Programs and projects.* Retrieved December 17, 2008, from http://www.nctsnet.org/nccts/nav.do?pid=ctr_top_focus_ctst#q2

National Consensus Project for Quality Palliative Care. (2009). *Clinical practice guidelines for quality palliative care* (2nd ed.). Retrieved June 22, 2010, from http://www.nationalconsensus project.org/guideline.pdf

National Funeral Directors Association. (2005). *U.S. Cremation Statistics.* Retrieved August 23, 2010, 2010, from http://www.nfda.org/consumer-resources-cremation/78-us-cremation-statistics.html

National Funeral Directors Association. (2009). *Statistics: Funeral service facts.* Retrieved August 13, 2009, from http://www.nfda.org/index.php/media-center/statisticsreports

National Highway Traffic Safety Administration (NHTSA). (2009). *Traffic safety facts: 2008 data: Speeding.* Retrieved June 23, 2010, from http://www.nrd.nhtsa.dot.gov/Pubs/811166.PDF

National Hospice and Palliative Care Organization (NHPCO). (2001). *Facts and figures on hospice care in America.* Retrieved January 28, 2010, from http://www.hawaii.edu/hivandaids/Facts%20and%20Figures%20on%20Hospice %20Care%20in%20America.pdf

National Hospice and Palliative Care Organization (NHPCO). (2008). *NHPCO reports growth in number of hospice patients served, 1.4 million, with a wider range of illnesses seen by providers.* Retrieved December 14, 2008, from http://www.nhpco.org/i4a/pages/index.cfm?pageid=5763

National Hospice and Palliative Care Organization (NHPCO). (2009). *NHPCO facts and figures: Hospice care in America.* Retrieved January 28, 2010, from http://www.nhpco.org/files/public/Statistics_Research/NHPCO_facts_and _figures.pdf

National Hospice and Palliative Care Organization (NHPCO). (2010). *NHPCO facts and figures: Hospice care in America.* Retrieved November 5, 2010, from http://www.nhpco.org/files/public/Statistics_Research/Hospice_Facts_Figures_ Oct-2010.pdf

National Institute of Mental Health. (2008). *Bipolar disorder.* Retrieved December 11, 2008, from http://www.nimh.nih.gov/health/publications/bipolar-disorder/complete-index.shtml

National Institute of Mental Health. (2009). *Men and depression: Diagnostic evaluation and treatment.* Retrieved February 5, 2010, from http://www.nimh.nih.gov/health/publications/men-and-depression/diagnostic-evaluation-and-treatment.shtml

National Organization for Victim Assistance (NOVA). (2008). *How to get help after a victimization: How to get help if you or someone you love has been a victim of crime.* Retrieved July 8, 2008, from http://www.trynova.org/victiminfo/victimizationhelp

National Organization of Parents of Murdered Children, Inc. (n.d.a). *Information for doctors and nurses.* Retrieved December 18, 2008, from http://www.pomc.com/doctors.cfm

National Organization of Parents of Murdered Children, Inc. (n.d.b). *Survivors of homicide victims.* Retrieved October 14, 2003, from http://www.pomc.com/survivor.cfm

National Quality Forum. (2006). *A national framework and preferred practices for palliative and hospice care quality.* Retrieved February 5, 2010, from http://www.qualityforum.org/Publications/2006/12/A_National_Framework_and_Preferred_Practices_for_Palliative_and_Hospice_Care_Quality.aspx

National Safety Council. (2009a). *Highlights from injury facts: Report on injuries in America.* Retrieved August 11, 2009, from http://www.nsc.org/news_resources/injury_and_death_statistics/Pages/HighlightsFromInjuryFacts.aspx

National Safety Council. (2009b). *Young drivers.* Retrieved August 11, 2009, from http://downloads.nsc.org/pdf/factsheets/Young_Drivers.pdf

Neff, K. (2004). Self-compassion and psychological well-being. *Constructivism in the Human Sciences, 9*(2), 27–37.

Neimeyer, R.A. (2000). Searching for the meaning of meaning: Grief therapy and the process of reconstruction. *Death Studies, 24*(6), 541–558.

Neimeyer, R.A. (2001). Meaning Reconstruction and Loss. In R.A. Neimeyer (Ed.), *Meaning Reconstruction and the Experience of Loss* (pp. 1–9). Washington, DC: American Psychological Association.

Neimeyer, R.A. (2006). *Lessons of loss: A guide to coping.* Memphis, TN: Center for the Study of Loss & Transition.

Neimeyer, R.A., Fortner, B., & Melby, D. (2001). Personal and professional factors and suicide intervention skills. *Suicide and Life-Threatening Behavior, 31*(1), 71–82.

Nelson-Gardell, D. & Harris, D. (2003). Childhood abuse history, secondary traumatic stress, and child welfare workers. *Child Welfare, 82*(1), 5–26.

Norlander, L. & McSteen, K. (2000). The kitchen table discussion: A creative way to discuss end-of-life issues. *Home Healthcare Nurse, 18*(8), 532–539.

Norris, F.H., Byrne, C.M., Diaz, E., & Kaniasty, K. (2001). *50,000 disaster victims speak: An empirical review of the empirical literature 1981–2001.* Retrieved July 1, 2010, from http://www.dhss.mo.gov/SpecialNeedsToolkit/General/disaster-impact.pdf

Nowatzki, N.R. & Kalischuk, R.G. (2009). Post-death encounters: Grieving, mourning, and healing. *Omega: Journal of Death and Dying, 59*(2), 91–111.

Nucleus Group. (2004). *Review of specific grief and bereavement services: Final report.* Department of Human Services, Victoria, Melbourne, Australia. Retrieved from http://www.health.vic.gov.au/palliativecare/archive/finalrep_grief.pdf

Nurse Advocate. (2008). *Warning nurses! Holding it all in can kill you!* Retrieved July 5, 2008, from http://allnurses.com/forums/f300/warning-nurses-holding-all-can-kill-you-292974.html

O'Connor, M.F. (2002–2003). Making meaning of life events: Theory, evidence, and research directions for an alternative model. *Omega: Journal of Death and Dying, 46*(1), 51–75.

Office of Minority Health. (2009). *American Indian/Alaska Native Profile.* Retrieved February 4, 2010, from http://www.omhrc.gov/templates/browse.aspx?lvl=2&lvlID=52

O'Leary, J. (2005). The trauma of ultrasound during a pregnancy following perinatal loss. *Journal of Loss & Trauma, 10*(2), 183–204.

Olvera, R.L. (2001). Suicidal ideation in Hispanic and mixed ancestry adolescents. *Suicide and Life-Threatening Behavior, 31*(4), 416–427.

One Hundred Eighth Congress of the United States of America at the Second Session. (2004). *Garrett Lee Smith Memorial Act.* Retrieved December 15, 2008, from http://frwebgate. access.gpo.gov/cgi-bin/getdoc.cgi?dbname =108_cong_bills&docid=f:s2634enr.txt.pdf

Orbach, I., Mikulincer, M., Sirota, P., & Gilboa-Schechtman, E. (2003). Mental pain: A multi-dimensional operationalization and definition. *Suicide and Life-Threatening Behavior, 33*(3), 219–230.

Organ Procurement and Transplantation Network (OPTN). (2010). *Donation and transplantation.* Retrieved March 19, 2010, from http://optn. transplant.hrsa.gov/about

Orpana, H.M. & Lemyre, L. (2004). Explaining the social gradient in health in Canada: Using the national population health survey to examine the role of stressors. *International Journal of Behavioral Medicine, 11*(3), 143–151.

Ortlepp, K. & Friedman, M. (2002). Prevalence and correlates of secondary traumatic stress in workplace lay trauma counselors. *Journal of Traumatic Stress, 15*(3), 213–222.

Ott, C.H. & Lueger, R.J. (2002). Patterns of change in mental health status during the first two years of spousal bereavement. *Death Studies, 26*(5), 387–411.

Packman, W., Horsley, H., Davies, B., & Kramer, R. (2006). Sibling bereavement and continuing bonds. *Death Studies, 30*(9), 817–841.

Pain & Policy Studies Group. (2008). *Achieving balance in state pain policy. A progress report card* (4th Edition). University of Wisconsin Paul P. Carbone Comprehensive Cancer Center. Madison, WI. Retrieved September 12, 2008, from http://www.painpolicy.wisc.edu/ Achieving_Balance/PRC2008.pdf

Papadatou, D., Bellali, T., Papazoglou, I., & Petraki, D. (2002). Greek nurse and physician grief as a result of caring for children dying of cancer. *Pediatric Nursing, 28*(4), 345–353.

Park, C.L. & Helgeson, V.S. (2006). Introduction to the special section: Growth following highly stressful life events – current status and future directions. *Journal of Consulting & Clinical Psychology, 74*(5), 791–796.

Parkes, C.M. (1970). The first year of bereavement: A longitudinal study of the reaction of London widows to death of husbands. *Psychiatry, 33*(4), 444–467.

Parkes, C.M. (2001). A historical overview of the scientific study of bereavement. In M.S. Stroebe, W. Stroebe, & R.O. Hansson (Eds.), *Handbook of bereavement* (25–45). Cambridge: Cambridge University Press.

Parkes, C.M. (2003). Acquainted with grief. *Illness, Crisis, & Loss, 11*(1), 37–46.

Parkes, C.M. (2005–2006). Symposium on Complicated Grief. *Omega: Journal of Death and Dying, 52*(1), 1-7.

Paulozzi, L.J., Saltzman, L.E., Thompson, M.P., & Holmgreen, P. (2001). *Surveillance for homicide among intimate partners – United States, 1981–1998.* MMWR Surveillance Summaries. Retrieved from http://www.cdc.gov/Mmwr/ preview/ mmwrhtml/ss5003a1.htm

Pearlman, R.A., Hsu, C., Starks, H., Back, A.L., Gordon, J.R., Bharucha, A.J., … Battin, M.P. (2005) Motivations for physician-assisted suicide: Patient and family voices. *Journal of General Internal Medicine, 20*(3), 234–239.

Pellegrino, E., De Jonge, K.E., Crawley, J.L., Cohen-Almagor, R., & Connolly, M.T. (2008). *United States studies: Ethical decision-making at the end of life.* Retrieved August 18, 2008, from http://www.wilsoncenter.org/index.cfm? topic_id=1427&fuseaction=topics.event_ summary&event_id=303954

Pennsylvania Department of Aging. (n.d.). *Understanding advance directives for health care: Living wills and powers of attorney in Pennsylvania.* Retrieved June 23, 2010, from http://www.lgbtheart.org/states/Pennsylvania-%20form.pdf

Perl, P., Greely, J.Z., & Gray, M.M. (2004). What proportion of adult Hispanics are Catholic? A review of survey data and methodology. *Journal for the Scientific Study of Religion, 45*(3), 419–436.

Peterson, E.M., Luoma, J.B., & Dunne, E. (2002). Suicide survivors' perceptions of the treating clinician. *Suicide and Life-Threatening Behavior, 32*(2), 158–166.

Pfaff, J.J., Almeida, O.P., Witte, T.K., Waesche, M.C., & Joiner, T.E., Jr. (2007). Relationship between quantity and frequency of alcohol use and indices of suicidal behavior in an elderly Australian sample. *Suicide & Life-Threatening Behavior, 37*(6), 616–26.

Pfeffer, C., Jiang, H., Kakuma, T., Hwang, J., & Metsch, M. (2002). Group intervention for children bereaved by the suicide of a relative. *Journal of the American Academy of Child and Adolescent Psychiatry, 41*(5), 505–513.

Pfeffer, C.R., Karus, D., Siegel, K., & Jiang, H. (2000). Child survivors of parental death from cancer or suicide: Depressive and behavioral outcomes. *Psychooncology, 9*(1), 1–10.

Pfefferbaum, B.J., DeVoe, E.R., Stuber, J., Schiff, M., Klein, T.P., & Fairbrother, G. (2005). Psychological impact of terrorism on children and families in the United States. *Journal of Aggression, Maltreatment, and Trauma, 9*(3–4), 305–317.

Phillips, D.P. (1979). Suicide, motor vehicle fatalities, and the mass media: Evidence toward a theory of suggestion. *American Journal of Sociology, 84*(5), 1150–1174.

Phipps, E., True, G., Harris, D., Chong, U., Tester, W., Chavin, S.I., & Braitman, L.E. (2003). Approaching the end of life: Attitudes, preferences and behaviors of African-American and White patients and their family caregivers. *Journal of Clinical Oncology, 21*(3), 549–554.

Physicians Postgraduate Press. (2001). Academic highlights: Trauma and stress: Diagnosis and treatment. *Journal of Clinical Psychiatry, 62*(11), 906–915.

Pickett, M., Barg, F.K., & Lynch, M.P. (2001). Development of a home-based family caregiver cancer education program. *Hospice Journal, 15*(4), 19–40.

Pirkis, J., Burgess, P., Blood, R.W., & Francis, C. (2007). The newsworthiness of suicide. *Suicide and Life-Threatening Behavior, 37*(3), 278–283.

Pitts, S.R., Niska, R.W., Xu, J., & Burt, C.W. (2008). *National Hospital Ambulatory Medical Care Survey: 2006 Emergency Department Summary.* Retrieved December 15, 2008, from http://www.cdc.gov/nchs/data/nhsr/nhsr007.pdf

Pollack, C.E. (2003). Intentions of burial: Mourning, politics, and memorials following the massacre at Srebrenica. *Death Studies, 27*(2), 125–42.

PollingReport.com. (2006). *Religion: CBS news poll.* Retrieved September 3, 2008, from http://www.pollingreport.com/religion.htm

Pompili, M., Lester, D., Leenaars, A.A., Tatarelli, R., & Girardi, P. (2008). Psychache and suicide: A preliminary investigation. *Suicide and Life-Threatening Behavior, 38*(1), 116–121.

Preuss, U.W., Schuckit, M.A., Smith, T.L., Danko, G.P., Bucholz, K.K., Hesselbrock, M.N., & Kramer, J.R. (2003). Predictors and correlates of suicide attempts over 5 years in 1,237 alcohol-dependent men and women. *American Journal of Psychiatry, 160*(1), 56–63.

Préville, M., Boyer, R., Hébert, R., Bravo, G., & Seguin, M. (2005). Correlates of suicide in the older adult population in Quebec. *Suicide and Life-Threatening Behavior, 35*(1), 91–105.

Price, S.K. (2008). Stepping back to gain perspective: Pregnancy loss history, depression, and parenting capacity in the Early Childhood Longitudinal Study, Birth Cohort (ECLS-B). *Death Studies, 32*(2), 97–122.

Prigerson, H., Ahmed, I., Silverman G.K., Saxena, A.K., Maciejewski, P.K., Jacobs, S.C., ... Hamirani, M. (2002). Rates and risks of complicated grief among psychiatric clinic patients in Karachi, Pakistan. *Death Studies, 26*(10), 781-792.

Prigerson, H.G., Bridge, J., Maciejewski, P.K., Beery, L.C., Rosenheck, R.A., Jacobs, S.C., ... Brent, D.A. (1999). Influence of traumatic grief on suicidal ideation among young adults. *American Journal of Psychiatry, 156*(12), 1994–1995.

Prigerson, H.G., Horowitz, M.J., Jacobs, S.C., Parkes, C.M., Aslan, M., Goodkin, K., ... Maciejewski, P.K. (2009). Prolonged grief disorder: Psychometric validation of a criterion proposed for DSM-V and ICD-II. *PLoS Medicine, 6*(8): e1000121.

Prigerson, H.G. & Jacobs, S.C. (2001). Traumatic grief as a distinct disorder: A rational, consensus criteria, and a preliminary empirical test. In M.S. Stroebe, R.O. Hansson, W. Stroebe, & H. Schut (Eds.), *Handbook of bereavement research: Consequences, coping and care* (613–647). Washington, DC: American Psychological Association.

Prigerson, H.G. & Maciejewski, P.K. (2005–2006). A call for sound empirical testing and evaluation of criteria for complicated grief proposed for DSM-V. *Omega: Journal of Death and Dying, 52*(1), 9–19.

Prigerson, H.G. & Vanderwerker, L.C. (2005–2006). Final remarks. *Omega: Journal of Death and Dying, 52*(1), 91–94.

Pruchno, R., Cartwright, F.P., & Wilson-Genderson, M. (2009). The effects of race on patient preferences and spouse substituted judgments. *International Journal of Aging and Human Development, 69*(1), 31–54.

Pryce, J.G., Shackelford, K.K., & Pryce, D.H. (2007). *Secondary traumatic stress and the child welfare professional.* Chicago, IL: Lyceum Books.

Puchalski, C.M. (2007-2008). Spirituality and the Care of Patients at the End-of-Life: An Essential Component of Care. *Omega: Journal of Death and Dying 56*(1), 33-46.

Racanelli, C. (2005). Attachment and compassion fatigue among American and Israeli mental health clinicians working with traumatized victims of terrorism. *International Journal of Emergency Mental Health, 7*(2), 115–124.

Rack, J.J., Burleson, B.R., Bodie, G.D., Holmstrom, A.J., & Servaty-Seib, H. (2008). Bereaved adults' evaluations of grief management messages: Effects of message person centeredness, recipient individual differences, and contextual factors. *Death Studies, 32*(5), 399–427.

Rando, T.A. (1993). *Treatment of complicated mourning.* Champaign, IL: Research Press.

Raphael, B. & Newman, L. (2000) *Disaster mental health response handbook: An educational resource for mental health professionals involved in disaster management.* Parramatta, North Sydney, NSW Institute of Psychiatry NSW Health.

Reese, D.J. & Raymer, M. (July, 2004). Relationships between social work involvement and hospice outcomes: Results of the National Hospice Social Work Survey. *Social Work, 49*(3), 415–422.

Reid, D., Field, D., Payne, S., & Relf, M. (2006). Adult bereavement in five English Hospices: Types of support. *International Journal of Palliative Nursing, 12*(9), 430–437.

Reid, J.K. & Reid, C.L. (2001). A cross marks the spot: A study of roadside death memorials in Texas and Oklahoma. *Death Studies, 25*(4), 341–356.

Reilly-Smorawski, B., Armstrong, A.V., & Catlin, E.A. (2002). Bereavement support for couples following death of a baby: Program development and 14-year exit analysis. *Death Studies, 26*(1), 21–37.

Religion Facts. (2009). *Christian beliefs about the afterlife.* Retrieved August 17, 2009, from http://www.religionfacts.com/christianity/beliefs/afterlife.htm

Reynolds, J.J. (2003–2004). Stillbirth: To hold or not to hold. *Omega: Journal of Death and Dying, 48*(1), 85–88.

Richardson, G.E. & Waite, P.J. (2002). Mental health promotion through resilience and resiliency education. *International Journal of Emergency Mental Health, 4*(1), 65–75.

Riches, G. & Dawson, P. (2002). Shoestrings and bricolage: Some notes on researching the impact of a child's death on family relationships. *Death Studies, 26*(3), 209–222.

Richman, J. (2006–2007). The role of psychotherapy and humor for death anxiety, death wishes, and aging. *Omega: Journal of Death and Dying, 54*(1), 41–51.

Rietjens, J.A., Hauser, J., van der Heide, A., & Emanual, L. (2007). Having a difficult time leaving: experiences and attitudes of nurses with palliative sedation. *Palliative Medicine, 21*(7), 643–649.

Riley, L.P., LaMontagne, L.L., Hepworth, J.T., & Murphy, B.A. (2007). Parental grief responses and personal growth following the death of a child. *Death Studies, 31*(4), 277–299.

Ritchie, E.C. (2003). Mass violence and early intervention: Best practice guidelines. *Primary Psychiatry, 8*(10), 43–52.

Roberts, S.B., Flannelly, K.J., Weaver, A.J., & Figley, C.R. (2003). Compassion fatigue among chaplains, clergy, and other respondents after September 11th. *Journal of Nervous and Mental Disease, 191*(11), 756–758.

Ron, P. (2002). Suicidal ideation and depression among institutionalized elderly: The influence of residency duration. *Illness, Crisis, & Loss, 10*(4), 334–343.

Rosen, E.J. (1990). *Families facing death: Family dynamics of terminal illness.* Lanham, MD: Lexington Books.

Rosenblatt, P.C. (2000). *Parent grief: Narratives of loss and relationship.* Philadelphia: Brunner/Mazel.

Rosenblatt, P.C. (2008). Recovery following bereavement: Metaphor, phenomenology, and culture. *Death Studies, 32*(1), 6–16.

Ross, K.L. (2008). *The generalized structure of moral/ethical dilemmas.* Retrieved July 5, 2008, from www.friesian.com/dilemma.htm

Rossi, N.E., Bisconti, T.L., & Bergeman, C.S. (2007). The role of dispositional resilience in regaining life satisfaction after the loss of a spouse. *Death Studies, 31*(10), 863–883.

Roy, A. (2001). Consumers of mental health services. *Suicide and Life-Threatening Behavior, 31*(suppl), 60–83.

Roy, A. (2003). Characteristics of drug addicts who attempt suicide. *Psychiatry Research, 121*(1), 99–103.

Rubel, B. (2008). Suicide in the military. *Tragedy Assistance Program for Survivors (TAPS) magazine, 14*(2), 28–29.

Rubel, B. (2009). *But I didn't say goodbye: Helping children and families after a suicide* (2nd ed.). Kendall Park, NJ: Griefwork Center.

Rubel, B. (2011). *The bereavement support group guide: How to start one and be the facilitator.* Kendall Park, NJ: Griefwork Center. IN PRESS.

Rubel, B. & McCown, A. (2007). *Compassion fatigue: Vicarious trauma.* VA: U.S. Department of Justice, Office of Justice Programs.

Rubin, S.S. & Malkinson, R. (2001). Parental response to child loss across the life cycle: Clinical research perspectives. In M.S. Stroebe, R.O. Hansson, W. Stroebe, & H. Schut (Eds.), *Handbook of bereavement research: Consequences, coping and care* (219–240). Washington, DC: American Psychological Association.

Rudd, M.D., Berman, A.L., Joiner, T.E., Jr., Nock, M.K., Silverman, M.M., Mandrusiak, … Witte, T. (2006). Warning signs for suicide: Theory, research, and clinical applications. *Suicide and Life-Threatening Behavior, 36*(3), 255–262.

Rurup, M.L., Onwuteaka-Philipsen, B.D., & Van Der Wal, G. (2005). A "suicide pill" for older people: Attitudes of physicians, the general population, and relatives of patients who died after euthanasia or physician-assisted suicide in the Netherlands. *Death Studies, 29*(6), 519–534.

Ruskin, R., Sakinofsky, I., Bagby, R.M., Dickens, S., Sousa, G. (2004). Impact of patient suicide on psychiatrists and psychiatric trainees. *Academic Psychiatry, 28*(2), 104–110.

Russell, S.T. (2003). Sexual minority youth and suicide risk. *American Behavioral Scientist, 46*(9), 1241–1257.

Sabin-Farrel, R. & Turpin, G. (2003). Vicarious traumatization: Implications for the mental health of health workers. *Clinical Psychology Review, 23*(3), 449–480.

Sahraian, A., Fazelzadeh, A., Mehdizadeh, A.R., & Toobaee, S.H. (2008). Burnout in hospital nurses: A comparison of internal, surgery, psychiatry and burns wards. *International Nursing Review, 55*(1), 62–67.

Samaritans. (2009). *Reporting suicide: Reporting tips.* Retrieved August 22, 2009, from http://www.samaritans.org/media_centre/media _guidelines/guide_to_reporting_suicide.aspx

Sanders, C. (2001). A woman of many abilities. *Illness, Crisis, & Loss, 9*(1), 50–54.

Sandler, I.N., Wolchik, S.A., & Ayers, T.S. (2008). Resilience rather than recovery: A contextual framework on adaptation following bereavement. *Death Studies, 32*(1), 59–73.

Santa-Emma, P.H., Roach, R., Gill, M.A., Spayde, P., & Taylor, R. (2002). Development and implementation of an inpatient acute palliative care service. *Journal of Palliative Medicine 5*(1), 93-100.

Saxe, G.N., Ellis, B.H., & Kaplow, J.B. (2007). *Collaborative treatment of traumatized children and teens: The trauma systems therapy approach.* New York, NY: Guilford Press.

Schaal, S., Elbert, T., & Neuner, F. (2009). Prolonged grief disorder and depression in widows due to the Rwandan genocide. *Omega: Journal of Death and Dying, 59*(3), 203–219.

Sears, J.T. (Ed.). (2005). *Gay, lesbian, and transgender issues in education: Programs, policies, and practices.* Binghamton, NY: Harrington Park Press.

Segal, D.L., Mincic, M.S., Coolidge, F.L., & O'Riley, A. (2004). Attitudes toward suicide and suicidal risk among younger and older persons. *Death Studies, 28*(7), 671–678.

Shalev, A.Y. (1996). Stress versus traumatic stress. From acute homeostatic reactions to chronic psychopathology. In B.A. van der Kolk, A.C. McFarlane, & L. Weisaeth (Eds.), *Traumatic stress: The effects of overwhelming experience on mind, body, and society* (77–101). New York, NY: Guilford Press.

Shapiro, E.R. (1994). *Grief as a family process: A developmental approach to clinical practice.* New York, NY: Guilford Press.

Shapiro, E.R. (2008). Whose recovery, of what? Relationships and environments promoting grief and growth. *Death Studies, 32*(1), 40–58.

Shear, K., Frank, E., Houck, P.R., & Reynolds, C.F. (2005). Treatment of complicated grief: A randomized controlled trial. *Journal of the American Medical Association, 293*(21), 2601–2608.

Shneidman, E. (1993). *Suicide as psychache: A clinical approach to self-destructive behavior.* Northvale, NJ: Jason Aronson.

Shneidman E. (1999). The psychological pain assessment scale. *Suicide and Life-Threatening Behavior, 29*(4), 287–294.

Siebert, A. (2005). *The resiliency advantage: Master change, thrive under pressure, and bounce back from setbacks.* San Francisco, CA: Berrett-Koehler.

Silverdale, N. & Katz, J. (2003). Changes in attitudes and practice toward dying people after completion of a U.K.-based distance learning death and dying course. *Illness, Crisis, & Loss, 11*(2), 183–196.

Silverman, G.K., Jacobs, S.C., Kasl, S.V., Shear, M.K., Maciejewski, P.K., Noaghiul, F.S., & Prigerson, H.G. (2000). Quality of life impairments associated with diagnostic criteria for traumatic grief. *Psychological Medicine, 30*(4), 857–862.

Simon, A., Kar, M., Hinz, J., & Beck, D. (2007). *Attitudes towards terminal sedation: An empirical survey among experts in the field of medical ethics.* BMC Palliative Care. Retrieved August 17, 2008, from http://www.biomedcentral.com/1472-684X/6/4

Simon, R.I. (2007). Gun safety management with patients at risk for suicide. *Suicide and Life-Threatening Behavior, 37*(5), 518–526.

Simpson, G. & Tate, R. (2007). Suicidality in people surviving a traumatic brain injury: Prevalence, risk factors, and implications for clinical management. *Brain Injury, 21*(13–14), 1335–1351.

Smith, J.C. (2002). *Stress management: A comprehensive handbook of techniques and strategies.* New York, NY: Springer.

Smith, M. & Segal, J. (2009). *Supporting a grieving person: Helping others through grief, loss, and bereavement.* Retrieved February 5, 2010, from http://www.helpguide.org/mental/helping_grieving.htm

Smith, T.J. (2003). We can reduce the cost of in-hospital end-of-life care. *Oncology Times, 25*(11), 4–6.

Somer, E., Buchbinder, E., Peled-Avram, M., & Ben-Yizhack, Y. (2004). The stress and coping of Israeli emergency room social workers following terrorist attacks. *Qualitative Health Research, 14*(8), 1077–1093.

Somhlaba, N.Z. & Wait, J.W. (2008). Psychological adjustment to conjugal bereavement: Do social networks aid coping following spousal death? Omega: *Journal of Death and Dying, 57*(4), 341–366.

Speece, M.W. & Brent, S.B. (1984). Children's understanding of death: A review of three components of a death concept. *Child Development, 55*(5), 1671-1686.

Spradlin, S.E. (2003). *Don't let emotions run your life: How dialectical behavior therapy can put you in control.* Oakland, CA: New Harbinger Publications.

Sprang, G., Clark, J.J., & Whitt-Woosley, A. (2007). Compassion fatigue, compassion satisfaction, and burnout: Factors impacting a professional's quality of life. *Journal of Loss and Trauma, 12*(3), 259–280.

Squidoo. (n.d.). *Help a child cope with loss and grief.* Retrieved September 12, 2009, from http://www.squidoo.com/children-grief#module3502613

Stack, S. (2005). Suicide in the media: A quantitative review of studies based on nonfictional stories. *Suicide and Life-Threatening Behavior, 35*(2), 121–134.

Stack, S. & Wasserman, I. (2009). Gender and suicide risk: The role of wound site. *Suicide and Life-Threatening Behavior, 39*(1), 13–20.

Stamm, B.H. (2002). Measuring compassion satisfaction as well as fatigue; Developmental history of the compassion satisfaction and fatigue test. In C.R. Figley (Ed.), *Treating compassion fatigue* (107–122). New York, NY: Routledge.

Steinbrook, R. (2008). *Physician Assisted Death – From Oregon to Washington State.* Retrieved August 13, 2009, from http://content.nejm.org/cgi/content/full/359/24/2513

Stewart, A.E., Harris Lord, J., & Mercer, D.L. (2000). A survey of professionals' training and experiences in delivering death notifications. *Death Studies, 24*(7), 611–631.

Stillion, J.M. & Noviello, S.B. (2001). Living and dying in different worlds: Gender differences in violent death and grief. *Illness, Crisis, & Loss, 9*(3), 247–259.

Stith Butler, A., Panzer, A.M., & Goldfrank, L.R. (Eds.). (2003). *Preparing for the psychological consequences of terrorism: A public health strategy.* Washington, DC: National Academies Press. Available at http://www.nap.edu/openbook.php?record_id=10717&page=R1

St John, A., Cooke, M., & Goopy, S. (2006). Shrouds of silence: Three women's stories of prenatal loss. *Australian Journal of Advanced Nursing, 23*(3), 8–12.

Straub, S.H. & Roberts, J.M. (2001). Fear of death in widows: Effects of age at widowhood and suddenness of death. *Omega: Journal of Death and Dying, 43*(1), 25–41.

Stroebe, M. & Schut, H. (1999). The dual process model of coping with bereavement: Rationale and description. *Death Studies, 23*(3), 197–224.

Stroebe, M.S. & Schut, H. (2001). Models of coping with bereavement: A review. In, M.S. Stroebe, R.O. Hansson, W. Stroebe, & H. Schut (Eds.), *Handbook of Bereavement Research: Consequences, coping, and care* (375–404). Washington, DC: American Psychological Association.

Stuart, C., Waalen, J.K., & Haelstromm, E. (2003). Many helping hearts: An evaluation of peer gatekeeper training in suicide risk assessment. *Death Studies, 27*(4), 321–333.

Substance Abuse and Mental Health Services Administration (SAMHSA). (2009). *Emergency mental health and traumatic stress: Tips for teachers: Questions to help children talk about a disaster.* Retrieved August 23, 2009, from http://mentalhealth.samhsa.gov/cmhs/EmergencyServices/questions.asp

Suicide Prevention Action Network (SPAN) USA. (2010). *American Foundation for Suicide Prevention: Veterans and military suicide prevention.* Retrieved July 8, 2010, from http://www.spanusa.org/index.cfm?fuse action=home.viewPage&page_ID=7ECD7BB 1-C613-FA47-9E53D64729C8A88C

Sulmasy D.P., He M.K., McAuley R., & Ury, W.A. (2008). Beliefs and attitudes of nurses and physicians about do not resuscitate orders and who should speak to patients and families about them. *Critical Care Medicine, 36*(6), 1817–1822.

Sveen, C.A. & Walby, F.A. (2008). Suicide survivors' mental health and grief reactions: A systematic review of controlled studies. *Suicide and Life-Threatening Behavior, 38*(1), 13–29.

Taku, K., Calhoun, L.G., Cann, A., & Tedeschi, R.G. (2008). The role of rumination in the coexistence of distress and posttraumatic growth among bereaved Japanese university students. *Death Studies, 32*(5), 428–444.

Tan, H.M., Braunack-Mayer, A., & Beilby, J. (2005). The impact of the hospice environment on patient spiritual expression. *Oncology Nursing Forum, 32*(5), 1049–1055.

Taubman-Ben-Ari, O. & Weintroub, A. (2008). Meaning in life and personal growth among pediatric physicians and nurses. *Death Studies, 32*(7), 621–645.

Tedeschi, R.G. & Calhoun, L.G. (2004). Posttraumatic growth: Conceptual foundations and empirical evidence. *Psychological Inquiry, 15*(1), 1–15.

Tedeschi, R.G. & Calhoun, L.G. (2008). Beyond the concept of recovery: Growth and the experience of loss. *Death Studies, 32*(1), 27–39.

Teno, J.M., Bird, C., & Mor, V. (2002). *The prevalence and treatment of pain in U.S. nursing homes.* The Center for Gerontology and Health Care Research, Brown University, RI. Retrieved December 4, 2008, from http://www. chcr.brown.edu/dying/factsondying.htm

Thomas, R., Wilson, D.M., Justice, C., Birch, S., & Sheps, S. (2008). A literature review of preferences for end-of-life care in developed countries by individuals with different cultural affiliations and ethnicity. *Journal of Hospice and Palliative Care Nursing, 10*(3), 142–161.

Tomer, A., Eliason, G., & Smith, J. (2000). The structure of the revised death anxiety scale in young and old adults. In A. Tomer (Ed.), *Death attitudes and the older adult: Theories, concepts, and applications* (pp. 109–122). Philadelphia, PA: Brunner-Routledge.

Tomer, A., Eliason, G., & Wong, P.T. (2007). *Existential and spiritual issues in death attitudes.* Mahwah, NJ: Lawrence Erlbaum Associates.

Torke, A.M., Garas, N.S., Sexson, W., & Branch, W.T. (2005). Medical care at the end of life: Views of African American patients in an urban hospital. *Journal of Palliative Medicine, 8*(3), 593–602.

Trémeau, F., Staner, L., Duval, F., Corrêa, H., Crocq, M.A., Darreye, A., ... Macher, J.P. (2005). Suicide attempts and family history of suicide in three psychiatric populations. *Suicide and Life-Threatening Behavior, 35*(6), 702–713.

Truog, R.D. & Miller, F.G. (2008). The dead donor rule and organ transplantation. *New England Journal of Medicine, 359*(7), 674–675.

Tsui, M.S. & Cheung, F.C. (2003). Dealing with terrorism: What social workers should and can do. *Social Work, 48*(4), 556–557.

Tuval-Mashiach, R. & Shalev, A. (2005). Epidemiology of psychological reactions of adults to ongoing terror in Israel. In E. Somer & A. Bleich (Eds.), *Mental health in terror's shadow: The Israeli experience* (929–954). Tel Aviv: Ramot (Hebrew).

Ujda, R.M. & Bendiksen, R. (2000). Health care provider support and grief after a perinatal loss: A qualitative study. *Illness, Crisis, & Loss, 8*(3), 265–285.

Ullman, S.E. & Najdowski, C.J. (2009). Correlates of serious suicidal ideation and attempts in female adult sexual assault survivors. *Suicide and Life-Threatening Behavior, 39*(1), 47–57.

Ungar, L. & Florian, V. (2004). What helps middle-aged widows with their psychological and social adaptation several years after their loss? *Death Studies, 28*(7), 621–641.

United Network for Organ Sharing (UNOS). (2009). *How the transplant system works: Matching donors and recipients.* Retrieved August 16, 2009, from http://www.unos.org/resources/factsheets.asp?fs=1

United States Department of Labor: Bureau of Labor Statistics. (2010). *Injuries, Illnesses, and fatalities: Census of fatal occupational injuries (CFOI) – current and revised data.* Retrieved July 1, 2010, from http://www.bls.gov/iif/oshcfoi1.htm

Uren, T.H. & Wastell, C.A. (2002). Attachment and meaning-making in perinatal bereavement. *Death Studies, 26*(4), 279–308.

U.S. Army Behavioral Health Technology Office. (2007). *Army Suicide Event Report (ASER).* Retrieved December 12, 2008, from http://media.mcclatchydc.com/smedia/2008/05/29/19/ArmySuicide.source.prod_affiliate.91.pdf

U.S. Public Health Service. (1999). *The Surgeon General's call to action to prevent suicide.* Washington, DC: Department of Health & Human Services. Retrieved October 7, 2003, from http://www.surgeongeneral.gov/library/calltoaction/calltoaction.htm

Valentine, C. (2007). The "moment of death." *Omega: Journal of Death and Dying, 55*(3), 219–236.

Vanderwerker, L.C. & Prigerson, H.G. (2004). Social support and technological connectedness as protective factors in bereavement. *Journal of Loss and Trauma, 9*(1), 45–57.

Van Orden, K.A., Joiner, T.E., Jr., Hollar, D., Rudd, M.D., Mandrusiak, M., & Silverman, M.M. (2006). A test of the effectiveness of a list of suicide warning signs for the public. *Suicide and Life-Threatening Behavior, 36*(3), 272–287.

Vargas, T. (2008). *As families opt for cremation, industry expands services, choices.* Retrieved January 27, 2010, from http://www.washingtonpost.com/wp-dyn/content/article/2008/09/06/AR2008090602853.html

Varna, J.M. (2004). *ASNA independent study activity: Compassion fatigue.* Retrieved September 12, 2008, from http://findarticles.com/p/articles/mi_qa4090/is_200403/ai_n9465515/?tag=content;col1

Vermont Ethics Network. (n.d.-a). *Worksheet 1 – Values questionnaire.* Retrieved August 26, 2010, from http://www.vtethicsnetwork.org/WorkSheet1.htm

Vermont Ethics Network. (n.d.-b). *Worksheet 2 – medical situations and their treatment.* Retrieved August 26, 2010, from http://www.vtethicsnetwork.org/Worksheet2.htm

Violanti, J.M. & Gehrke, A. (2004). Police trauma encounters: Precursors of compassion fatigue. International *Journal of Emergency Mental Health, 6*(2), 75–80.

VITAS Healthcare Corporation. (2004). *National survey on death, dying, and hospice care in America.* Retrieved August 17, 2008, from http://www.bendixenandassociates.com/studies/VITAS%20National%20Survey%20on%20Death,%20Dying,%20and%20Hospice%20Care%20in%20America%202004.pdf

Voice of America. (2008). *U.S. Army suicide rate continues to rise.* Retrieved July 30, 2008, from http://www.voanews.com/english/archive/2008-05/2008-05-29voa64.cfm?CFID=25240943&CFTOKEN=95149601

Volpe, J.S. (1996). *Traumatic stress: An overview.* Retrieved from http://www.aaets.org/article1.htm

von Gunten, C.F. (2005). Intervention to manage symptoms at the end of life. *Journal of Palliative Medicine, 8*(Suppl 1), S88–94.

Wada, K. & Park, J. (2009). Integrating Buddhist psychology into grief counseling. *Death Studies, 33*(7), 657–683.

Wagner, B., Knaevelsrud, C., & Maercker, A. (2005). Internet-based treatment for complicated grief: Concepts and case study. *Journal of Loss and Trauma, 10*(5), 409–432.

Wallace, M. & O'Shea, E. (2007). Perceptions of spirituality and spiritual care among older nursing home residents at the end of life. *Holistic Nursing Practice, 21*(6), 285–289.

Walsh, F. (2003). Family resilience: A framework for clinical practice-theory and practice. *Family Process, 42*(1), 1–18.

Walsh, F. & McGoldrick, M. (1988). Loss and the family life cycle. In C.J. Falicov (Ed.), *Family transitions: Continuity and change over the life cycle* (pp. 311–336). New York, NY: Guilford.

Walsh, F. & McGoldrick, M. (1991). Loss and the family: A systemic perspective. In F. Walsh & M. McGoldrick (Eds.), *Living beyond loss: Death in the family* (pp. 1–29). New York, NY: Norton.

Walsh, S.M. & Hogan, N.S. (2003). Oncology nursing education: Nursing students' commitment of "presence" with the dying patient and the family. *Nursing Education Perspectives, 24*(2), 86–90.

Washington Secretary of State Sam Reed. (2009). *November 4, 2008 General Election.* Retrieved August 13, 2009, from http://vote.wa.gov/elections/wei/Results.aspx?RaceTypeCode=M&JurisdictionTypeID=2&ElectionID=26&ViewMode=Results

Wass, H. (2004). A perspective on the current state of death education. *Death Studies, 28*(4), 289–308.

Webb, T.E. (2001). Assessing a crisis of faith and making a pastoral crisis intervention. International Journal of Emergency Mental Health, 3(3), 181–186.

Webb, T.E. (2004). Crisis of faith vs. spiritual cry of distress. *International Journal of Emergency Mental Health, 6*(4), 217–222.

Wee, D.F. & Myers, D. (2002). Stress response of mental health workers following disaster: The Oklahoma City bombing. In C.R. Figley (Ed.), *Treating compassion fatigue* (57–83). New York, NY: Routledge.

Wee, D.F. & Myers, D. (2003). Compassion satisfaction, compassion fatigue, and critical incident stress management. *International Journal of Emergency Mental Health, 5*(1), 33–37.

Weeks, O.D. & Johnson, C. (Eds.). (2001). *When all the friends have gone: A guide for aftercare providers.* Amityville, NY: Baywood.

Werth, J.L., Jr., Gordon, J.R., & Johnson, R.R., Jr. (2002). Psychosocial issues near the end of life. *Aging and Mental Health, 6*(4), 402–412.

Westefeld, J.S., Homaifar, B., Spotts, J., Furr, S., Range, L., & Werth, J.L., Jr. (2005). Perceptions concerning college student suicide: Data from four universities. *Suicide and Life-Threatening Behavior, 35*(6), 640–645.

Wickie, S.K. & Marwit, S.J. (2000–2001). Assumptive world views and the grief reactions of parents of murdered children. *Omega: Journal of Death and Dying, 42*(2), 101–113.

Wicks, R. (2006). *Overcoming secondary stress in medical and nursing practice: A guide to professional resilience and personal well-being.* New York, NY: Oxford University Press.

Wicks, R., Parsons, R., & Capps, D. (Eds.). (2003). *Clinical handbook of pastoral counseling: Volume 3.* Mahwah, NJ: Paulist Press.

Wijngaards-de Meij, L., Stroebe, M., Stroebe, W., Schut, H., Van Den Bout, J., Van Der Heijden, P.G., & Dijkstra, I. (2008). The impact of circumstances surrounding the death of a child on parents' grief. *Death Studies, 32*(3), 237–252.

Williams, J., Hackworth, S.R., & Cradock, M.M. (2002). Medical crisis and loss clinic: Novel approach to family transitions. *Illness, Crisis, & Loss, 10*(4), 356–366.

Willis, L.A., Coombs, D.W., Drentea, P., & Cockerham, W.C. (2003). Uncovering the mystery: Factors of African American suicide. *Suicide and Life-Threatening Behavior, 33*(4), 412–429.

Wilsey, S.A. & Shear, M.K. (2007). Descriptions of social support in treatment narratives of complicated grievers. *Death Studies, 31*(9), 801–819.

Winter, L., Dennis, M.P., & Parker, B. (2007–2008). Religiosity and preferences for life-prolonging medical treatments in African-American and White elders: A mediation study. *Omega: Journal of Death and Dying, 56*(3), 273–288.

Winter, L., Parker, B., & Schneider, M. (2007). Imagining the alternatives to life prolonging treatments: Elders' beliefs about the dying experience. *Death Studies, 31*(7), 619–631.

Wolchik, S.A., Ma, Y., Tein, J.Y., Sandler, I.N., & Ayers, T.S. (2008). Parentally bereaved children's grief: Self-system beliefs as mediators of the relations between grief and stressors and caregiver-child relationship quality. *Death Studies, 32*(7), 597–620.

Wolfelt, A.D. (2009). *The handbook for companioning the mourner: Eleven essential principles.* Fort Collins, CO: Companion Press.

Wood, D. (2005). S*potlight on nursing: Watching for and overcoming compassion fatigue.* Retrieved September 12, 2008, from http://www.travelnursing.com/News.aspx?ArticleID=14601

Worden, J.W. (1991). *Grief counseling and grief therapy: A handbook for the mental health practitioner* (2nd ed.). New York, NY: Springer.

Worden, J.W. (2002). *Grief counseling and grief therapy: A handbook for the mental health practitioner* (3rd ed.). New York, NY: Springer.

World Health Organization (WHO). (1998). WHO *Definition of palliative care.* Retrieved August 28, 2008, from http://www.who.int/cancer/palliative/definition/en

World Health Organization (WHO). (2007). *Palliative Care: Cancer control: Knowledge into action: WHO guide for effective programmes.* Retrieved January 29, 2010, from http://www.who.int/cancer/media/FINAL-Palliative%20Care%20Module.pdf

World Health Organization (WHO). (2008). *Cancer: Palliative Care.* Retrieved August 28, 2008, from http://www.who.int/cancer/palliative

Wortmann, J.H. & Park, C.L. (2008). Religion and spirituality in adjustment following bereavement: An integrative review. *Death Studies, 32*(8), 703–736.

Wu, A.M. & Tang, C.S. (2009). The negative impact of death anxiety on self-efficacy and willingness to donate organs among Chinese adults. *Death Studies, 33*(1), 51–72.

Xu, J., Kochanek, K.D., Murphy, S.L. & Tejada-Vera, B. (2010). *Deaths: Final data for 2007.* Retrieved November 4, 2010, from http://www.cdc.gov/NCHS/data/nvsr/nvsr58/nvsr58_19.pdf

Yang, S. & Chen, S.F. (2002). A phenomenographic approach to the meaning of death: A Chinese perspective. *Death Studies, 26*(2), 143–175.

Yang, S. & Rosenblatt, P.C. (2007). Couple rage and emotional distancing when a partner is dying. *Journal of Loss and Trauma, 12*(4), 305–320.

Yasien-Esmael, H. & Rubin, S.S. (2005). The meaning structures of Muslim bereavements in Israel: Religious traditions, mourning practices, and human experience. *Death Studies, 29*(6), 495–518.

Ybarra, M.L. & Eaton, W.W. (2005). Internet-based mental health interventions. *Mental Health Services Research, 7*(2), 75–87.

Yeolekar, M.E., Mehta, S., & Yeolekar, A. (2008). End of life care: Issues and challenges. *Journal of Postgraduate Medicine, 54*(3), 173–175.

Ying, Y-H.. & Chang, K. (2009). A study of suicide and socioeconomic factors. *Suicide and Life-Threatening Behavior, 39*(2), 214–226.

Yoder, K.A., Whitbeck, L.B., Hoyt, D.R., & LaFromboise, T.D. (2006). Suicidal ideation among Amerian Indian youths. *Archives of Suicide Research, 10*(2), 177–190.

Young, E. (2007–2008). Figures of grief: Metaphors from a bereavement writing group. *Omega: Journal of Death and Dying, 56*(4), 359–367.

Zamperetti, N., Bellomo, R., & Ronco, C. (2008). Bioethical aspects of end-of-life care. *European Journal of Anaesthesiology, 42*(Suppl), 51–57.

Zettel-Watson, L., Ditto, P.H., Danks, J.H., & Smucker, W.D. (2008). Actual and perceived gender differences in the accuracy of surrogate decisions about life-sustaining medical treatment among older spouses. *Death Studies, 32*(3), 273–290.

Zinner, E.S. (2000). Being a man about it: The marginalization of men in grief. *Illness, Crisis, & Loss, 8*(2), 181–188.

INDEX

Page references followed by *fig* indicate an illustrated figure; followed by *t* indicate a table.

A

abortions, 104

acceptance of death, 5–6, 39

accidental deaths

    demographics of, 8–10

    intervention for bereaved children/adolescents following, 183–185

    notifying survivors after sudden or, 10–16

    rituals for sudden or, 125

"act of God," 113

acute phase of coping, 40

acute workplace stress, 194

addiction (or drug dependence), 84, 85*t*

adolescents

    developmental understanding of death by, 176–177

    suicide among, 139–140

    See also bereaved adolescents; children

advance care planning

    advance directives, 73–75

    case study on, 86–87

    discussions for, 78, 80

    end-of-life decision making worksheets, 77*fig*, 79*fig*

    ethical issues related to, 83–86

    factors influencing decision-making process, 75–76, 78, 97

    Five Wishes document for, 80

    overview of, 73

    POLST document for, 80–82*fig*

    Web resources on, 88

advance directives

    description of, 73

    informed consent, 75

    laws governing the use of, 74–75

    living will, 73–74

    medical power of attorney, 74

    personal insights into, 74

African Americans

    complicated grief rates among, 106

    death anxiety among elderly, 5

    death and dying attitudes by, 75

    end-of-life treatment decisions by, 75–76, 97

    homicide deaths and, 114

    suicide rates of, 133

    See also racial/ethnicity differences

aftercare services, 25

age differences

    motor vehicle traffic deaths and, 10

    suicide and, 132–133

Aging with Dignity, 80

aging population, 101

    See also older adults

AIDS-related deaths, 2–3, 103, 162–163

Alaska Native suicide rates, 133

Alberta Mental Health Board, 132

alcohol-suicide relationship, 141

Allchin, 1

Allina End of Life Project, 78

altruistic suicide, 135

American Association of Colleges of Nurses (AACN), 54

American Association of Suicidology, 147, 148*t*

American Cancer Society, 55

American Foundation for Suicide Prevention, 136

American Indian suicide rates, 133

American Red Cross, 119, 121

anger

    anticipatory grief and, 43

    as stage of dying, 39

anomic suicide, 135–136

anticipatory grief, 43–44

artificial organ support, 78

Asian Americans, 97

assessments

    comprehensive hospice, 62

    depression, 146

    of family beliefs about pain management, 45

    initial hospice, 62

    palliative care, 62

    suicidal behaviors, 144–147

assessment tools

    Beck Anxiety Inventory, 146

    Beck Depression Inventory, 146

    Beck Hopelessness Scale, 146

    Mental Pain Scale, 146

    Psychological Pain Assessment Scale, 146

    Reasons for Living Inventory, 146

    Scale of Suicide Ideation, 146

Western Schools® offers over 2,000 hours to suit all your interests – and requirements!

Cardiovascular
Cardiovascular Nursing: A Comprehensive Overview
Cardiovascular Pharmacology
A The 12-Lead ECG in Acute Coronary Syndromes

Clinical Conditions/Nursing Practice
A Advanced Assessment
Ambulatory Surgical Care (2nd ed.)
Asthma: Nursing Care Across the Lifespan
Clinical Care of the Diabetic Foot
A Complete Nurses Guide to Diabetes Care (2nd ed.)
Chronic Obstructive Lung Disease
Death, Dying, & Bereavement (2nd ed.)
Diabetes Essentials for Nurses
Essentials of Patient Education
Fibromyalgia in Women
Genetic & Inherited Disorders of the Pulmonary System
Helping the Obese Patient Find Success
Holistic & Complementary Therapies
Home Health Nursing (3rd ed.)
Humor in Health Care: The Laughter Prescription (2nd ed.)
Management of Systemic Lupus Erythematosus
Multiple Sclerosis: Nursing Strategies to Improve Patient Outcomes
Orthopedic Nursing: Caring for Patients with Musculoskeletal Disorders (2nd ed.)
Pain & Symptom Management
Pain Management: Principles and Practice
A Palliative Practices: An Interdisciplinary Approach
   — Issues Specific to Palliative Care
   — Specific Disease States and Symptom Management
   — The Dying Process, Grief, and Bereavement.
Pharmacologic Management of Asthma
Pneumonia in Adults
Pulmonary Rehabilitation
Seizures: A Basic Overview
Wound Management and Healing

Critical Care/ER/OR
Acute Respiratory Distress Syndrome (ARDS)
Adult Acute Respiratory Infections (UPDATED 1st ed.)
Auscultation Skills (4th ed.)
   — Heart Sounds
   — Breath Sounds
Basic Nursing of Head, Chest, Abdominal, Spine and Orthopedic Trauma
A Case Studies in Critical Care Nursing
Critical Care & Emergency Nursing
Fire Risk Reduction for Operative and Invasive Procedures
Hemodynamic Monitoring
Lung Transplantation
A Practical Guide to Moderate Sedation/Analgesia
Principles of Basic Trauma Nursing
Traumatic Brain Injury

Geriatrics
Alzheimer's Disease: A Complete Guide for Nurses
Alzheimer's Disease and Related Disorders
Cognitive Disorders in Aging
Depression in Older Adults
Early-Stage Alzheimer's Disease
Geriatric Assessment
Healthy Aging
Nursing Care of the Older Adult (2nd ed.)
Psychosocial Issues Affecting Older Adults (2nd ed.)
Substance Abuse in Older Adults

Infectious Diseases
Avian (H5N1) Influenza (2nd ed.)
H1N1 Flu (2nd ed.)
Hepatitis C: The Silent Killer (2nd ed.)
HIV/AIDS
Infection Control Training for Healthcare Workers
Influenza: A Vaccine-Preventable Disease (UPDATED 2nd ed.)
MRSA
Pertussis: Diagnosis, Treatment, and Prevention
Tuberculosis Across the Lifespan
West Nile Virus (3rd ed.)

Oncology
Cancer in Women (2nd ed.)
Cancer Nursing
Chemotherapy and Biotherapies
Lung Cancer (UPDATED 2nd ed.)

Pediatrics/Maternal-Child/Women's Health
A Assessment and Care of the Well Newborn
Birth Control Methods and Reproductive Choices
Birth Defects Affecting the Respiratory System
Childhood Obesity
Diabetes in Children (2nd ed.)
Effective Counseling Techniques for Perinatal Mood Disorders
Fetal and Neonatal Drug Exposure
Induction of Labor
Manual of School Health (3rd ed.)
Maternal-Newborn Nursing
Menopause: Nursing Care for Women Throughout Mid-Life
A Obstetric and Gynecologic Emergencies
   — Obstetric Emergencies
   — Gynecologic Emergencies
Pediatric Health & Physical Assessment
Perinatal Mood Disorders: An Overview
Pregnancy Loss
Respiratory Diseases in the Newborn
Women and Cardiovascular Disease
Women's Health: Contemporary Advances and Trends (3rd ed.)

Professional Issues/Management/Law
Documentation for Nurses
Ethical Issues in Children's Health Care
Protecting Patient Safety: Preventing Medical Errors
Management and Leadership in Nursing
Ohio Nursing Law Affecting Daily Practice
Surviving and Thriving in Nursing

Psychiatric/Mental Health
A ADHD in Children and Adults
Adoptive Families: Trends and Therapeutic Interventions
Asperger's Syndrome
Attention Deficit Hyperactivity Disorders Throughout the Lifespan
Basic Psychopharmacology
Behavioral Approaches to Treating Obesity
A Bipolar Disorder
A Child/Adolescent Clinical Psychopharmacology (2nd ed.)
A Childhood Maltreatment
A Clinical Psychopharmacology
Clinical Neuropsychology: Applications in Practice
A Collaborative Therapy with Multi-stressed Families
Counseling Substance Abusing or Dependent Adolescents
Depression: Prevention, Diagnosis, and Treatment
Disaster Mental Health
A Ethnicity and the Dementias
A Evidence-Based Mental Health Practice
Grief, Bereavement, and Mourning in Children and Adults
Group Work with Substance Abusing & Dually Diagnosed Clients
A Growing Up with Autism
Harm Reduction Counseling for Substance Abusing Clients
Identifying and Assessing Suicide Risk in Adults
A Integrating Traditional Healing Practices into Counseling
A Integrative and Comprehensive Trauma Treatment
A Integrative Treatment for Borderline Personality Disorder
Intimate Partner Violence: An Overview
A Mental Disorders in Older Adults
A Mindfulness and Psychotherapy
A Multicultural Perspectives in Working with Families
Multidimensional Health Assessment of the Older Adult
A Obsessive Compulsive Disorder
Post-Divorce Parenting: Mental Health Issues and Interventions
Posttraumatic Stress Disorder: An Overview
A Problem and Pathological Gambling
Psychiatric Nursing: Current Trends in Diagnosis (2nd ed.)
Psychiatric Principles & Applications
A Psychosocial Adjustment to Chronic Illness in Children and Adolescents
A Psychosocial Aspects of Disaster
A Schizophrenia
Schizophrenia: Signs, Symptoms, and Treatment Strategies
Serious Mental Illness: Comprehensive Case Management
Substance Abuse (UPDATED 1st ed.)
Suicide
A Trauma Therapy
A Treating Explosive Kids
A Treating Substance Use Problems in Psychotherapy Practice
A Treating Victims of Mass Disaster and Terrorism
Understanding Attachment Theory
Understanding Loss & Grief: Implications for Healthcare Professionals

Visit our website at www.WesternSchools.com for course descriptions and additional CE offerings!